Storying Later Life

Storying Later Life

ISSUES, INVESTIGATIONS, AND INTERVENTIONS IN NARRATIVE GERONTOLOGY

EDITED BY

GARY KENYON, ERNST BOHLMEIJER,

AND WILLIAM L. RANDALL

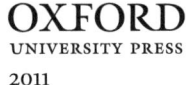

OXFORD
UNIVERSITY PRESS
2011

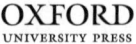

OXFORD
UNIVERSITY PRESS

Oxford University Press, Inc., publishes works that further
Oxford University's objective of excellence
in research, scholarship, and education.

Oxford   New York
Auckland   Cape Town   Dar es Salaam   Hong Kong   Karachi
Kuala Lumpur   Madrid   Melbourne   Mexico City   Nairobi
New Delhi   Shanghai   Taipei   Toronto

With offices in
Argentina   Austria   Brazil   Chile   Czech Republic   France   Greece
Guatemala   Hungary   Italy   Japan   Poland   Portugal   Singapore
South Korea   Switzerland   Thailand   Turkey   Ukraine   Vietnam

Published by Oxford University Press, Inc.
198 Madison Avenue, New York, New York 10016
www.oup.com

Oxford is a registered trademark of Oxford University Press

Library of Congress Cataloging-in-Publication Data
Storying later life : issues, investigations, and interventions in narrative gerontology/edited by
Gary Kenyon, Ernst Bohlmeijer, and William Randall.
p. cm.
Includes bibliographical references and index.
ISBN 978-0-19-539795-6 (hbk. : alk. paper) 1. Geriatric psychiatry. 2. Narrative therapy.
3. Gerontology—Biographical methods. 4. Reminiscing in old age. 5. Autobiographical memory.
I. Kenyon, Gary M., 1949– II. Bohlmeijer, Ernst, 1965– III. Randall, William Lowell, 1950–
RC451.4.A5S772 2011
618.97'689—dc22
2010015287
ISBN-13: 978-0-19-539795-6
ISBN-10: 0-19-539795-9

9 8 7 6 5 4 3 2

Printed in the United States of America on acid-free paper

Contents

Foreword   IX
Acknowledgments   XI
Preface   XIII
Contributors   XIX

PART 1   ISSUES

Chapter 1   Narrative Foreclosure in Later Life:
Possibilities and Limits   *3*
Mark Freeman

Chapter 2   Memory, Metaphor, and Meaning: Reading for
Wisdom in the Stories of Our Lives   *20*
William L. Randall

Chapter 3   Narrative Events and Biographical Construction
in Old Age   *39*
Jaber F. Gubrium

Chapter 4   Inventing Yourself: How Older Adults Deal with
the Pressure of Late-Modern Identity Construction   *51*
Frits de Lange

Chapter 5   In Waves of Time, Space, and Self:
The Dwelling-Place of Age in Virginia
Woolf's *The Waves*   *66*
Rishi Goyal and Rita Charon

Chapter 6   The Narrative Frame in Discourse on Aging:
Understanding Facts and Values Behind Public Policy   *84*
Phillip G. Clark

PART 2   INVESTIGATIONS

Chapter 7   The Power of Stories Left Untold: Narratives
of Nazi Followers   *101*
Stephan Marks

Chapter 8   Young Bodies, Old Bodies, and Stories
of the Athletic Self   *111*
Cassandra Phoenix

Chapter 9   The Raging Grannies: Narrative Construction
of Gender and Aging   *126*
Linda Caissie

Chapter 10   Narrative and Gender Differences: How Men and
Women Interpret Their Lives   *143*
*Patricia O'Neill, James E. Birren, and
Cheryl Svensson*

Chapter 11   Telling Stories: How Do Expressions of
Self Differ in a Writing Group Versus
a Reminiscence Group?   *159*
Kate de Medeiros

Chapter 12   *Mnëmë* and *Anamnësis*: The Contribution of
Involuntary Reminiscences to the Construction
of a Narrative Self in Older Age   *177*
Philippe Cappeliez and Jeffrey Dean Webster

Chapter 13   Achieving Narrative Coherence Following Traumatic
War Experience: The Role of Social Support   *195*
Karen Burnell, Peter Coleman, and Nigel Hunt

Chapter 14   Using Self-Defining Memories in Couples Therapy
with Older Adults   *213*
Jefferson A. Singer and Beata Labunko Messier

PART 3   INTERVENTIONS

Chapter 15   On Suffering, Loss, and The Journey To Life:
Tai Chi as Narrative Care   *237*
Gary Kenyon

Chapter 16   Older Adults in Search of New Stories: Measuring the
                 Effects of Life Review on Coherence and Integration in
                 Autobiographical Narratives   *252*
                 Thijs Tromp

Chapter 17   Reminiscence Interventions: Bringing Narrative
                 Gerontology into Practice   *273*
                 Ernst Bohlmeijer and Gerben Westerhof

Chapter 18   Life Review Using Autobiographical Retrieval: A Protocol
                 for Training Depressed Residential Home Inhabitants in
                 Recalling Specific Personal Memories   *290*
                 Bas Steunenberg and Ernst Bohlmeijer

Chapter 19   "Green and Gray": An Educational Program to Enhance
                 Contact Between Younger and Older Adults by Means of
                 Lifestories   *307*
                 Gerben J. Westerhof

Chapter 20   Implementation of Narrative Care in The Netherlands:
                 Coordinating Management, Institutional, and Personal
                 Narratives   *319*
                 Gerdienke M. Ubels

Chapter 21   Asking the Right Questions: Enabling Persons with
                 Dementia to Speak for Themselves   *338*
                 Marie-Elise van den Brandt-van Heek

Chapter 22   The Ripple Effect: A Story of the Transformational
                 Nature of Narrative Care   *354*
                 Daphne Noonan

                 Afterword
                 Toward a Narrative Turn in Health Care   *366*
                 Ernst Bohlmeijer, Gary Kenyon, and William L. Randall

                 Index   381

Foreword

Writing, reading, telling, and listening to people's accounts of their lives—
these activities are receiving increasing attention. The details of individuals'
narratives are adding much to our understanding of human experience and
the forces in society that shape it. They also add to our understanding of the
interactions between individuals and the cultures of the times in which they
grew up and grew old.

In the past, lifestories were considered unworthy of scholarly study, as
contributing nothing of significance to science. This, too, is changing. The
ways in which people experience their lives and interpret the events that they
have lived through are known to influence their behavior and decisions. We
can expect future research to examine how life experiences are filed within
the nervous system itself as well as ways of tracing developmental influences
on them.

Another aspect of life narratives is that they contribute to the unveiling
and understanding of historical epochs. We could characterize this as
"bottom-up history"—the history of events from the perspective of the
people who have lived them, in contrast to "top-down history"—history
from the perspective of the leaders. Many details of major historical events
have been lost, since most of the people who experienced them were
illiterate at the time.

The emerging field of *narrative gerontology* is well captured in this book.
Scholars and academics from various disciplines and countries provide a
rich perspective on its breadth and depth. The scope of the subject matter
ranges from the uses of narrative in improving the lives of individuals and
releasing their potential to the functions that narrative gerontology can
serve in a variety of professions and in society at large. In a sense, narrative

gerontology makes key contributions in both science and professional effectiveness, and taps the value of lifelong experience and wisdom.

Interest in narrative gerontology is multidisciplinary, cutting across the humanities, the social sciences, and the professions. Several fields of professional practice, from social work to medicine, play a role in helping clients tell their lifestories. Indeed, reviewing and improving the stories that we tell ourselves about who we are have beneficial effects on our well-being.

During the information age, societies have become more efficient, but at the same time, less personal. Individuals are often placed in effective roles yet with fewer personal contacts. This book reveals the value of looking in greater detail and from multiple perspectives at the *inside* of life. It provides a window into important issues and opens the door to further studies of individual lives.

James E. Birren

Acknowledgments

For my wife Liz, thank you for your support and practical wisdom, and for my Tai Chi friends at York Manor and Windsor Court. GK

For Monique: Your stories daily inspire my stories and your stillness daily inspires my stillness. EB

For the staff and fellow patrons of my favorite coffee shop, where my chapter in this volume was composed and where any other of the editing tasks I undertook were carried out, thank you for the sanctuary you provided. WR

All three of us owe an enormous debt of gratitude to our colleague Beth McKim for so generously coming to our rescue in the final weeks of preparing this manuscript for publication with her marvelous and much-needed attention to editorial detail. A warm thank you is also in order to Lori Handelman, our editor at Oxford University Press, for her enthusiasm for and support of this project from the start.

Preface

A basic assumption of narrative gerontology is that the biographical side of human life is as complicated and as critical to fathom as, for instance, the biological side, about which gerontology has acquired an impressive range of knowledge. An appreciation for the biographical or narrative dimensions is equally essential, however, if we want to seek a balanced and more optimistic perspective on what aging is about. And it is essential for honoring the dignity, humanity, and uniqueness of the lives of older persons.

In the foreword to the volume, *Narrative Gerontology: Theory, Research, and Practice*, veteran gerontologist James Birren proposes that, for the science of aging, the twenty-first century could become "the century of the liberation of personal accounts of lives, the telling of our lifestories" (2001, p. ix). A key purpose of the present volume is to trace the story of narrative gerontology itself: past, present, and future. It is a story that demonstrates the prophetic nature of Birren's words, for in the study of aging, the past 10 years have witnessed a significant increase in interest in the life-as-story metaphor. Besides a rise in the number of graduate students and faculty who are engaged in research in this area, special issues of various scholarly journals have also been devoted to its exploration, among them *Generations* and the *Journal of Aging Studies*. What is more, a biennial series of international, interdisciplinary conferences called *Narrative Matters* (in 2002, 2004, 2006, 2008, and 2010) have helped bring attention to the storied nature of human life on several levels, aging included. In fact, nearly half of the contributors to this volume have made presentations at these events, including Mark Freeman and Rita Charon as keynote speakers in 2004 and 2008, respectively. Finally, and particularly pleasing to us as editors, are the various invitations we have received to give lectures or workshops to a broad range of audiences on narrative gerontology and related topics—in particular, on *narrative care*, about which we will say more in a moment.

The conceptual roots of narrative gerontology lie in the publication of *Metaphors of Aging in Science and the Humanities* (Kenyon, Birren, & Schroots, 1991). Following this collection came *Aging and Biography: Explorations in Adult Development* (Birren, Kenyon, Ruth, Schroots, & Svensson, 1996), and then the book just mentioned, *Narrative Gerontology: Theory, Research, and Practice* (Kenyon, Clark, & de Vries, 2001). Featured in these volumes is work by colleagues who have been active in developing their own insights related to narrative. As the editors of the present volume, we deeply value the rich, long-standing collaborations we have enjoyed with a number of these thinkers. Above all, we value the singular and enduring contribution of Jim Birren.

The story of the present collection began with the meeting of Bill Randall and Ernst Bohlmeijer in Florida in 2005 at the annual conference of the *International Institute for Reminiscence and Life Review*. Following this, Bill and Gary were invited by Ernst to come to The Netherlands on at least two occasions to address events that he was instrumental in organizing. In the wake of them, Ernst was invited to St Thomas University, where Bill and Gary teach and where, one day over coffee, the idea for this book was born. The collaboration among the three of us as editors has already resulted in rich learning in our professional and personal stories alike. Indeed, we have found that when one works from a narrative perspective, the two stories—professional and personal—are closely connected. It is a special experience to collaborate with colleagues whom one also considers friends, as we have found, for instance, in hiking along the seaside trails of rural New Brunswick or among the rolling dunes on the edge of the North Sea—"The Dutch Alps," as we like to call them.

The expansion and deepening of interest in narrative gerontology is evidenced in the three key areas that are well represented in this collection: *issues*, or theoretical questions; *investigations*, or research inquiries; and *interventions*, or applications in practice. At each of these levels of discourse, the narrative metaphor is rich with implications. On the first level, that of theory, it inspires a host of intriguing insights and questions concerning human nature and human development. Among others, the following four are perhaps especially significant. First, the story metaphor opens our eyes to meaningful moments in a person's life that, from a traditional medical perspective, may go unnoticed, as Gary Kenyon explores in his chapter on Tai Chi as a form of narrative care. Second, if evolving stories are indeed the principal vehicle by which we make meaning of our experiences and through which we develop our self-identities, then with Mark Freeman we can ask which factors bring this capacity to a premature halt, to "narrative foreclosure." Third, as Phillip Clark inquires, how are personal stories influenced by public policies? And fourth, as Frits de Lange wonders, what are the limits and possible negative side effects of the narrative metaphor?

On the second level, that of research, the narrative metaphor has important scientific implications. Indeed, stories are the foremost research tools and "data" within a hermeneutically based science. The systematic analysis of the stories that people tell about their lives highlights the motivations behind specific behaviors, as in the case of The Raging Grannies, discussed by Linda Caissie, or, more darkly, the case of people's willing participation in the phenomenon of Nazi Germany, as explored by Stephan Marks. Karen Burnell, Peter Coleman, and Nigel Hunt open up new perspectives on the organization of various forms of care and support in relation to trauma. The narrative lens also helps provide us with in-depth insight into the physical aspects of aging, in the sense that it inquires into the relationship we have with our own bodies and the meaning which that relationship holds for us. Cassie Phoenix explores this relationship through her study of older athletes, while Rishi Goyal and Rita Charon do so by employing an approach characteristic of literary gerontology in their analysis of a novel by Virginia Woolf.

Finally, on the third level of discourse, that of intervention, the narrative metaphor contributes to the amelioration and transformation of the care we offer older persons. Many important decisions regarding care simply cannot be made without knowing the stories of patients and without seeing "clients" or "patients" as co-creators of these decisions (Gass, 2001). Care is fundamentally related to the question of how to live a good life, and the answer to this question is highly subjective. In many ways, effective and ethical care should incorporate and build on the notion of older adults as storying agents. From this perspective, developing policies for the implementation of narrative insights within eldercare becomes absolutely crucial, as, for instance, Gerdienke Ubels considers. So is the creation of narrative-based interventions that provide training for present and future caregivers, as argued persuasively by Gerben Westerhof. With respect to intervention, what is particularly noteworthy about this volume is that it profiles the concept of narrative care—above all, the notion of narrative care as *core* care. To call it "core care" is to say that acknowledging and respecting a person's lifestory is ultimately as important as the provision of food or shelter or medication. As a physician-colleague, a geriatrician, recently remarked in discussing the challenges of the present-day health care system, narrative care "reminds me of why I became a doctor in the first place."

Compared with other countries and contexts, gerontologists in The Netherlands have been particularly progressive in putting narrative gerontology into practice, and this volume presents a range of these innovative initiatives. These and other recent interventions raise issues that suggest new directions for narrative gerontology theory. To take just one example, we are learning more and more about the dynamics of "the stories we are" (Randall, 1995), even when we are in such extreme circumstances as trauma, terminal illness, or advanced dementia. Indeed, narrative gerontology helps to undo the "warehousing" of persons with dementia by seeing them as still biographically active, as still having narrative agency, even if they can no longer tell their stories in ordinary language or in words at all. Such insights have close affinity, of course, with those that inform the field of narrative medicine (Goyal & Charon, this volume).

What we find exciting is the increase in topics, contexts, and populations to which a narrative perspective is being applied in terms of practice. Besides trauma and dementia, as just mentioned, the list includes widowhood, body image, Holocaust survivors, war veterans, palliative care, chronic pain, suffering, frailty, and depression. Explorations of or references to several such topics are found in the pages that follow.

A narrative approach is particularly appropriate to the exploration of such topics as memory and meaning, spirituality and wisdom, as well as the links among them—links with which Bill Randall and Gary Kenyon are each in their respective ways concerned. A narrative approach lends itself to inquiring into all of these topics, for it allows us a unique perspective on the *inside* of aging. In other words, we are able to ask our fellow travelers what it is like to experience these phenomena and to ask what meaning a particular experience has for them. A number of chapters focus on memory and meaning by way of innovative applications of reminiscence, life writing, and life review, with the objective of improving the quality of life of older adults in a range of settings. Excellent examples in this case are the contributions by Kate de Medeiros, Bas Steunenberg and Ernst Bohlmeijer, Bohlmeijer and Gerben Westerhof, Jefferson Singer and Beata Labunko Messier, and Thijs Tromp. Another new development in this volume is the chapter by Philippe Cappeliez and Jeff Webster, who explore the seldom-studied topic of involuntary reminiscence and link it to the scholarly literature on reminiscence in general.

All of this is in significant contrast, we believe, to what has been the more common approach within the social sciences in general, and gerontology in particular, where the chosen method often provides only an *outside* view of aging, a limitation that results in a partial and, ultimately, decremental story of human aging—in a "narrative of decline" (Gullette, 2004). At the same time, the ontological map of our lifestory is much broader than our individual narrative, as demonstrated in several of the chapters in this book. In other words, while each of us has or is a unique inside story out of which, or amid which, we create meaning, we are simultaneously and paradoxically part of a network of larger stories that we live within, what Gubrium calls the "shared contextuality of... biographical material" (Gubrium, this volume, p. 43; see also Burnell, Coleman, & Hunt, and O'Neill, Birren, & Svensson, this volume).

Still, narrative gerontology does not espouse any one method in particular. While narrative gerontologists share a passion for lifestories, and for the richness and effectiveness of the life-as-story metaphor, the present volume, as with the works that have preceded it, reflects a wide range and combination of methodologies. It contains examples of both theoretical and empirical approaches, both qualitative and quantitative research, both background inquiry and frontline intervention, and social constructionist or sociological perspectives along with individualist or psychological ones.

The beauty of gerontology as a field is that it is inherently multidisciplinary. It thus reflects a scholarly curiosity that lends itself to flexibility in choice of method. In this respect, a novel development in this volume is that several chapters in the intervention section show the attempt to use empirical–experimental approaches to provide evidence for the effectiveness of narrative care. A key reason for doing this, of course, is to translate the story of narrative care into language that will be of use to administrators and managers so that they will implement particular programs and, in the process, come to realize that narrative care is indeed core care (Ubels, this volume).

A great variety is reflected in this book. Its international dimension is evident not only in the range of countries that its contributors represent but also in the fact, for instance, that Phillip Clark, a researcher from the United States, writes about Canadian public policy. In addition, the contributors employ different voices and different styles in their writing, they originate in different disciplines and intellectual paradigms, and they are not all gerontologists as such. What is more, they represent a range of understandings of "narrative" itself. All of this only adds to the richness of the volume.

Toward the end of the book we have included two chapters that are particularly powerful, even inspirational. The contributions by Daphne Noonan and Marie-Elise van den Brandt-van Heek both concern frontline practice. In our view, they speak for themselves in the way they demonstrate how narrative practice and narrative care are creative processes that focus on individual lifestories. In other words, in narrative, there is no such thing as "one size fits all." The magic of a biographical encounter occurs in the mutual presence of one person to another. Both Noonan and van den Brandt-van Heek have caught the vision of narrative care, have intuitively accepted its relevance, and are following their instincts as they run with it in their respective contexts. Along with the contributions by Caissie, with her research on the Raging Grannies, and by O'Neill, Svensson, and Birren, who use guided autobiography to challenge gender-role stereotypes in later life, they are representative of the new generation of narrative gerontologists whom we have sought to feature in this volume.

Our afterword consists of a commentary on the contribution of narrative gerontology to contemporary health care. Clearly, narrative gerontology takes in a broader spectrum of topics and themes than is encompassed by health care as such or by intervention in general. Nonetheless, the reformulation of health care has become an urgent and ever-growing issue in our world. In the dialogue concerning that issue, narrative gerontology—especially by way of the concept of narrative care—can play a central and vital role.

Gary Kenyon

William L. Randall

Ernst Bohlmeijer

REFERENCES

Birren, J. (2001). Foreword. In G. Kenyon, P. Clark, & B. de Vries (Eds.), *Narrative gerontology: Theory, research, and practice* (pp. vii–ix). New York: Springer.

Birren, J., Kenyon, G., Ruth, J.-E., Schroots, J., & Svensson, T. (Eds.). (1996). *Aging and biography: Explorations in adult development.* New York: Springer.

Gass, D. (2001). Narrative knowledge and health care of the elderly. In G. Kenyon, P. Clark, & B. de Vries (Eds.), *Narrative gerontology: Theory, research, and practice* (pp. 215–236). New York: Springer.

Gullette, M. (2004). *Aged by culture.* Chicago: University of Chicago Press.

Kenyon, G., Birren, J., & Schroots, J. (Eds.). (1991). *Metaphors of aging in science and the humanities.* New York: Springer.

Kenyon, G., Clark, P., & de Vries, B. (Eds.). (2001). *Narrative gerontology: Theory, research, and practice.* New York: Springer.

Randall, W. (1995). *The stories we are: An essay on self-creation.* Toronto: University of Toronto Press.

Contributors

James E. Birren, PhD, is Professor and Dean Emeritus of Gerontology at the University of Southern California, Los Angeles, California, USA.

Ernst Bohlmeijer, PhD, is Associate Professor of Clinical Health Psychology at the University of Twente, Enschede, The Netherlands.

Karen Burnell, PhD, is a Research Associate in the Department of Mental Health Sciences at University College London, London, United Kingdom.

Philippe Cappeliez, PhD, is Professor in the School of Psychology, University of Ottawa, Ottawa, Ontario, Canada.

Linda Caissie, PhD, is Assistant Professor of Gerontology at St Thomas University, Fredericton, New Brunswick, Canada.

Rita Charon, MD, PhD, is Professor of Clinical Medicine at Columbia University, New York, New York, USA.

Phillip G. Clark, ScD, is Professor and Director of the Program in Gerontology and the Rhode Island Geriatric Education Center at the University of Rhode Island, Kingston, Rhode Island, USA.

Peter Coleman, PhD, is Professor of Psychogerontology at the School of Psychology, University of Southampton, Southampton, United Kingdom.

Frits de Lange, PhD, is Professor of Ethics at Protestant Theological University, Kampen, The Netherlands.

Kate de Medeiros, PhD, is the Brookdale Leadership in Aging Fellow at the Copper Ridge Institute in Sykesville, Maryland, USA, and is Assistant Professor in the Department of Psychiatry and Behavioral Sciences at the Johns Hopkins University School of Medicine in Baltimore, Maryland, USA.

Mark Freeman, PhD, is Professor of Psychology at College of the Holy Cross, Worcester, Massachusetts, USA.

Rishi Goyal, MD, MPhil, is Chief Resident in Emergency Medicine at New York Presbyterian Hospital, New York, New York, USA.

Jaber F. Gubrium, PhD, is Professor and Chair of Sociology at University of Missouri, Columbia, Missouri, USA.

Nigel Hunt, PhD, is Associate Professor in the Institute of Work, Health, and Organisations at the University of Nottingham, Nottingham, United Kingdom.

Gary Kenyon, PhD, is Professor of Gerontology at St Thomas University in Fredericton, New Brunswick, Canada.

Stephan Marks, PhD, is Director of the History and Memory Project at the University of Education, Freiburg, Germany.

Beata Labunko Messier, MA, is a Research Associate at Connecticut College, New London, Connecticut, USA.

Daphne Noonan, MEd, is Manager of Therapeutic Recreation at York Care Centre, Fredericton, New Brunswick, Canada.

Patricia O'Neill, JD, is a PhD candidate at the Oxford Institute of Ageing, Oxford University, Oxford, United Kingdom.

Cassandra Phoenix, PhD, is Lecturer in Qualitative Research at the University of Exeter, Exeter, United Kingdom.

William L. Randall, EdD, is Professor of Gerontology and Director of the Centre for Interdisciplinary Research on Narrative at St Thomas University in Fredericton, New Brunswick, Canada.

Jefferson A. Singer, PhD, is Professor of Psychology at Connecticut College, New London, Connecticut, USA.

Bas Steunenberg, PhD, is Assistant Professor of Clinical Health Psychology at the University of Utrecht, Utrecht, The Netherlands.

Cheryl M. Svensson, PhD, is an Instructor at the Davis School of Gerontology, University of Southern California, Los Angeles, California, USA.

Thijs Tromp, PhD, is Manager of Reliëf Christian Association of Health Care Institutions in Utrecht, The Netherlands.

Gerdienke M. Ubels, MA, is Senior Policy Advisor for ActiZ, the Dutch National Association of Residential and Home Care Organizations for the Elderly, Utrecht, The Netherlands.

Marie-Elise van den Brandt-van Heek, Drs, is a psychologist in nursing homes for the elderly in The Hague, Netherlands; she also works for

Reliëf Christian Association of Health Care Institutions in Utrecht, The Netherlands.

Jeffrey Dean Webster, MEd, is an Instructor in the Psychology Department of Langara College in Vancouver, British Columbia, Canada.

Gerben J. Westerhof, PhD, is Associate Professor in Psychology at the University of Twente, Enschede, The Netherlands.

Part 1   Issues

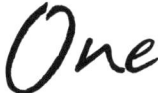

NARRATIVE FORECLOSURE IN LATER LIFE:

POSSIBILITIES AND LIMITS

Mark Freeman

NARRATIVE AND BEYOND

This chapter is an attempt to find a suitable answer to a vexing, very disturbing question that has been with me for some time. Before posing this question, however, some background is in order. A number of years ago, I came across several instances, in both my research and my personal life, in which people had gathered the conviction that the stories of their lives were essentially over. I called the phenomenon "narrative foreclosure," and while it certainly wasn't restricted to later life, there was no questioning its salience during this phase of the life course—particularly in those cultural climates in which later life might be seen as little more than an opportunity to "pass the time" until it runs out (Freeman, 2000a; Randall & McKim, 2008; see also Coleman, 1999; McAdams, 2006). There was a critical edge to this early work on the phenomenon as well as a measure of hope: insofar as narrative foreclosure was a function of individuals having internalized cultural narratives of decline, there would be a way, in principle at least, of breaking their coercive spell and thereby reopening the stories at hand.

Some subsequent work dealing with narrative foreclosure served to moderate these claims. For it was clear that in some cases the weight of the personal past was so oppressively burdensome and the resultant immobility so seemingly irrevocable that, on the face of it, there seemed to be no way of revivifying one's story. For these people, it was too late, or so it felt; the ending was a foregone conclusion—there would be, there could be, no moving on. For this reason, suicide might seem like the only viable option: if it is impossible to imagine a future that is any different from the present, the conviction may emerge that the ending is to be hastened, seized ahead of time. It should be emphasized that, even in such dire circumstances, there may still remain a measure of hope—if not necessarily for the foreclosed person him- or herself. The therapeutic challenge in this context is precisely to "convince" the individual that even if he or she believes that the future will be no different than the present, this very belief may well be unfounded. The burden will be lessened in due time; the pain will subside. Along the lines being drawn here, one's belief that it is "too late" may be premature. Indeed, strictly speaking, one might argue, it is never too late. There is always room to move, to change the course of things. I shall have more to say about these issues in the pages to come.

But how was I to think about those instances of narrative foreclosure that were a function neither of prevailing cultural storylines nor of one's unshakable convictions about the dead end of the future but instead of the irrefutable fact of one's inevitable decline due to physical and/or mental deterioration? I am thinking of dementia especially, and I have quite specific reasons for raising this question. I can put it in even simpler terms: How might one think about the phenomenon of narrative foreclosure in those circumstances when there truly *is* no hope, when it would appear that there is no possibility at all of opening up the future and revivifying the lifestory? Vexing indeed, and troubling.

This afternoon I will be heading to my mother's assisted living residence. And very likely I will be greeted by a rush of delight (albeit somewhat muted) and then shortly thereafter by a litany of questions and painful lamentations: "Do I live here?" "How long have I lived here?" "I've been here for several years?" And then it hits her, as it does almost every time I see her. "Oh, my God. Oh, my God. Oh, what a person becomes. Sometimes you just live too long." There was a time when I could challenge some of these utterances by extracting whatever sense of possibility I could. Things are different now, I would essentially explain, but there was still room for some measure of meaning, maybe even for a kind of fulfillment that was more difficult to come by earlier on. In the first piece I wrote about her situation, I in fact spoke of "dementia's tragic promise" (2008a): due to the progressive demise of memory and self, there seemed to emerge a kind of openness to the present moment—a good meal, a piece of music, a family gathering— that was, on some level (dare I say it), enviable. But this phase was relatively short-lived, and the way things stand now, the very idea of envy seems impertinent if not outrageous. My mother is biding her time. And although we still do what we can to help fashion enjoyable moments, they are few and far between. She is frequently bewildered and lost, and despite the fact that there are some enjoyable moments still, they are not at all a part of the story, such as it is, that she can tell about her life. She forgets these moments, as she does all the activities in which she has been engaged throughout the day. And so when I ask how her day has been, she generally tells me that she's done nothing at all. "There's nothing doing here. They don't have any activities at all." This can lead to dreadful questions of the sort she asked me just last week: "So, how do you feel about leaving me in a place like this?"

Should I stop asking her how her day has gone? Perhaps. As awful as it may be to admit, I have also come to be somewhat ambivalent about even going to spend time with her—not because of what it does to me (though it does plenty) but because of what it does to her. My very presence almost always elicits confusion, and then questions, and then either horror (given what she has become) or resentment (given that she is all alone, in a place that feels utterly unfamiliar, where there seems to be absolutely nothing to do) or some other dark emotion. There is a good chance that none of this would have emerged had I not come for a visit. What is to be done?

Before providing an answer to this question, let me recount my own path of exploring the idea of narrative foreclosure. In doing so, I shall focus on both the possibilities and limits—that is, on how ostensibly foreclosed narratives might be reopened and why, in certain circumstances, it may be all but impossible to do so. Indeed, it is precisely in such circumstances that we see the limits of narrative itself.

FORECLOSURE 1: DEAD ENDS

In my initial foray into the idea of narrative foreclosure, I wrote about the story of an aging artist who, having struggled to hit his artistic stride throughout most of his life, had arrived at the tragic conclusion that it simply would not, and could not, happen (Freeman, 2000a).[1] In his eyes, it was too late for opening up a new chapter; he was getting on in years, and with the (imagined) ending now in sight, there was little left to do but carry on fatalistically, knowing—or at least believing—that there really was nothing to be done. Especially tragic in this case was the fact that this very conviction had poisoned the entire story of his life: the excitement he had once felt as an up-and-comer now seemed silly and self-indulgent; the deep truths that he had once discovered, or thought he had discovered, came to seem like illusions. There was simply no way that something truly authentic and good could have culminated in his sorry state.

What I went on to suggest in light of this man's life was that he had unwittingly internalized certain cultural storylines that served to undermine his creativity. One was about what I called the "Artist/God," whose achievements all but transcend the earthly world. For a multitude of reasons, this artist had proved to be all too human, which in turn meant that he would be forever destined to fall short of the mark. Indeed, he would continue to be a "Wandering Self," trying one path to greatness, then another, only to find that each of them was "less an avenue than a blind alley." These storylines, coupled with his own conviction that time was running out, had cast him in the role of victim—of a community where no one seemed to know anything about Real Art; of an art world that too often seemed to privilege cheap, showy gimmicks over authentic creativity; of an era that privileged engineers and technology-types over the likes of romantic throwbacks like him.

His predicament is a painful one. On one level, his deep doubt about the possibility of his own artistic self-realization leads to his telling a story of the past that, for all of its putative triumphs, cannot help but appear silly and delusional: as he looks backward, he sees a grandiose young man so taken with his own fantasies that he mistook them for realities. From this angle, his past has become tainted, poisoned; the ending is foisted onto the beginning, excising whatever goodness there might actually have been. At the same time, there emerges the suspicion that, when it came right down it, there probably wasn't much there to begin with. From this second angle, therefore, he is finally able to see the past for what it truly was, shorn of consolations, defenses, self-protective fictions about his potential. Both of these angles of vision, redoubled by his self-perception as a man past his prime, lead to a profound sense of disappointment, stasis, and felt impossibility.

Consider the process of reading works of literature in this context. In the case of mysteries and suspense novels especially, only after we have finished reading are we able to understand why things happened as they did. The ending reverberates backward: what had heretofore been open and at least partially indeterminate comes together, bringing a measure of interpretive closure and fulfillment. There can be surprise and pleasure too, particularly if the ending is unanticipated: what had seemed to lead in one direction may turn out to have led in quite another. As a kind of corollary to this idea, it is also the case that, insofar as we already know, or believe we know, how a given work will end, there may be little motivation to continue reading. This is essentially what happened in this man's case. Because he "knows" how the story will end, his own motivation, creativity, and narrative desire have been sapped. He therefore remains immobilized, frozen in his artistic tracks. The only way to move forward, I had surmised, would be to identify and name the storylines at hand and see how pervasive they had been in structuring his very desires and expectations about what was possible and what was not. Only then would he be able to reopen the story of his life and restart the creative process. It is not at all clear that he would be able to do so. By all indications, his story was in the process of congealing and hardening, perhaps irretrievably.

FORECLOSURE 2: THE POINT OF NO RETURN

In more recent work (Freeman, 2010), I presented the story of another artist, who had also been in the throes of narrative foreclosure and had managed to reopen her story in just this way. Her story was rather different, however. At one point in her career, this woman had been part of an art scene that was terrifically exciting. As a member of a well-known group of artists who shared many of her artistic ideas and aims, she had been able to gain entry into the art world in a way that was comparatively problem-free. Eventually, however, she grew uncomfortable with the art she was doing; it seemed too boisterous and loud, and ran counter to some of the ideas she was beginning to explore. So it was that she began "working against everything" she had learned in school. It was time to not only fashion her own artistic identity but also lay bare the most elemental ingredients of art itself. In true postmodern fashion, she became fascinated with how paintings were "constructed," her aim being to eliminate from her work anything and everything that was inessential and thereby discover what paintings required for their very existence. Important though this process of eliminative stripping-down was, it eventually yielded a disturbing realization: if she continued in this reductive mode of painting, there would soon be nothing left at all. She therefore came to realize—or to believe—that *nothing* was essential to a work of art, that there *was* no foundational rationale whatsoever for a painting's existence. Perhaps, moreover, there was no identifiable reason for her, or anyone else, to paint. Here she was, creating essentially use-less objects that had no discernible rationale, no reason for being. There would eventually be an artistic breakdown, a point of no return. She would be rendered mute, reduced to silence (see Freeman, 2000b).

It was precisely at this point of no return that she had to ask herself, as honestly as she could, whether in fact she had anything to say as an artist. If she did, she could return to painting and begin to reinsert some substance into her art. If she didn't, she would simply have to do something else altogether. Upon arriving at the conclusion that she was indeed an artist after all, unlike the man I had written about earlier, she was able to see how she had unwittingly been held captive by certain quite specific ideas and assumptions circulating through the art world at the time. Upon seeing this, she was able free herself from their tenacious hold and thereby create once again. Much of the work she had done in her reductive phase, she realized, had been about certain perceptual "issues" being addressed in the art world. At the time, being capable of addressing these issues seemed important, indeed critical, to her success as an artist. But there was also something overly calculated and "manipulative" about this work, and she eventually came to feel that, somehow, she had strayed from the true path and had become a kind of accomplice to an overly intellectualized approach to creating art. Only in hindsight could she see what had happened. And it was only now, with this understanding, that she could begin to do something more real, more in tune with her true interests and passions.

This woman had thus undergone a dual process of "demystification" and "desocialization": in addition to clearing away the previously obscure sources of her artistic foreclosure, she had to undo the regressive work of those social forces that had been operative in her own near-demise. In her case, there was ultimately a happy measure of triumph. Her work became "additive," even "operatic"; she could once again feel that sort of ecstatic connectedness that sometimes emerges "when it all fuses." What's more, this connectedness would extend to viewers as well, her refound authenticity having been made manifest in the work itself. Her story was reopened and her creativity, remobilized. She too had been living a life whose contours owed their very existence to cultural discourses and storylines—to an element of *narrative force*, as it might be called (see Freeman, 2010)—that for a time she had been unable to identify and name. Unlike the man described in the previous section, however, she eventually managed to break the spell of this force and thereby set in motion her own *narrative freedom*—which is to say, the freedom to chart her own artistic and personal path. Her story was thus a story of hope, of *possibility*, in the face of what had once seemed to be insurmountable odds. In this respect, it serves as an apt illustration of the fact that, even when one has reached what feels like a point of no return, it may nevertheless be possible to move creatively into the future (see Langer, 2009).

FORECLOSURE 3: IRREVOCABILITY

But is it always possible? In some other work, also related to the idea of narrative foreclosure, I followed a different, and decidedly more tragic, line of thinking through exploring some of the work of Primo Levi (Freeman, 2003). Given the harrowing precision of Levi's account of the concentration camp experience, I take the liberty here of drawing directly on some of his own words. In a chapter entitled "Shame" from his book *The Drowned and the Saved* (1989), Levi states that there is a tendency to think of the moment of liberation as a one of supreme relief, even joy. Unfortunately, however, Levi insists, this story is largely false. Far from there being relief, there was instead newfound suffering. For it would suddenly become clear that they had been living "at an animal level," their "days [having] been encumbered from dawn to dusk by hunger, fatigue, cold, and fear; any space for reflection, reasoning, experiencing emotions was wiped out." What had also become clear, Levi adds, is that "[w]e had not only forgotten our country and our culture, but also our family, our past, the future we had imagined for ourselves, because like animals, we were confined to the present moment" (p. 75).

Narrative becomes a double-edged sword in this context. On the one hand, it presents a positive possibility here, an opportunity to move beyond the animal-like confines of the present moment. With the distance conferred by time, Levi is able to see, all too clearly, the full measure of his own dimin-ishment. And it was this seeing, from afar, that had caused so much pain. Indeed, Levi maintains, it was exactly this "turning to look back at the 'perilous water'" that led to so many suicides following Liberation. There were numerous reasons for this tragic outcome. Foremost among them was the conviction that they hadn't done enough against the "system" at hand. Levi and his fellow camp inmates would occasionally witness the strength of resistors, some of whom were hanged publicly. "This is a thought that then barely grazed us," Levi writes, "but that returned 'afterward': you too could have, you certainly should have" (pp. 77–78).

For some, there could also be the shame of having failed their fellow prisoners. "Few survivors feel guilty about having deliberately damaged, robbed, or beaten a companion," Levi notes. "By contrast, however, almost everybody feels guilty of having omitted to offer help" (p. 78). There were, of course, good reasons for their behaving the way they did at the time; they did what they could to survive. Nevertheless, "shame there was and is, concrete, heavy, perennial" (p. 81).

There is one additional dimension of shame that Levi addresses toward the end of his chapter. He calls it "the shame of the world," and it was tied to "the misdeeds that others and not they had committed, and in which they felt involved, because they sensed that what had happened around them and in their presence, and in them, was irrevocable. Never again could it be cleansed" (p. 86). It is this sense of the "irrevocable" that needs to be underscored here, the felt impossibility of ever "cleansing," rectifying, undoing what had—and had not—been done.

Levi himself was not a believer. He does note that believers generally fared better throughout their ordeal in the camps. He speaks of "the saving force of their faith," and suggests that "[t]heir universe was vaster than ours, more extended in space and time, above all more comprehensible: they had a key and a point of leverage, a millennial tomorrow so that there might be a sense to sacrificing themselves, a place in heaven or on earth where justice and compassion had won, or would win in a perhaps remote but certain future" (p. 146). Levi was denied all of this meaning and solace, this *hope*. But what he was not denied—and what he *could* not deny—was the conviction of his having participated, in some way, in the very crimes that had been perpetrated against him. More than shame was at work. Shame is something one might be able to work through and beyond; it is a malady of the self, and lends itself to some measure of change. What Levi had experienced, I suggest, would more appropriately be considered *sin*. It was a malady of the soul, and could not become an object of change, of reconstruction. Hence the depth of the tragedy: there is here what one might plausibly call religious experience, in a radically negative form, but there are no religious resources available to allow for the possibility of self-forgiveness or redemption. The damage is done. It's too late.

The form of narrative foreclosure reflected in Levi's story is a particularly pernicious one. There are no unwittingly internalized cultural storylines to be exposed, as in the stories of the two artists. Devoid of those resources that might have allowed Levi a measure of reprieve from his shame, he is held captive by his past. So much for "liberation": having been freed physically from the confines of the camps and mentally from the confines of the present moment, he has been imprisoned once again, with no prospect whatsoever of release.

Narrative, so often portrayed as a source of solace, comfort, and positive self-regard, a balm to soothe the wounds of one's life (e.g., Gazzaniga, 1998; Ross & Wilson, 2000), can generate wounds of its own. Looking backward, one can sometimes see certain features of the past for the very first time; and while the result can be great joy and gratitude, it can also be the deepest pain and regret. The tragic irony of Levi's situation is that in this narrative seeing he returned to his moral self, his human self. To see the moral depravity and animality of his own behavior, and to suffer from it as much as he did, is itself a sign of virtue, even a kind of transcendence. A fully *human* being, he recognized, surpasses the condition of animality. One notable way of doing so is precisely through narrative—that is, by moving beyond the confines of the present, with its more immediate impulses, wishes, and needs, and gathering a broader view of things. Herein lies the irony: Only through Levi's deep and abiding humanity could he become witness to his own inhumanity. If only he could have received some consolation from this. But he cannot. He is in prison once again. The prison is his narrative. The narrative is his prison.

FORECLOSURE 4: EXISTENTIAL DESPAIR

Again, is there any hope in this sort of situation? Is there any prospect of reopening the story? The classic example of such narrative transformation is found in Tolstoy's novella *The Death of Ivan Ilych* (1960/1886; see also Freeman, 1997, 2010). Having sustained a minor injury during the course of some routine redecorating only to see it ramify into a horrid and ever-intensifying sense of disease, Ivan Ilych, faced suddenly with the reality of his imminent death, looks back on his ostensibly good life only to find wreckage. Upon beginning to recall "the best moments of his pleasant life," it was suddenly the case that "none of those best moments of his pleasant life now seemed at all what they had then seemed." Indeed, "[a]s soon as the period began which produced the present Ivan Ilych"—the beginning of his awful end—"all that had then seemed joys now melted before his sight and turned into something trivial and often nasty. And the further he departed from childhood and the nearer he came to the present the more worthless and doubtful were the joys" (p. 144). Thus he can only conclude: "It is as if I had been going downhill while I imagined I was going up. And that is what it really was. I was going up in public opinion, but to the same extent life was ebbing away from me. And now it is all done and there is only death" (pp. 144–145). With "only death" remaining, here too, the damage has been done. It is too late, or so it seems; foreclosure thus appears to be complete, fixed, unchangeable.

Alongside Ivan Ilych's recognition "of how his illness had progressed and grown worse," he also saw that the further back he looked the more life there had been. There had been more of what was good in life and more of life itself. The two merged together: "Just as the pain went on getting worse and worse, so my life grew worse and worse," he thought. "There is one bright spot there at the back, at the beginning of life, and afterwards all becomes blacker and blacker and proceeds more and more rapidly—in inverse ratio to the square of the distance from death," thought Ivan Ilych. And the example of a stone falling downward and with increasing velocity entered his mind. Life, a series of increasing sufferings, flies further and further toward its end—the most terrible suffering. "I am flying... . He shuddered, shifted himself, and tried to resist, but was already aware that resistance was impossible" (p. 147). Was there anything to be done but wait until the end, hurtling ever more speedily and fiercely toward him?

And then the question emerges that is at one and the same time the source of Ivan Ilych's deepest despair as well as his eventual salvation: "'What if my whole life has really been wrong?'" (p. 148). In Primo Levi's case, the sense of irrevocability had reached a fever pitch in its own right, and this despite the fact that his own sphere of culpability was limited largely to those years of his life he spent in the camps. In Ivan Ilych's case, the sphere in question is his entire life, the result being that as he looked candidly at all that had transpired, "There was nothing to defend... . 'But if that is so,' he said to himself, 'and I am leaving this life with the consciousness that I have lost all that was given me and it is impossible to rectify it—what then?'" (p. 149). There was no question but that "he was lost, that there was no return, that the end had come, the very end" (p. 150).

On the face of it, this is the foreclosure of foreclosures. Unlike the three other cases we have explored, there would appear to be nary a hope of reopening the story at hand. The reason is simple enough: Ivan Ilych is on the brink of death, his entire life has been a colossal mistake, and he not only *feels* that time is running out, he *knows* it is. But even here, in this most extreme case, Tolstoy suggests that there stills exists the possibility of reopening an ostensibly foreclosed narrative. After struggling desperately in the "black sack" of his imminent death, he falls through the "black hole" into which he had been thrust, catches sight of the light at the bottom of the hole, "and it was revealed to him that though his life was not what it should have been, this could still be rectified" (p. 151). His son kisses his hand and Ivan Ilych feels sorry for him. His wife, with undried tears, comes up to him and he feels sorry for her too. Now, "he must act so as not to hurt them and free himself from these sufferings." Alongside the emergence of the sorry truth of his life is the emergence of goodness, in the form of unprecedented care and sympathy for the others who surround him. There is a new ending: "In place of death there was light" (p. 152). The spell, and horror, of foreclosure is broken.

FORECLOSURE, FINITUDE, AND FINALITY

In Ilych's case, both his life and his lifestory were in the process of ending; death was imminent, and up until the final moments, there seemed to be precious little to be done about it. In other cases, as we have seen, narrative foreclosure may have less to do with the reality of imminent death than with the conviction that it is simply too late to live meaningfully. This conviction, I have suggested, is often not the individual's alone. It may also be a societal conviction, tied to extant myths and images of aging, for instance, or to the existence of cultural institutions that fail to support the continued development of the narrative function. Indeed, another way of speaking about narrative foreclosure is in terms of a breakdown of the narrative function, an inability to see one's experience as having any significance beyond itself. Its ill effects may extend to any and all people whose futures have become stripped of new possibilities, emptied of new opportunities for self-renewal. As we have also seen throughout this chapter, there may remain reasons for hope even in such dire circumstances; new possibilities can and sometimes do emerge, even in the eleventh hour, and what one assumes to be utterly irrevocable may in fact not be. But here I want to return to the question posed at the very beginning of the chapter: How might we think about those instances of narrative foreclosure that are a function neither of prevailing cultural narratives about aging nor of one's unshakable convictions about the dead end of the future but instead of the irrefutable fact of one's inevitable decline due to physical and/or mental deterioration? In some circumstances, there can *be* no reopening of one's lifestory. Indeed, in some circumstances, there really *is* no lifestory "to speak of"—not at least for the person whose story it was, for there may remain only the most minimal sense of what that life was about. There is not much room for hope here. And we are up against the limits not only of reopening a foreclosed narrative but also of narrative itself.

It is time to return to my mother's story. By way of providing some additional context for understanding her story, I shall refer briefly to three recent pieces of work which, taken together, chart the trajectory of her condition over the course of recent years. Having been diagnosed with dementia when the process was already well under way, she struggled mightily against the reality of her increasing infirmity in the earlier phases of the condition. Sometimes, she would do so in a lighthearted way. At one point, for instance, she spoke of being afflicted by "CRS" (Can't Remember Shit) syndrome. More often, however, she would become vehement, and occasionally very angry, about her own limitations as well as those sometimes placed upon her. "I know I can still drive just fine," she would say. "I've always taken care of my own papers." "I've never been late with a check." And when I would question these abilities, as was sometimes necessary, her response would be swift and sharp: "I'm not an imbecile." "You're treating me like a child." Long after it was feasible, she proclaimed one day that "I want to get some kind of job," maybe office managerial work, of the sort she had pursued following my father's death. And when I tried to explain to her that things were different now, that some of the things she used to do so well would be much tougher, she would either reject the idea out of hand or simply be mystified by it. Time to move on to another topic, quickly.

She was also highly critical of her assisted living residence during this earlier phase. She deplored the bus trips for ice cream, the never-ending Bingo games (which she still deplores), and the fact that the place was "dead" by 8 o'clock at night. She was also upset by all the walkers and wheelchairs everywhere, not to mention the very old and fragile people who were using them. And for good reason: as I was able to write some years ago (Freeman, 2008a), "[My mother] doesn't look like them at all; she's attractive and moves briskly, still confident in her step" (p. 170). It's painful to read those words now, not even four years later. Suffice it to say that she looks very different at this point and moves extremely slowly, often needing a wheelchair herself; and her "step," far from being confident, is instead hesitant and unsure. She shuffles, her eyes often fixed in a dull stare, sometimes holding onto the wall for balance. But back then, she stood out from the crowd, seemed to know it on some level, and thoroughly resented where she had landed, both literally and figuratively. "What do you want?," I had asked her one day. "I want to be a person," she answered. When she lived on her own, she was a "free agent" who could come and go as she pleased. And in her own mind, she still was that person, or at least a close relative. "There is a story that can be told about this person," I wrote.

> It is the story of a child whose parents were too poor to keep her and who therefore sent her off to a children's home—which she had quite loved—for a couple of years. It is the story of a teenager, a bit shy but the smartest in the whole class; of a young woman, competent and hardworking, going it alone, while her husband was away in India during the war; of a middle-aged woman, prematurely widowed, who, after years of being a homemaker, had to go out into the work world once more, where she excelled, rising to the position of office manager, in charge of lots of people and able to make the whole outfit run smoothly and efficiently. This story still seems to be with her. How dare anyone suggest that she could no longer balance a checkbook! She had balanced books for a living, and was damn good at it! On one level, the continued presence of this story is surely a good thing. But it is also the source of much of her current frustration and sorrow. (2008a, p. 171)

It was in light of these issues that I entertained the idea of "deconstructing the cultural story" (2008a, p. 175), my suggestion being that a portion of my mother's response to her current situation might plausibly be considered the "product of a culture that, in a distinct sense, refuses to admit the reality of decline, and death, into its midst" (pp. 175–176). What I also suggested was the existence of a "dual narrative… operating behind the scenes of consciousness." First, there was "the narrative of the vital, self-sufficient Individual, who resists the kind of fragility, vulnerability, and dependency that growing old sometimes brings in tow." It was surprising to learn how pervasive and potent this narrative was, and how resistant it was to being modified. Second, there was what I termed "the narrative of inexorable decline," which, in a distinct sense, operates in tandem with—and is on some level parasitic upon—the first.

> Old people, with their walkers and their wheelchairs, surround my mother. People sit in the lobby, slumped over, dozing, waking briefly when there are passersby. Some of them do seem to have little to do, little left to live for: their story *is* over—or at least that is how they see it. And part of the reason *why* they see it this way may be linked back to the image of that vital self just considered. They are the inverted image of that self, beyond vitality, beyond self-sufficiency—in some ways, my mother has suggested, beyond personhood itself. She is vehemently *not*-them. The nightly Bingo that they play downstairs, in open view, really gets to her. At the end of the day, there are only mindless games, camaraderie created by random numbers. Time for them is not to be lived, but passed. There is no story to be told after such days; they are just like the one before and the one before that. My mother sometimes seems to resent these "non-persons" with their non-stories. In her eyes, they have crossed the line, and the image of them sitting there, night after night, is painful to behold. I suppose one could say that, on some level, they exist in the moment. And it's quite possible that they are less troubled by their existence than she is hers. But this is hardly an occasion for envy. (2008a, pp. 176–177)

And yet, as I noted earlier, there was a period of time following this earlier phase in which there emerged an enviable kind of "self-forgetfulness": attending a concert, sitting outside on a beautiful day, having a good meal with some good wine, she would be transfixed, more than ever, it seemed. Hence my reference to "dementia's tragic promise": gone, for the moment, is the nagging narrative that had so frustrated her; she is freed, temporarily, of her burdens; with the continued attenuation of self, of ego, she can experience the nourishment of what is Other. "The world has returned, and it has done so at precisely the same moment that the (autobiographical) self and its narrative have 'disappeared'" (p. 173). I even cautiously entertained the possibility that this sort of experience might be related to mystical experience, which, "in their quite different ways of moving beyond narrative, offers a kind of deliverance, a reprieve from the anxiety and pressure of the autobiographical self. Whether this process of autobiographical unselfing has the redemptive outcome we are hoping for," I went on to say, "only time will tell" (p. 183).

And it did. After a brief period of intensification, in which my mother was indeed able occasionally to experience a kind of ecstatic oneness with the world, this oneness was transformed into a kind of nothingness, coupled at times with moments of horror in the face of her own self-dissolution (see Freeman, 2008b). It was in the face of this subsequent phase of her condition that I began to wonder whether she had essentially left narrative behind— whether, that is, she had moved into a mode of being shorn of any sense of her own history and story, of past and future, indeed, of her very identity. I would often get panicky phone calls from her at this time (there would usually be an aide by her side, helping her to reach me). Where was she? It was her first day at her new apartment (she would say); why wasn't there anyone around to help her get settled? She could recognize some of the things in her apartment, but the apartment itself was utterly unfamiliar. How did all of her things get there? Who brought them? I myself came to assume the rather strange role of being her lifeline to reality itself. In the midst of her dislocations, she needed something to hold onto, some piece of familiarity, some source of recognition; and that something was me. It was a good thing I arrived at her apartment when I did, she said to me during one of these dislocations; had I not done so, she would have screamed. So much for the alleged virtues of "being in the moment," "living in the present," the quasi-mysticism of the dissolving demented self. The experience of ecstatic oneness, I realized, "still requires a self, in contact enough with the world as to be able to draw nourishment from it… . To be fully present to the world, there needs to be a being, there, to witness it and savor it, an 'I' who sees and feels, a self actively engaged with reality" (2008b, p. 140). It wasn't happening. I feared that I was losing her, and for good reason. In her words, there is sometimes "Nothing, absolutely nothing."

My mother still has many such moments, moments in which she becomes so dislocated and untethered that it seems as if she might flee reality altogether. There are more phone calls: "Okay, Mark, if you could please call me, I would appreciate it, honey, because I'm bewildered and I'm in a fog. So if you could do that, I would appreciate it. Thank you." "Mark? I'm trying to get in touch with you; I don't know what the story is. So, if you can call me, I would appreciate it, honey. OK? I think you have my number. All right. Bye." If it's serious enough, I will try my best to get over to her apartment. "Welcome to my new abode," she said to me recently. "What do you mean, ma?" And then it begins again: "I just moved in today.

I don't know how things got here so fast." "You've been here for a while, ma." "How long have I been here?" "About three years." "In this apartment?" "You've been in this apartment for over a year now. You used to be in one upstairs." "Oh, my God." "When did I get here?" "About three years ago, ma." "Huh." "*How long?*" "It's about three years now, ma." And so the conversations go. She means it quite literally when she says, "I don't know what the story is."

What's striking in this context, however, is her memory that there *is* a story. Despite severe memory loss, there are occasionally flashes of awareness, recognition. In fact, this past New Year's Day seemed to mark a change. I called her late afternoon to see how she was feeling, and she immediately spoke about having woken up confused from a nap. "I've lost big chunks of my memory," she said. "I've lost big chunks of my life." As for what this feels like, at times: "Moron." "I don't have a brain." "I'm like a child now." "No, you're not," I protest; "you're a full-grown adult." "But mindless." "Dumb." "I have to be put in a nursery with infants, to be watched. Brainless. I don't have a brain anymore." "*Oh, what a person becomes.*" There can be empathy too, or something like it: "What you must feel like when you leave, to see your poor mother like this." And the refrain: "Oh, my God. Oh, my God." Sometimes it's all just "amazing." But it can also be "horrifying" and "terrifying."

Through it all, she is relatively devoid, it seems, of deep feeling about the situation. She doesn't cry, which she did in the past; her response is more cerebral, even intellectual. It also doesn't seem particularly personal; there is loss, to be sure, but it's not so much "hers" as it is an awareness of human loss, human demise, the fate of people and their stories. There is still some sense of identity, but it is highly diffuse, even, strangely enough, impersonal. As I recently (2009) put the matter, she seems to have a memory of how to be *a* person if not *this* person. She seems, in other words, to have a kind of generic idea of what being a person means. The phrases I referred to earlier—"I want to be a person" and "Oh, what a person becomes"—reflect this awareness, as do her lamentations about being brainless, mindless, or like a child. Even now, there is an image in view of who and what she once was. But unlike the earlier years, when she would fight mightily to hold onto this image, there's no holding on anymore. She no longer knows "the story." But she does seem to know that it's over. Recall the sentence I referred to earlier: "Sometimes," she says, "you just live too long."

Is there anything to be done? Can I somehow "talk her through" this? More to the point still: Is there any possibility at all of opening up her story, in whatever way, once again? Strictly speaking, I think the answer is "no." Among other reasons, any story that might be reopened is destined to fade into oblivion once again at the next dislocation or panicky awakening from an afternoon nap. What's more, given that she has only the most minimal sense of the future, it's hard to imagine what it is that she might live *for*, if by "for" we are referring to some purpose, some motivating source of meaning and value. She seems to know this too; her days are much the same, and she can feel this sameness, this tedious ongoing endlessness. And even when Something Significant disrupts the flow, even when her days are—from an outsider's perspective—quite full, the story, such as it is, remains much the same: because she can't remember what's gone on, it seems to her that *nothing* goes on, ever. "Events," therefore, of the sort that would ordinarily go to narrative, fade and dissipate. I once explained this to her. After she had complained, yet again, about there being nothing to do where she lives, I told her that, actually, she did quite a bit; the director of her program and the aides told me so. "You do lots of things, ma. You just don't remember doing them." It was after one of these (largely useless) explanations that she asked, "So, what's the point?" She had of course arrived at an important insight. Of what value is experience itself, she had essentially asked, if it can no longer achieve "memorability" and has been divested of its place in the narrative order?

What I want to suggest, in closing, is that even here, in this limited case, the possibility of keeping narrative open and alive still remains—if not for *her* then for those of us who have been entrusted with her care and well-being. This means doing what we can to ensure that, even in the absence of memorability, there still remains some measure of meaning and value— *moral* value—in her experience. She is not particularly bothered at this point by sitting around and doing nothing. If we were strict empiricists about the matter, therefore, we could just leave her to her own devices and move on. That is, we could rest comfortable with her foreclosure and direct our energies and care elsewhere. Along with her, we would simply be asking, "What's the point?" If truth be known, we occasionally *do* ask this question— particularly when, after what had seemed to be a worthwhile and fulfilling experience, there is not even a trace of a memory. But it is important, I believe, to resist this sort of utilitarian thinking and to help her find moments that are not only pleasurable or meaningful but that, linked together, serve still to fashion a *life* that is dignified and worthwhile. She will not be the one to forge these links, and she will not be the one to look back on the trajectory of her late life to discern its value and worth. We will be. This means keeping narrative open and alive evermore.

NOTE

[1] The case history information used in this chapter was gathered as part of a research project funded by the Spencer and MacArthur Foundations, conducted at the University of Chicago under the direction of Mihaly Csikszentmihalyi, J.W. Getzels, and Stephen P. Kahn.

REFERENCES

Coleman, P. (1999). Creating a life story: The task of reconciliation. *The Gerontologist, 39*, 133–139.

Freeman, M. (1997). Death, narrative integrity, and the radical challenge of self-understanding: A reading of Tolstoy's *Death of Ivan Ilych. Ageing and Society, 17*, 373–398.

Freeman, M. (2000a). When the story's over: Narrative foreclosure and the possibility of self-renewal. In M. Andrews, S. Sclater, C. Squire, and A. Treacher (Eds.), *Lines of narrative: Psychosocial perspectives* (pp. 81–91). London: Routledge.

Freeman, M. (2000b). Modernists at heart? Postmodern artistic breakdowns and the question of identity. In D. Fee (Ed.), *Pathology and the postmodern: Mental illness as discourse and experience* (pp. 116–140). Beverly Hills, CA: Sage.

Freeman, M. (2003). Too late: The temporality of memory and the challenge of moral life. *Journal für Psychologie, 11*, 54–74.

Freeman, M. (2008a). Life without narrative? Autobiography, dementia, and the nature of the real. In G.O. Mazur (Ed.), *Thirty year commemoration to the life of A.R. Luria* (pp. 129–144). New York: Semenko Foundation.

Freeman, M. (2008b). Beyond narrative: Dementia's tragic promise. In L.-C. Hyden & J. Brockmeier (Eds.), *Health, illness, and culture: Broken narratives* (pp. 169–184). London: Routledge.

Freeman, M. (2009). The stubborn myth of identity: Dementia, memory, and the narrative unconscious. *Journal of Family Life, 1*. Retrieved March 19, 2009, from http://www.journaloffamilylife.org/mythofidentity

Freeman, M. (2010). *Hindsight: The promise and peril of looking backward.* New York: Oxford University Press.

Gazzaniga, M. (1998). *The mind's past.* Berkeley, CA: University of California Press.

Langer, E. (2009). *Counterclockwise: Mindful health and the power of possibility.* New York: Ballantine.

Levi, P. (1989). *The drowned and the saved.* New York: Vintage International.

McAdams, D. (2006). *The redemptive self: Stories Americans live by.* New York: Oxford University Press.

Randall, W., & McKim, A. (2008). *Reading our lives: The poetics of growing old.* New York: Oxford University Press.

Ross, M., & Wilson, A. (2000). Constructing and appraising past selves. In D. Schacter & E. Scarry (Eds.), *Memory, brain, and belief* (pp. 231–258). Cambridge, MA: Harvard University Press.

Tolstoy, L. (1960). *The death of Ivan Ilych and other stories.* (A. Maude, Trans.). New York: New American Library (original work published 1886).

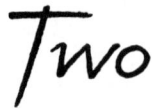 *Two*

MEMORY, METAPHOR, AND MEANING: READING

FOR WISDOM IN THE STORIES OF OUR LIVES

William L. Randall

> *Memory itself is only a metaphor, a dim surrogate for past time that can never be recovered, never embodied, never made to sit still.*
> —Daniel Albright (1994, p. 39)

> *Metaphor, though never to be found at Delphi, is… a priest of interpretation; but what it interprets is memory.*
> —Cynthia Ozick (1989, p. 282)

LIVES AS TEXTS

My father has been an avid reader all his life, though of some books more than others. My mother once quipped that while Louis L'Amour had authored over 50 novels of the Wild West, Dad had read "all 200 of them." More recently, the focus of his devotion has been *Blue Highways: A Journey into America*, by William Least Heat Moon (1982). The book recounts Moon's meanderings along the roads less traveled of rural USA in search of peace of mind following a breakup with his lover. It's a soulful weave of local history, chats with characters encountered en route, and musings on the human condition that usually cruise beneath the radar of academic theory. To read it (as a man, at least) is to sense a resonance with one's own journey, one's own story—as autobiography is adept at allowing us to do.

Since I first lent him my copy of it some 10 years ago, Dad (now 91) has read the book a dozen times. It's become something of a Bible for him. Often, I'll return home in the evening to find a message on my answering machine: "This is your father, and I'm reading from The Book... ." He then recites some passage that, though he's read it several times before, has caught his eye afresh, as if at last he can appreciate its significance or finds it voicing some insight which, that very day, perhaps, he had been pondering in connection with his own experience. Whatever parallel he feels between the passage and the past, I can't presume to grasp what is happening inside him. As a gerontologist, I can only wonder what brand of *postformal thought*, indeed, what *wisdom* is at work within his aging brain as a particular section elicits a particular reaction: a penny to drop, a door to open, a question to stir—and with each one, I like to think, a deepening and expanding of his inner world.

Colleagues in "literary gerontology" (Wyatt-Brown, 2000; see also Goyal & Charon, this volume) can explain far better than I this ability of books to act as *aides-mémoire*, to offer metaphors for patterns in our past and alternative interpretations of experiences that have puzzled us for years and, in general, to serve as stimuli for making meaning. But my interest here is less in literature itself than in memory—specifically, *autobiographical* memory, which is "what we usually mean by the term memory in everyday usage" (Rubin, 1996, p. 1). It is not that the literary text "contains" the meaning—least of all, *the* meaning—and that the reader is but an empty vessel waiting to be filled. Rather, meaning gets made in the intimate "transaction" between the text per se and the text of memory in the reader's mind (Rosenblatt, 1978), and then *re*made with each rereading (Lesser, 2002). If you will, the outer text exerts a metaphorical effect upon the inner one; yet without the inner text, the outer one is dead.

Where aging is concerned, it is what happens in this inner text—our *texistence*—that fascinates me most, whether it be books that act as the catalysts or other things instead. What fascinates me is that elusive interpretive activity that my colleague Beth McKim and I call "reading our lives" (Randall & McKim, 2008). Inspiring our reflections on "the poetics of growing old" are scholars such as Mark Freeman (this volume), several of whose publications are devoted to probing "the poetics of selfhood" (1999). Encouraging us as well are psychologists like Dan McAdams and Ruthellen Josselson, much of whose work grapples with the complex links between identity and narrative (Brockmeier & Carbaugh, 2001; McAdams, Josselson,

& Lieblich, 2006). The conviction to which Beth and I have kept returning is that "our lives" are experienced and understood by us not as strings of raw events but as stories; as vast, open-ended texts; as flesh-and-blood *novels* that are unfolding over time, continually thickening with potential for meaning. And (with a nod to Socrates) it behooves us, eventually, to examine them.

MEMORY, METAPHOR, AND MEANING

My aim in this chapter is to dip deeper into a theme that has been surfacing for me as particularly intriguing. Though not exactly new to narrative psychology, it seldom features in the discourse of mainstream gerontology, which makes it all the more vital to consider if we are to enhance our understanding of the inside of aging, or "biographical aging" (Ruth & Kenyon, 1996). The theme in question concerns the intricate interplay between memory, metaphor, and meaning. It concerns the metaphorical potential in the memories we have formed about our lives and the metaphorical dynamics of "development" itself (Freeman, 1994). Three quotations set the stage for the thesis that has been building in my mind.

The first comes from Freeman's book *Rewriting the Self* (1994): "The process of autobiographical reflection [is] a fundamentally metaphorical one: a new relationship is being created between the past and present, a new poetic configuration, designed to give greater form to one's previous—and present—experience. The text of the self is thus being rewritten" (p. 30). The second is from Donald Polkinghorne's important volume, *Narrative Knowing and the Human Sciences* (1988). "Experience makes connections and enlarges itself," he writes, "through the use of metaphorical processes that link together experiences similar but not exactly the same" (p. 16). The third is from *Reminiscence and the Self in Old Age,* by gerontologist Edmund Sherman (1991): "metaphor enables us to take experiences and construct them into larger meaningful wholes," leading, says Sherman, "to valuable new linkages or integrations with other life experiences" (p. 87).

Before I outline my thesis, let me say a word about the three key concepts that figure in it. First, I view memory (autobiographical memory, that is) in hermeneutical or textual terms. Such terms, however, have been largely ignored by psychologists of aging, who have attended more to the *mechanics* of memory—for example, speed of retrieval and accuracy of recall—than to the *meanings* our memories may possess for us. Concerning the latter, memories are textual entities. They are hardly straight recordings of actual occurrences, devoid of bias or interpretation and with all of the details intact.

They are *stories*—big or little, long or short—that we weave (and re-weave) around original occurrences to invest them with personal significance. Or at least that fraction of events that we manage to retain, inasmuch as most of us forget far more than we ever remember. The point is, they are not those events themselves, but narrativized summaries of them—in a real sense, metaphors *for* them—whose form when we recount them reflects the narrative environments we have lived within across the years, each with its repertoire of "narrative templates" for interpreting experience (Abbott, 2002, p. 7). Composed in part through our relationships with others, our memories are thus odd blends of fact and fictionalization that are perhaps more fairly seen as *facsimiles* or *factions*. They are edited, interpreted renditions of past episodes (positive or negative) as viewed through the lens of our agendas in the present in light of our expectations for the future. And as our present changes, plus our expectations for the future, so will our perceptions of the past. No reading of any part of it is therefore ever final, impervious to further reinterpretation. There is, literally, no end of meaning to be gleaned from it. Says Polkinghorne: "The realm of meaning has great plasticity" (1988, p. 16). "The past" is a moving target, an open text, despite our tendency to perceive it as solid and settled: *the past is past and that's that.* In short, memory is a process, not a thing. Not that it is thereby flawed for failing to afford us pure, unchanging access to "what actually happened," as computer analogies for memory can tempt us to expect (Randall, 2007). On the contrary, this is how memory works, how it *must* work, if it is to serve us as the basis for a sense of Self that is substantial enough yet supple enough to navigate our ever-changing lives (Randall, 2010).

As for metaphor, the topic is both vast and vexed. Not only have literary theorists wrestled with it, but so too have thinkers in philosophy and theology, psychology and medicine, education and linguistics, not to mention gerontology, especially *narrative* gerontology, with its explicit employment of the metaphor of *life-as-story* (Kenyon, Clark, & de Vries, 2001). To borrow from Ricoeur (1977), "the rule of metaphor" extends in all directions. It infuses our speech, informs our beliefs, and underlies our learning. It fuels our capacity for empathy and, for better or worse, shapes our sense of self (see Kövecses, 2002; Lakoff & Johnson, 1980; Sacks, 1979; Turner, 1996). A major challenge, then, is to define what *metaphor* even means.

For my purposes here, the perspective of autobiography scholar James Olney (1981) can serve as a guide. In *Metaphors of Self*, he writes, "Metaphor is essentially a way of knowing.... To a wholly new sensational or emotional experience, one can give sufficient organization only by relating it to the already known, only by perceiving a relation between this experience and another experience already placed, ordered, and incorporated. This," notes Olney, "is the psychological basis of the metaphorizing process: to grasp the unknown through the known" (p. 30). Very broadly then, "far from being a strange device found only in poetry and esoteric prose" (Thomas, 1969, p. 25), metaphor—or the *metaphorizing process*—is a tool for making meaning, "a means of entering the unknown through the gateway of the known" (Kenyon, Birren, & Schroots, 1991, p. 8). What intrigues me here, however, is the role of metaphor in inviting us to enter the territory of our own memory in more meaning-filled ways.

A central premise of narrative psychology and narrative gerontology alike, of course, is that we are meaning-making beings. However, the study of personal meaning—of "meaning in life" or "existential meaning" (Reker & Chamberlain, 2000)—has thus far focused more on the sources or dimensions of such meaning, or on the measuring of it, than on the meaning-making *process*, including its narrative complexities (see Cohler, 1993). This seems curious, insofar as surely a central source—perhaps *the* source—of the meaning that we make is, in the end, our own stories, above all, perhaps, in later life: "the narrative phase par excellence" (Freeman, 1997, p. 394). Furthermore, in later life making meaning is critical, it can be argued, to our continuing development, our *narrative* development. Simply put, the older we get, the more meaning we require in order to cope with, and grow through, the losses and challenges (physical, financial, emotional) that later life can bring. Such challenges may well fuel what an acquaintance of mine, recently retired, once described as "the late-life crisis." While not a crisis of *identity* per se perhaps, later life can certainly confront us with a crisis of self-understanding. "Who am I and what is my story, now that I'm no longer employed or needed or able?" At bottom, this is "a crisis of meaning" (Missine, 2003, p. 113; see also Cohler, 1993). And the problem—-the tragedy perhaps—is that many older adults enter the final phase of life with too meager a sense of meaning at their disposal, too narrow or thin a story. As loved ones die and their social circle shrinks, they therefore risk internalizing the "narrative of decline" (Gullette, 2004) by which aging as such is routinely construed (see Caissie, this volume; Phoenix, this volume). In consequence, they may succumb to "narrative foreclosure" (Freeman, 2000; this volume). Though their life itself continues on, in their minds their story has all but ended, with no new chapters deemed likely to open up and no re-readings or reinterpretations deemed possible to entertain.

Roughly worded, then, my thesis runs like this: memory yields its meaning through metaphor—which is to say, through metaphorical association. And the subtle, symbiotic process that weaves the three together is essential to the continuing evolution of our story-world and, with that world, our wisdom (see Randall & Kenyon, 2001). There are five steps I want to take to sketch this thesis out—"sketch out," not "spell out," being the operative phrase, for complex matters are at issue here. First, memories convey metaphors. Second, metaphors evoke memories. Third, the meanings seeded in our memories are continually being reconfigured, as we tell and retell our stories, examine and reexamine them, over time. Fourth, later life itself provides the very kinds of inner and outer conditions that can, in fact, facilitate this reconfiguration, thus intensifying the potential for making meaning. Finally, whatever else it is, wisdom is inseparable from the process of self-understanding, which in turn can be understood in terms of the intricate, dynamic links between memory, metaphor, and meaning.

MEMORIES CONVEY METAPHORS

As structures for meaning rather than raw recordings of "the facts," memories contain metaphors, or have metaphors running through them, or are the *medium* for metaphors. Simply put, our memories are generally "about something." On some level, there are reasons we have formed them, obscure though those reasons remain. Otherwise, one could argue, our inner editor would not have retained them in the first place. "We store in memory only images of value," writes memoirist Patricia Hampl (1999). "*This,* we say somewhere within us, is something I'm hanging on to" (p. 29)—for better or worse, that is, since we "often… cleave to things because they possess heavy negative charge. Pain," Hampl reminds us, "has strong arms" (p. 29). While we can rarely gauge beforehand what *this* will end up being, what we hang onto, one might say, is what seemed significant to the self we were living at the time. These memories are episodes—incipient ones, at least—in some internal storyline that we entertained about our lives.

Not that all of our memories will be equally significant to our sense of self. But surely good candidates in this respect would be the "signature stories" (Kenyon & Randall, 1997) and the "self-defining memories" (Singer & Blagov, 2004; Singer & Messier, this volume) around which our sense of self so often revolves. Included in these are memories that make up the so-called reminiscence bump: that clustering of key events between the ages of, say, 18 and 30 when our adult identity is taking shape in earnest: when, typically, we are leaving home, pursuing an education, establishing a career, finding a partner, and starting a home of our own (Rubin, Rahhal, & Poon, 1998). Such recollections often figure centrally in our *lifestory*, namely the "internalized and evolving personal myth," as McAdams defines it, "that functions to provide life with unity and purpose" (1996, p. 132). In many cases, surely, they can assume mythic proportions inside our imagination as, later in life, we think our way back to how it is we became who we are. We thus may make them pivotal to our memoir (should we write one), as if they carried clues to our innermost nature, to why we value what we value and believe what we believe, to our abiding "life themes" (Csikszentimihalyi & Beattie, 1979). At the core of each such memory, as perhaps of many of our dreams, may lie some guiding metaphor of self (Olney, 1981) on which we would do well to reflect.

METAPHORS EVOKE MEMORIES

Memories convey metaphors. At the same time, metaphors evoke memories. Memory researcher Craig Barclay (1994) discusses how certain metaphors elicit certain recollections. As examples, *my life as a journey* (Kenyon, 1991) and *my life as a tree with branching points* (Birren & Deutchman, 1991) will invariably trigger different sets of memories—or the same ones interpreted from different angles—than *my life as a roller coaster*, on the one hand, or *a box of chocolates* on the other. Each invites a different selection and emplotment of our life's events, a different line of storying our self—indeed, a different self. Barclay (1994) calls these "protoselves" (pp. 69–71). For him, in fact, there is no continuous, centered self within us but, depending on the context or the people we are interacting with, only a great array of possible ones: self-as-failure, self-as-survivor, self-as-martyr, self-as-hero, self-alone-against-the-world. Echoes autobiography scholar, Paul John Eakin (1999), "There are many stories of self to tell and more than one self to tell them" (p. xi).

Therapists, especially *narrative* therapists, exploit such possibilities routinely when urging clients to articulate the metaphors implicit in their self-talk (or their dreams), to critique the limiting stories they have been living by to date, and to envision healthier self-narratives instead (White & Epston, 1990; Freedman & Combs, 1996; Kropf & Tandy, 1998). To borrow the phrase that Birren uses in connection with *guided autobiography* (Birren & Deutchman, 1991, pp. 86–87), clients "trade in and trade up" the metaphors by which they define their identity for more nuanced and more positive ones instead. For adult educators, group facilitators, life coaches, and the like, the use of "guided imagery" can also inspire us to reconnect with long-submerged parts of our past and to imagine the future for which we yearn: *You are strolling down a tree-lined path on a summer afternoon. You arrive at a sunlit meadow. In the center sits a fountain. You toss in a coin. What will be your wish?* As noted already, novels, movies, plays, biographies—stories of any kind—can serve as extended metaphors for dimensions of our lives that otherwise linger at the edges of awareness. Through their plots, their characters, their themes, we hear echoes of our own stories. If only temporarily, they expand our inner memory text, rendering more of our selves available as sources of personal meaning.

MEANING DEVELOPS OVER TIME

In one of the journals that she published in her later years, novelist-poet May Sarton (1977) noted that "the past is always changing, is never static, never 'placed' forever like a book on a shelf. As we grow and change," she says, "we understand things… in new ways" (p. 95). To some extent, Sarton's experience is familiar to us all, whether or not we keep a journal of our thoughts. The "new ways" she alludes to, though, are the consequence of two key features of our life in time: the changing "horizon of self-understanding" (Berman, 1994) and the changing relationship between part and whole.

The first feature I have touched upon already. Our perceptions of the past are colored by our experiences in the present, which in turn are filtered through our expectations for the future. Harry Berman (1994), drawing on the journals of Sarton and other older women to probe the internal complexities of aging—what he calls "hermeneutical gerontology" (p. xxiv)—observes that, in reading Sarton's work, "we repeatedly witness her attempts to sum up the story of her life based on an assessment of what lies behind and what lies ahead." However, "the events of her life again and again force a revision of the story" (p. 181). Polkinghorne says something similar: "We are in the middle of our stories and cannot be sure how they will end"; as a result, "we are constantly having to revise the plot as new events are added to our lives" (1988, p. 150).

The second feature concerns our habit of viewing the part in terms of the whole: "we make sense of the present," says Berman (1994), "in terms of our working theory of the kind of story we are in" (p. 180). Our perception of the situation we are facing in the moment depends in part on what we sense our story as a whole is all about. Is losing my keys an isolated incident in an otherwise smoothly ticking life or simply one more sign that my story is the tale of a loser, from beginning to end? In this part-whole dynamic, though, lies potential for positive change. "As the horizon of self-understanding shifts," he writes, "it may become apparent that we were not in the middle of the story we thought we were in the middle of" (p. 180). He goes on: "Perhaps we thought our life was a tragedy and all along, unbeknownst to us, it was a romance. Or perhaps we thought our life was almost over, at least in terms of the future holding anything new, and it turned out there was a lot more to it" (p. 180). In other words, our story opens up.

Philosopher Stuart Charmé (1984), in discussing Sartre's concept of "existential psychoanalysis"—specifically, his notion of our "fundamental project"—adds to our understanding here by defining a fundamental project as "an evolving totality" (p. 45) and as "a systematic structure of inter-related meanings" (p. 46) that "resembles a literary text in some important way" (p. 51). Just as our understanding of every sentence in a novel is contingent on our understanding of where the story as a whole is headed, so "each element in the developing totality [of a person's life] is comprehensible only in relation to the rest of the changing whole" (p. 46). As the whole enlarges, the meaning of each part of it—each memory, for example—is (so to speak) updated. Yet previous updatings are never entirely discarded. Traces will persist, such that further layers of significance inevitably accrue. "My past is always changing," Charmé says (p. 45)—always *thickening*, I would add. Thus "the meaning of the past is something that develops throughout life" (p. 4).

Autobiographical activities like writing in our journal, compiling a memoir, or quietly reflecting on our lives, turning things over in our minds, can serve what is, ultimately, a metaphorical function. They take us from the known (from the seemingly settled past) to novel ways of seeing things: the *un*known. They serve, therefore, as antidote to narrative foreclosure by helping us "re-genre-ate" our past (for example, from tragedy to romance), to "restory" it (Kenyon & Randall, 1997), to "rewrite" it (Freeman, 1994). As alluded to already, the therapeutic process also invites such reconfiguration—consciously and intentionally, in fact. But soulful conversation with a confidant or friend can have a comparable effect, if less enduring or on a lesser scale; and so, conceivably, can spiritual confession. The experience of telling part or all of our narrative to a compassionate listener can awaken us to new ways of framing old experiences (Chandler & Ray, 2002). The telling takes us to a new place, allowing us to distance ourselves a little from the story that we have been living by thus far, to identify themes and patterns within it that escaped our awareness before, and to inch our way toward a larger, healthier, more self-affirming story instead. A "wiser" story, one might say, may evolve, though not the "whole" story surely, for this cannot be told. Even a full-length autobiography is merely a metaphor for the life it purports to represent. The point is, the entire process, to which there is no intrinsic end, is a metaphorical one, a straining from known to unknown. Notes one source, "we tell a story in order to find a story" (Winquist, 1980, p. 43). Consequently, our narrative development knows no bounds. While biologically we are bound by 120 years (or so), biographically or narratively, no such limits pertain. There are no barriers to how far we can grow.

AGING AS OPPORTUNITY TO GROW

With age, I am arguing, we require sufficient inner reserves of meaning—sufficient "biographical capital" (Mader, 1996)—to cope with the changes that aging carries with it. We require what Beth and I have dubbed "a good, strong story" (Randall & McKim, 2008, p. 118). What I wish to argue now is that certain changes associated with aging can actually *facilitate* the making of meaning. Before I note them, though, I need to be clear. I am certainly not proposing that a condition like dementia represents such a change, if only we viewed it from the necessary angle. That said, some scholars are tentatively suggesting that, while dementia seems indeed to impede one's capacity for making meaning, especially *new* meaning, one can still be biographically active, still capable of narrative development to some degree. If so, the story of dementia is not the total tragedy we assume it to be. It has another side.

With its onset, friends and family are implicitly invited to assume (or *re*sume) their role as *co-authors* of the affected person's narrative, by remembering it and honoring it on his or her behalf. As such, they serve as keepers of the story that the individual him- or herself is unable to articulate in clear, unconfabulated fashion, thereby supplying some of the meaning that has otherwise gone missing (see Crisp, 1995; Basting, 2003; Noonan, this volume). In essence, responsibility shifts to others for the meaning-making process and for repairing the fabric of collective life whose cohesion the dementia has threatened (Freeman, this volume). In an age when the interdependence of all life and all people is increasingly accepted, surely such expressions of narrative care must be acknowledged and encouraged.

The example of dementia aside, in the wake of retirement, the death of a spouse, or any other of the several losses that can come with later life, there is one change by which aging is commonly accompanied: an increase in disposable time. Concurrent with this comes a degree of detachment from the workaday world, a movement that later life itself invites us to enjoy or, alternatively, that is foisted upon us against our will. Either way, despite controversy surrounding "disengagement theory," plus countervailing emphases on "activity theory" (and with it, "successful aging"), for many people, aging still entails a tendency to turn inward, and this is not automatically a negative trend. One can be active not just in outer and observable ways but in inner ways as well. One can be engaged in responding to the age-old exhortation to inquire within, in tackling the "philosophic homework" (Schacter-Shalomi & Miller, 1995, p. 124–126) that later life, aided by the prospect of our dying, sets before us as a key developmental task. And, conveniently, later life allows us both the time and the space—a certain distance, say, from previous involvements—to tackle such tasks in earnest. Among them are stepping back and taking stock; reviewing our life and (ideally) valuing it, overall, as meaningful; assimilating painful or problematic events into the plot of our life-narrative (Coleman, 1999); recontextualizing negatives into positives; writing a "generativity script" (McAdams, 1996, 2006); making amends wherever possible; and saying "I'm sorry," "I forgive you," or simply "goodbye."

Ironically, given changes in the brain itself, such complex assignments may actually be easier, not harder, to undertake. Gerontologist Gene Cohen (2005), in *The Mature Mind*, identifies four "attributes of the brain," for instance, that "lay the foundation for an optimistic view of human potential in the second half of life" (p. 3). First, "the brain is continually resculpting itself in response to experience and learning"; second, "new brain cells *do* form throughout life," a phenomenon known as *neurogenesis*; third, "the brain's emotional circuitry matures and becomes more balanced with age"; and fourth, "the brain's two hemispheres are more equally used by older adults" (p. 4). One result of such changes, he argues, is that with age we experience an increased "inner push" (p. 75) toward "autobiographical expression" (p. 22). In other words, "the autobiographical drive among older people"—the impulse to tell stories about their lives—"is related to a rearrangement of brain functions that makes it easier to merge the speech, language, and sequential thinking typical of the left hemisphere with the creative, synthesizing right hemisphere" (p. 23). Paradoxically, then, physical aging—otherwise equated with inevitable "decline" (Gullette, 2004)—may in the end enable us to (actively) *grow* old and not just (passively) *get* old: to engage in "conscious aging" (Randall & Kenyon, 2001). At once, it provides us with the *means* (changes in the brain), the *opportunity* (more time and space), and the *motive* (the prospect of death and the inner push to autobiographical expression). In addition, it supplies us with ample *material* to work with: an ever-thicker text of memories and stories whose metaphorical potential, and thus meaning-potential, increases correspondingly and awaits our conscious exploration.

AGING, METAPHOR, AND WISDOM

Wisdom, too, is a complex topic that thus far is underexamined by gerontologists themselves. When it is examined, the prevailing approach has been to cast it in practical-ethical-cognitive terms—as, for example, "a highly developed body of factual and procedural knowledge and judgments concerning the fundamental pragmatics of life" (Baltes & Smith, 1990, p. 87). For all its merits, what an approach like this eclipses is a corresponding emphasis on somewhat more elusive matters with which, rightly or wrongly, conceptions of wisdom have usually been linked, among them self-understanding or self-knowledge. But if wisdom has to do with self-knowledge, and if self is inseparable from the stories through which we conceive it, then, like memory and meaning, wisdom also has a narrative dimension (see Randall & McKim, 2008, pp. 223–242). And it is ultimately not a thing, not a "body of knowledge," but a process. To grow in wisdom, whatever else that process may entail, is to grow in (ironic) awareness of the narratives we have woven round our life's events. It is to open ourselves to the layers of significance those narratives possess. To borrow from Hampl (1999), wisdom involves not merely *telling* our stories (which, itself, we may have seldom really done) but "to listen to what our stories tell us" (p. 33).

Commenting on an obscure memory from her childhood that she writes about in an essay entitled "Memory and Imagination," Hampl says that "I can read this little piece as a mystery which drops clues to the riddle of my feelings" (p. 29). Bearing this possibility in mind invites us to ask what is *in* our own stories, what do they *mean* to us, and why have we held onto them in the first place, and not the hundreds of other stories we might have formed instead—our untold stories, as it were. It opens us to play with alternative interpretations of what are otherwise familiar memories—our more self-defining ones, for instance, whether positive or negative in nature. Such openness is fostered by a process that Sally Chandler and Ruth Ray (2002) call "dynamic reminiscence" (p. 77) and by programs of "creative reminiscence"that Ernst Bohlmeijer and colleagues have designed for older clients who suffer from depression (Bohlmeijer et al., 2005; Steunenberg & Bolhmeijer, this volume). And it is central to the life-writing groups led by Thomas Cole and Kate de Medeiros (Cole & de Medeiros, 2001; see also de Medeiros, 2007; this volume), in which participants delve into puzzling or painful life events (a breakup, the death of a parent, an experience of abuse) through a variety of genres: first-person narration, third-person narration, a short story, a letter, a poem. In *Beyond Nostalgia,* a book based on her research with older women involved in a life-writing group, Ray (2000) offers us this intriguing observation on what such explorations have to do with wisdom: "Wise people," she says, "watch themselves tell life stories, learn from others' stories, and intervene in their own narrative processes to allow for change by admitting new stories and interpretations into their repertoire" (p. 29).

Once again, what seem to assist us on the path of wisdom are changes in the brain itself. Cohen (2005) makes a connection between "rearrangements" in the functioning of the aging brain and the emergence of what psychologists, building on the work of Piaget, call *postformal thought*. Especially relevant here is an aspect of postformal thought that psychologist Giselle Labouvie-Vief has made the focus of her research on "qualitative differences in how younger and older adults interpret text" (1990, p. 69). Specifically, "the younger individual often reads text analytically, examining aspects of internal structure and keeping inferences to such intratextual processes. For the older adult, however, the interest of text often lies not in the delineation of a particular action-event sequence but rather in the fact that it signifies truths about the human condition." That is, "inferencing is based on a symbolic processing style in which inner and psychological processes rather than purely logical ones are important" (p. 74). In short, "the more mature individual construes text not only logically but also psychologically and symbolically" (p. 69). Indeed, in later life, "the symbolic emerges... in a uniquely mature form," and may come to be accepted "as an independent source of knowing in its own right" (p. 74). Overall, Labouvie-Vief advocates a vision of wisdom that avoids the "*logos* bias... in most major theories of intellectual development" (p. 65) and sees it instead as "integrated thought"—the integration, that is, of *logos* and *mythos* (p. 74; see also Labouvie-Vief, 2000).

The concept of "metaphoric competence" is relevant here as well. Thirty years ago, Howard Gardner and Ellen Winner (1979) identified a "set of competencies" that appear to be involved in it, among them "the capacity to paraphrase a metaphor, to explain the rationale for the metaphor's effectiveness, to produce a metaphor appropriate to a given context, to evaluate the appropriateness of several competing metaphoric expressions" (pp. 126–127). At the time, Gardner and Winner were preoccupied with how such competence evolves in the minds of children in the context of education, inasmuch as new concepts are only truly "learned" when they can be linked with what has been learned already. However, a cluster of issues is intriguing to consider here in conjunction with postformal thought and symbolic thought, with generic memory and pattern recognition, not to mention with "instrumental reminiscence," where memories of challenges encountered in the past are drawn upon to deal with comparable challenges in the present (Wong, 1995, p. 25). For instance, how might our metaphoric competence continue to develop in later life? What are the dynamics of this development and what types of narrative environments—what types of listening—might stimulate it more? And what is the role of religion in inspiring and informing it, given the heritage of metaphor, myth, and master narratives in which religious traditions are typically rich? Might the observed trend of many older adults becoming more spiritual with age be attributable, in part, less to the power of religion itself than to their greater openness to the symbolic in general?

Finally, neurologist Elkhonon Goldberg (2005), whose views run parallel to Cohen's, sees wisdom as "inherently connected with… a certain kind of memory," namely "generic memory" (p. 107). Incidentally, Ulrich Neisser (1986) proposed something similar with his concept of "repisodic memory" (p. 79). We will likely recall few specific instances of ordering a meal in a restaurant, yet given repeated such episodes (repisodes), we will have a spread-out sense—a script, as it were—of what "ordering a meal" involves. Similarly, generic memories, says Goldberg (2005), "are *memories for patterns*" (p. 125); and the capacity for "pattern recognition," he insists, "comprises a very important element of wisdom." In other words, "a person endowed with wisdom has the ability to recognize an unusually large number of patterns, each encompassing a whole class of important situations" (p. 149). No doubt, Goldberg has in mind more complex, emotional-relational situations than ordering a meal in a restaurant; among them, raising a child, managing a marriage, or making decisions on ethically ambiguous issues. But the key in any case is that "the amount of these generic memories accumulates with age" (p. 149).

The capacities to see patterns in our memories and sense the significance of metaphors and symbols are intertwined, with aging itself as the common thread. Together, they suggest that, in viewing wisdom in terms of the narrative complexity of self-understanding, the links among memory, metaphor, and meaning are essential to consider. To such links the aged poet John Hall Wheelock seemed instinctively attuned. "As life goes on," he wrote, "it becomes more intense, because there are tremendous numbers of associations and so many memories" (cited in Sarton, 1977, p. 231).

There are further issues to be entertained, of course, in fathoming the memory–metaphor–meaning connection and the connection with wisdom in turn. Included is the impact on our capacity to read our lives in later life—on our "autobiographical consciousness" (Brockmeier, 2002, p. 457)— of our level of literacy overall, including our *literary* literacy, or "literary competence" (Culler, 1997) and, with it, our metaphoric competence. Are we in the habit of reading, period? If so, what types of texts? What is more, and as we know is invariably significant in terms of any topic we investigate as gerontologists, there is the impact of our gender and culture, our education and profession, our marital status and health status… the list goes on.

Allow me to conclude my musings with a quotation from Christina Baldwin (2005), author of assorted publications on the wisdom that resides within our own stories—on our "ordinary" wisdom, as it were (Randall & Kenyon, 2001). "Each of us is born into life a blank page," she writes, "and every person leaves life a full book" (Baldwin, 2005, p. ix). The "blank page" image is disputable, of course, given the larger stories into which we are we are born (family, culture, gender) and by whose plotlines and themes so much in our narratives is inevitably shaped. That said, Baldwin's metaphor returns me to the example of my father. Not that he is normal for his age-group—as a white, educated, comparatively healthy, highly literate male, far from it. But his *book* is nearly full. At 91, he knows full well that few new chapters (except the one entitled "Death and Beyond") are apt to open up. Does this, though, make him narratively foreclosed? His affinity with *Blue Highways* suggests otherwise. It suggests that his *story* remains an open work, by virtue of his continuing capacity to reflect upon his life, to appreciate fresh patterns of significance, and thus to journey deeper—and wiser—into the complex text of his own remembered past. Is this mere *navel-gazing*, as the saying goes, or something more profound? With apologies for the pun, might I suggest that we see it as *novel-grazing* instead: the savoring and exploring of the many-layered narrative that, in memory and imagination, is synonymous with our life?

REFERENCES

Abbott, H. (2002). *The Cambridge introduction to narrative*. New York: Cambridge University Press.

Albright, D. (1994). Literary and psychological models of the self. In U. Neisser & R. Fivush (Eds.), *The remembering self: Construction and accuracy in the self-narrative* (pp. 19–40). New York: Cambridge University Press.

Baldwin, C. (2005). *Storycatcher: Making sense of our lives through the power and practice of story*. Novalto, CA: New World Library.

Baltes, P., & Smith, J. (1990). Toward a psychology of wisdom and its ontogenesis. In R. Sternberg (Ed.), *Wisdom: Its nature, origins, and development* (pp. 87–120). New York: Cambridge University Press.

Barclay, C. (1994). Composing protoselves through improvisation. In U. Neisser & R. Fivush (Eds.). *The remembering self: Construction and accuracy in the self narrative* (pp. 55–77). New York: Cambridge University Press.

Basting, A. (2003). Reading the story behind the story: Context and content in stories by people with dementia. *Generations: The Journal of the American Society on Aging, 23*(3), 25–29.

Berman, H. (1994). *Interpreting the aging self: Personal journals of later life.* New York: Springer.

Birren, J., & Deutchman, D. (1991). *Guiding autobiography groups for older adults: Exploring the fabric of life.* Baltimore: Johns Hopkins University Press.

Bohlmeijer, E., Valenkamp, M., Westerhof, G., Smit, G., & Cuijpers, P. (2005). Creative reminiscence as an early intervention for depression: Results of a pilot project. *Aging & Mental Health, 9*(4), 302–304.

Brockmeier, J. (2002). Possible lives. *Narrative Inquiry 12*(2), 455–466.

Brockmeier, J., & Carbaugh, D. (Eds.). (2001). *Narrative and identity: Studies in autobiography, self, and culture.* Amsterdam: John Benjamins.

Chandler, S., & Ray, R. (2002). New meanings for old tales: A discourse-based study of reminiscence and development in later life. In J. Webster & B. Haight (Eds.), *Critical advances in reminiscence work: From theory to application* (pp. 76–94). New York: Springer.

Charmé, S. (1984). *Meaning and myth in the study of lives: A Sartrean perspective.* Philadelphia: University of Pennsylvania Press.

Cohen, G. (2005). *The mature mind: The positive power of the aging brain.* New York: Basic Books.

Cohler, B. (1993). Aging, morale, and meaning: The nexus of narrative. In T. Cole, W. Achenbaum, P. Jakobi, & R. Kastenbaum (Eds.), *Voices and visions of aging: Toward a critical gerontology* (pp. 107–133). New York: Springer.

Cole, T., & de Medeiros, K. (2001). *Life stories: Aging and the human spirit.* [Video]. Washington, DC: Old Dog Productions. (Available from New River Media: www.nrmedia.com.)

Coleman, P. (1999). Creating a life story: The task of reconciliation. *The Gerontologist, 39*(2), 133–139.

Crisp, J. (1995). Making sense of the stories that people with Alzheimer's tell: A journey with my mother. *Nursing Inquiry, 2,* 133–140.

Csikszentimihalyi, M. & Beattie, O. (1979). Life themes: a theoretical and empirical exploration of their origins and efforts. *Journal of Humanistic Psychology, 19*(1), 45–63.

Culler, J. (1997). *Literary theory: A very short introduction.* New York: Oxford University Press.

de Medeiros, K. (2007). Beyond the memoir: Telling life-stories using multiple literary forms. *Journal of Aging, Humanities, and the Arts, 1*(3), 159–167.

Eakin, P. (1999). *How our lives become stories: Making selves.* Ithaca, NY: Cornell University Press.

Freedman, J., & Combs, G. (1996). *Narrative therapy: The social construction of preferred realities.* New York: W. W. Norton.

Freeman, M. (1994). *Rewriting the self: History, memory, narrative.* London: Routledge.

Freeman, M. (1997). Death, narrative integrity, and the radical challenge of self-understanding: A reading of Tolstoy's *Death of Ivan Ilych. Ageing and Society, 17,* 373–398.

Freeman, M. (1999). Life narratives, the poetics of selfhood, and the redefinition of psychological theory. In W. Maiers, B. Bayer, B. Esgalhado, R. Jorna, & E. Schraube (Eds.), *Challenges to theoretical psychology* (pp. 245–250). Toronto: Captus University Publications.

Freeman, M. (2000). When the story's over: Narrative foreclosure and the possibility of self-renewal. In M. Andrews, S. Slater, C. Squire, & A. Treacher (Eds.), *Lines of narrative: Psychosocial perspectives* (pp. 81–91). London: Routledge.

Gardner, H., & Winner, E. (1979). The development of metaphoric competence: Implications for humanistic disciplines. In S. Sacks (Ed.), *On metaphor* (pp. 121–139). Chicago: University of Chicago Press.

Goldberg, E. (2005). *The wisdom paradox: How your mind can grow stronger as your brain grows older*. New York: Gotham.

Gullette, M. (2004). *Aged by culture*. Chicago: University of Chicago Press.

Hampl, P. (1999). *I could tell you stories: Sojourns in the land of memory*. New York: W. W. Norton.

Kenyon, G. (1991). Homo viator: Metaphors of aging, authenticity and meaning. In G. Kenyon, J. Birren, & J. J. F. Schroots (Eds.), *Metaphors of aging in science and the humanities* (pp. 17–35). New York: Springer.

Kenyon, G., Birren, J., & Schroots, J. (Eds.). (1991). *Metaphors of aging in science and the humanities*. New York: Springer.

Kenyon, G., Clark, P., & de Vries, B. (Eds.). (2001). *Narrative gerontology: Theory, research, and practice*. New York: Springer.

Kenyon, G., & Randall, W. (1997). *Restorying our lives: Personal growth through autobiographical reflection*. Westport, CT: Praeger.

Kövecses, Z. (2002). *Metaphor: A practical introduction*. New York: Oxford University Press.

Kropf, N., & Tandy, C. (1998). Narrative therapy with older clients: The use of a "meaning making" approach. *Clinical Gerontologist, 18*(4), 3–16.

Labouvie-Vief, G. (1990). Wisdom as integrated thought: Historical and developmental perspectives. In R. Sternberg (Ed.), *Wisdom: Its nature, origins, and development* (pp. 52–83). New York: Cambridge University Press.

Labouvie-Vief, G. (2000). Positive development in later life. In T. Cole, R. Kastenbaum, & R. Ray (Eds.), *Handbook of the humanities and aging* (2nd ed.), (pp. 365–380). New York: Springer.

Lakoff, G., & Johnson, M. (1980). *Metaphors we live by*. Chicago: University of Chicago Press.

Lesser, W. (2002). *Nothing remains the same: Rereading and remembering*. Boston: Houghton Mifflin.

Mader, W. (1996). Emotionality and continuity in biographical contexts. In J. Birren, G. Kenyon, J-E. Ruth, J. Schroots, & T. Svensson (Eds.), *Aging and biography: Explorations in adult development* (pp. 39–60). New York: Springer.

McAdams, D. (1996). Narrating the self in adulthood. In J. Birren, G. Kenyon, J-E. Ruth, J. Schroots, & T. Svensson, (Eds.), *Aging and biography: Explorations in adult development* (pp. 131–148). New York: Springer.

McAdams, D. (2006). *The redemptive self: Stories Americans live by*. New York: Oxford University Press.

McAdams, D., Josselson, R., & Lieblich, A. (Eds.) (2006). *Identity and story: Creating self in narrative.* Washington, DC: APA Books.

Missinne, L. (2003). The search for meaning of life in older age. In A. Jewel (Ed.), *Ageing, spirituality and well-being* (pp. 113–123). London: Jessica Kingsley.

Moon, W. L. H. (1982). *Blue highways: A journey into America.* New York: Fawcett Crest.

Neisser, U. (1986). Nested structure in autobiographical memory. In D. Rubin (Ed.), *Autobiographical memory* (pp. 71–81). New York: Cambridge University Press.

Olney, J. (1981). *Metaphors of self.* Princeton, NJ: Princeton University Press.

Ozick, C. (1989). *Metaphor and memory.* New York: A.A. Knopf.

Polkinghorne, D. (1988). *Narrative knowing and the human sciences.* Albany, NY: State University of New York Press.

Randall, W. (2007). From computer to compost: Rethinking our metaphors for memory. *Theory & Psychology, 17*(5), 611–633.

Randall, W. (2010). The narrative complexity of our past: In praise of memory's sins. *Theory & Psychology 20*(2), 1–23.

Randall, W., & Kenyon, G. (2001). *Ordinary wisdom: Biographical aging and the journey of life.* Westport, CT: Praeger.

Randall, W., & McKim, A. (2008). *Reading our lives: The poetics of growing old.* New York: Oxford University Press.

Ray, R. (2000). *Beyond nostalgia: Aging and life-story writing.* Charlottesville, VA: University Press of Virginia.

Reker, G., & Chamberlain, K. (Eds.) (2000). *Exploring existential meaning: Optimizing human development across the lifespan.* Thousand Oaks, CA: Sage.

Ricoeur, P. (1977). *The rule of metaphor: Multi-disciplinary studies of the creation of meaning in language.* (R. Czerny, Trans.) Toronto: University of Toronto Press.

Rosenblatt, L. (1978). *The reader, the text, the poem: The transactional theory of the literary work.* Carbondale, IL: Southern Illinois University Press.

Rubin, D. (1996). Introduction. In D. Rubin (Ed.), *Remembering our past: Studies in autobiographical memory* (pp. 1–15). New York: Cambridge University Press.

Rubin, D., Rahhal, T., & Poon, L. (1998). Things learned in early adulthood are remembered best. *Memory and Cognition, 26,* 3–19.

Ruth, J.-E., & Kenyon, G. (1996). Biography in adult development and aging. In J. Birren, G. Kenyon, J.-E. Ruth, J. Schroots, & T. Svensson (Eds.), *Aging and biography: Explorations in adult development* (pp. 1–20). New York: Springer.

Sacks, S. (Ed.) (1979). *On metaphor.* Chicago: University of Chicago Press.

Sarton, M. (1977). *Journal of a solitude.* New York: W. W. Norton. (Original work published 1973).

Schachter-Shalomi, Z., & Miller, R. (1995). *From age-ing to sage-ing: A profound new vision of growing older.* New York: Warner.

Sherman, E. (1991). *Reminiscence and the self in old age.* New York: Springer.

Singer, J., & Blagov, P. (2004). The integrative function of narrative processing: Autobiographical memory, self-defining memories, and the life story of identity. In D. Beike, J. Lampinen, & D. Behrend (Eds.), *The self and memory* (pp. 117–138). New York: Psychology Press.

Thomas, O. (1969). *Metaphor and related subjects.* New York: Random House.

Turner, M. (1996). *The literary mind.* New York: Oxford University Press.

White, M., & Epston, D. (1990). *Narrative means to therapeutic ends.* New York: W. W. Norton.

Winquist, C. (1980). *Practical hermeneutics: A revised agenda for the ministry.* Chico, CA: Scholars Press.

Wong, P. (1995). The processes of adaptive reminiscence. In B. Haight & J. Webster (Eds.), *The art and science of reminiscing: Theory, research, methods and applications* (pp. 23–35). Washington, DC: Taylor & Francis.

Wyatt-Brown, A. (2000). The future of literary gerontology. In T. Cole, R. Kastenbaum, & R. Ray (Eds.), *Handbook of the humanities and aging* (2nd ed., pp. 41–61). New York: Springer.

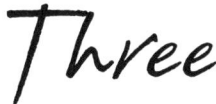

NARRATIVE EVENTS AND BIOGRAPHICAL

CONSTRUCTION IN OLD AGE

Jaber F. Gubrium

The editors of this volume have commented that the "biographical side of human life is as complicated and as critical to fathom as… the biological side" (p. xiii). If biology provides information and insight about life as it derives from the body, biography features the many dimensions of experience, from the knowing self to its diverse meanings, from the personal to the cultural. These are heady matters, as we live not only as embodied creatures, but as creatures that form and retain understandings. This applies across the life course, for the biographical meaning of childhood is as important to fathom as understandings of middle and old age (Holstein & Gubrium, 2000).

As a contribution to narrative gerontology, this chapter focuses on biographical construction in later life. It is concerned with everyday constructions, not the production of formal biographies. As ordinary members of our worlds, we continually represent ourselves and our experience to others, just as they represent their experience to us, mostly orally but occasionally in writing. This is eminently interpersonal, as representation orients to our selves in relation to the past, present, and future, as well as derives from those who construct our lives from their perspectives. It also is situational, as the lived contexts of biographical construction add to the mix. If traces of the interpersonal and the situational are persistent features of constructed lives, the analysis of lifestories usefully centers on narrative events (Bamberg, 2006; Bauman, 1986; Gubrium & Holstein, 2009; Ochs & Taylor, 1992).

STANLEY'S LESSONS AND THE PLAY OF BIOGRAPHICAL CONSTRUCTION

Before turning to exemplary material on the eventfulness of biographical construction in old age, consider the lessons that legendary interview subject Stanley provides. Stanley is a quite extraordinary everyday biographer, astute in the ways of narrative eventfulness. Years ago, sociologist Clifford Shaw (1930) published a biography of this delinquent boy he named "Stanley." The book, called *The Jack-Roller* and now a classic in the social sciences, was subtitled *A Delinquent Boy's Own Story*. The account ostensibly was Stanley's very own, the assumption being that it could be understood on its own terms. As Shaw comments in the first chapter, referring to what was to become a named method, "The case is published to illustrate the value of the 'own story' in the study and treatment of the delinquent child" (p. 1).

However, a close reading of the biography indicates that both interpersonal influences and social context are at play when Stanley represents himself. As Stanley refers to various narrative events in his life, it's clear that what is otherwise construed by Shaw as Stanley's "own story" is astutely organized in relation to the immediate and long-term challenges and consequences of biographical construction. Talking glowingly about his cellmate at the Illinois State Reformatory, Stanley flags the significance of constructing one's life in particular ways on distinct occasions.

> He [cell partner] was only seventeen, but older than me, and was in for one
> to ten years for burglaries. He delighted in telling about his exploits in crime,
> to impress me with this bravery and daring, and made me look up to him as
> a hero. Almost all young crooks like to tell about their accomplishments in
> crime. Older crooks are not so glib. They are hardened, and crime has lost its
> glamor and become a matter of business. Also, they have learned the dangers
> of talking too much [and] keep their mouths shut except to trusted friends.
> But Bill (my cell partner) talked all the time about himself and his crimes.
> I talked, too, and told wild stories of adventure, some true and some lies, for
> I couldn't let Bill outdo me just for lack of a few lies on my part. (p. 104)

The passage suggests that biographical construction on these occasions places a premium on the bravado from which social status derives. Construction has definitional consequences for self and others. The lesson is that biographical construction does something besides representing one's own experience, something related to the interpersonal expectations and representational rules of narrative occasions. Evidently, Stanley and others "do status" in communicating their experiences as "wild stories of adventure." They construct biographies not only befitting their personal experience but suitable to a preferred location in life.

Stanley also teaches a lesson about silence. Here and elsewhere in the book, he recounts the "dangers of talking too much." Besides everyday biography's situatedness, another important lesson is that the nonproduction of biographical material can characterize a narrative event. This goes against the grain of the common understanding in narrative inquiry that biographical production is healing or otherwise contributes to well-being. The moral from Stanley and other studies of everyday storytelling is that active representation can be as socially degrading, if not life threatening, as it is uplifting (see, for example, Wieder, 1974, and Anderson, 1999).

Taking Stanley at his word shows that the ordinary significance of accounts cannot be figured in strictly personal terms. Whether written or oral, biographical constructions do things, for us and to others. Stories have consequences for storytellers and their listeners, on which their eventfulness sheds considerable light. The consequences are not universal but relate to particular circumstances. As we turn to examples of how this applies in old age, it will become clear that simply "looking back" or "looking ahead" in later life is more complex than extended reflection, personal reminiscence, or communicating a positive or negative outlook on life.

The complexity centers on the interplay of the situated and interpersonal dimensions of everyday construction. The situation in question may center on the shared or big story of what it means to be able-bodied in a particular apartment setting. Or it may relate to the popular understanding of what it means to wind up in a nursing home for the rest of one's life. I'll turn to both of these below. Across these narrative environments are individual formulations found in the little stories of personal experience communicated with others. Complexity results from how big and little stories play out biographically in relation to each other on different narrative occasions (see Gubrium & Holstein, 2009, Chapter 11).

The words *play* and *interplay* are used deliberately. While the interpersonal and the circumstantial mediate everyday construction, neither fully determines the results. As the first of the following examples from the gerontological literature emphasizes, "poor dear" narratives in the circumstances in question are widely shared and yet recognizably play out in many ways on specific narrative occasions. The second example shows how individual particulars can contrastingly feature what is shared in common, to the point that what is shared is hardly recognizable in the differences. As nursing home resident Peter Rinehart's story will illustrate, biographical particulars can be amazingly at odds with what might be expected from the popular view of the circumstances.

"POOR DEAR" NARRATIVES

Arlie Russell Hochschild's (1973) research setting is an apartment building for the elderly, on which she reports in her book titled *The Unexpected Community*. Merrill Court, which is the pseudonym she assigns to the apartment building, is located near San Francisco Bay. It is not in any sense a nursing home, but it does have organized activities for residents. Hochschild worked there as an assistant recreation director while conducting fieldwork. The residents were independent, ate and slept in their own units, and came and went as they pleased or were able. Most were born and raised in the Southwest and Midwest and moved to California in later life.

It is significant that the title of Hochschild's book refers to the unexpected. The element of surprise derives from a common experience of living in urban apartment dwellings. These dwellings typically house individuals unknown to each other. Certainly, some might in time become acquainted, but they are just as likely to come and go anonymously. Individuals housed in apartment units down the hall or on the floor above or below don't much matter in the daily scheme of things. As strangers, residents might regularly pass each other in the hallways or the lobby or smile at one another in elevators. The social tide might occasionally turn into something more when neighborliness or friendships develop, setting the stage for community formation and culture of accounts. But in public places such as apartment buildings, this is rare or superficial.

As far as storytelling is concerned, Hochschild expected encounters in the setting to be bereft of common accounts. She didn't expect there to be a big story around which individual narratives coalesced or took account of. Instead, Hochschild expected residents' (littler) stories to be mostly private, unknown to others. As a result, at the start of her fieldwork, Hochschild was looking for the personal stories she might tap into, compare, and analyze. She didn't presume there would be a larger understanding that could challenge individual residents' accounts or, conversely, could tie things together for them in any way. Merrill Court, she originally figured, would be the site of little stories—individual narratives of coming of age somewhere far from their original homes.

As Hochschild continued her fieldwork, however, she found a setting ridden with shared understanding and related representation practices. Accounts of roles and relationships overshadowed individual tales of social isolation and anonymity. The social dimensions of personal narratives were captivating but also socially telling, she reports, which started to reveal the distinct shared contextuality of her biographical material:

> The book tells about their community as a mutual aid society, as a source of jobs, as an audience, as a pool of models for growing old, as a sanctuary and as a subculture with its own customs, gossip, and humor. It tells about friendships and rivalries within the community as well as relations with daughters, store clerks, nurses, and purse snatchers outside. (p. ix)

A key element of the unexpected big story in the setting is what Hochschild calls "the poor dear hierarchy." Figured as a common biographical anchor for individual constructions, it relates mainly to social status, but its use indicates that it has other narrative ramifications. The hierarchy centers on the assumption that, since the mostly female residents of Merrill Court are elderly, there's a good chance that they might become frail, infirm, or disabled. There's a persistent expectation that someone will need to go to a nursing home for a while and sometimes permanently. Those lucky enough to remain in good health, who are active and ambulatory, command considerable presence in the setting. They are visible in the lobby and other public spaces. The status associated with this becomes apparent narratively in terms of residents' related use of the term *poor dear* for those less fortunate.

In rounds of fieldwork, Hochschild heard many and varied stories about residents' conduct. Residents incessantly evaluated each other in terms of good or bad fortune, much of it related to the infirmities of aging. The words *poor dear* were used to describe those less able and, at times, the elderly in general, in comparison to those more advantaged. If much of this related to ill health, this could be extended to other disadvantages, such as insufficient income. Hochschild soon found that the words had vast narrative applicability, extending to all manner of status distinctions.

Poor dear did extensive status work of the sort Stanley flagged and could be counted on to indicate where those who used the phrase were placed in the broader scheme of things. "Poor dear" was the narrative key to a bigger story, one telling of hierarchy in the community. Referring to residents as "poor dears" was a way of narratively assigning a lower position in the hierarchy of luck. It was an important part of how little stories related to terms of reference shared with each other. The term *poor dear* figured as a common moral indicator, narratively specifying which residents were worthier and which less worthy in local reckoning.

Hochschild describes her emerging sense of the shared narrative relevance of this usage. I'll quote her at length to illustrate the big story that Hochschild eventually recognized, one resonating throughout the initially unexpected community. Note that the big story is not simply reproduced in individual accounts but creatively plays out in diverse constructions. Put differently, if there is a big story at Merrill Court, it is never the whole story. As Hochschild is careful to explain, the social logic that words can flag comes in different versions, applications, and proportions in practice. While *poor dear* marks status in general, it does so by way of diverse invocations. The eventfulness of usage shows that little stories take the big story in many directions in this most surprising of circumstances:

> At the monthly meetings of the countywide Senior Citizens Forum, to which Merrill Court sent two representatives, the term "poor dear" often arose with reference to old people. It was "we senior citizens who are politically involved versus those 'poor dears' who are active in recreation." Those active in recreation, however, did not accept a subordinate position relative to the politically active. On the other hand, they did not refer to the political activists as "poor dears." Within the politically active group there were those who espoused general causes, such as getting out an anti-pollution bill, and those who espoused causes related only to old age, such as raising Social Security benefits or improving medical benefits. Those in politics and recreation referred to the passive card players and newspaper readers as "poor dears." Old people with passive life styles in good health referred to those in poor health as "poor dears" and those in poor health but living in independent housing referred to those in nursing homes as "poor dears." Within the nursing home there was a distinction between those who were ambulatory and those who were not. Among those who were not ambulatory there was a distinction between those who could enjoy food and those who could not. Almost everyone, it seemed, had a "poor dear." (pp. 60–61)

What is biographically relevant in everyday life in this context works against the view that biography more or less reflects individual experience (see Georgakopoulou, 2006, Freeman, 2006, and Bamberg, 2006, for a recent debate on this issue). Accounts of lives, whether one's own or that of others, relate to locally shared formulations and the eventfulness of accounts. What one's place in life means individually is by some measure representationally commonplace at Merrill Court. Biography is tied to a shared narrative structure, which in turn is borrowed from broader cultural usage, the term *poor dear* having meaningful resonance throughout society. Yet its ordinary biographical complications feature the innumerable applications that creatively extend the shared notion of how some are "poor dears" and others are not.

BIOGRAPHICAL DIVERSITY IN LONG-TERM CARE

Lest it be figured that what is shared is ramified in various ways, consider how what is circumstantially commonplace can be contrastingly constructed. With the problem of biographical reproduction in mind, my research in the 1990s turned critically to a setting that is often assumed to congeal lifestories into a common narrative of despair—the nursing home (see Gubrium, 1993). If Hochschild found both shared and creatively extended elements in biographical usage at Merrill Court, my question was, would the nursing home, a "total" institution (Goffman, 1961), be even more influential in shaping residents' constructions into a common narrative? In particular, would the negative public resonances of the nursing home homogenize all biographical constructions into a single story of the nursing home experience? Would each narrative opportunity produce negative stories, in other words?

Critically responding to the public resonances of the nursing home, I deliberately offered to each resident in a series of interviews the opportunity to view themselves and their current circumstance through the lens of their lives as a whole (see Gubrium, 1993, for a detailed description of the study and some of its results). Rather than plunge directly into quality of life and care concerns, which I figured would unwittingly frame residents' account in terms of the popular conceptions of nursing home life, I began the first of each series of interviews with a resident with the request to tell me his or her lifestory. In follow-up interviews, I regularly referred back to what I knew about residents' experiences from initially hearing their stories. As a result, the interviews became narrative events not framed by default in terms of the popular version of the nursing home story. The working question was, would different horizons of meaning derived from the past diversely provide opportunities to speak of life?

The lifestories varied in detail. Some were lengthy and others were short. Some were told vividly and others conveyed in humdrum fashion. Some of the residents quickly became exhausted because they were frail, but most nonetheless wanted to go on and asked me to return so that they could "tell [me] the rest of it." I did return whenever asked to do so, and I persisted in attempting to maintain the lifestory, not the popular nursing home story, as the narrative context of their accounts. I was especially interested in the accounts of long-stayers, residents for whom the nursing facility had putatively become home. Such residents are continuing denizens of their worlds.

If anything, it is long-stayers whose stories might be homogenized by the popularization of their circumstances. Short-stayers are passersby in the nursing home scene, typically temporarily in residence for physical and occupational therapy or for postsurgical recovery.

Here I focus on the stories of two residents, Myrtle Johnson and Peter Rinehart, the extracts of which are taken from material gathered in interviews with them. Their accounts contrast mightily in how they represent what they presently share in common. The difference persisted across repeated interviews, prompted by my regular references to their lives as a whole. The difference and the persistence were typical of other residents, whose stories I eventually categorized into types of biographical construction in the circumstance. While Johnson's and Rinehart's narratives carry idiosyncratic elements, their stories can be viewed as having features shared with those of other residents of their narrative type. If, as we will see, Johnson's story is indeed a narrative of despair and does broadly reproduce the public image of the nursing home experience, Rinehart's story is a narrative of equanimity, whose accounts feature a horizon of meaning quite at odds with the public image.

The first of the two residents, Myrtle Johnson, was a 94-year-old widowed African American woman who had lived in the nursing home for a year. She suffered from Parkinson's disease and arthritis, and had difficulty maintaining balance. According to Johnson, falls had been the bane of old age for her and were the main reason she was placed in a nursing home. Her comments on the present quality of her life and her care in the home offer a stark contrast with the quality of her life in her earlier years.

Like some other accounts, her story loudly echoes the big story in question. Residents such as Johnson reflected on their lives, which they reported to have been filled with hard work, enjoyment, and kindness toward others, and grimly wondered how God could have planned this outcome for their lives. Some shook their heads tellingly as they related their story, lamenting how "it's come to this." I eventually used this phrase to identify a type of biographical construction, one with plots and themes that convey stories of having once been useful and now fated to be useless. In these accounts, the current quality of nursing home life engulfs the lifestory.

In one of the interviews, as Johnson compares an earlier useful life with a life now hardly worth living, she refers to suicide. But she links that with those who don't have the faith to sustain themselves in the circumstances. If it weren't for her faith in God, Johnson explains, hers would be the story of those who take their lives because life is no longer worth living. This happens to them because, she points out, "it's come to this." The following extract from one of the interviews is illuminating. It flags a biography constructed in terms of before and after. Tragic destiny permeates both her own and others' similar stories:

> But I worked hard all my life. And I enjoyed life. I'll say that what I enjoyed the most was when I lived on a farm in Missouri. Now that's where I enjoyed myself the most because I was able to get and do things, you know, help others. If there's one thing I don't like, it's just sittin'. That's what I have to do now. But then I try to make the best of it. But I would say that when I was able to be up and around and work is when I enjoyed myself the most… .

> Of course I'm not happy sitting here this way. But then it's part of life and you've got to… I say I've often thought about it, just since I've been passing between the chair and the bed. What use is it?

> You know, I can realize why some people commit suicide. They don't have faith. People that have faith in God don't commit suicide. But I can see why when people are in my position and don't have faith in the Lord, they commit suicide. I've thought about that so much. You know, you often say, "Well, why did so-and-so do so-and-so?" Well, if you sit down and study about it, you can figure that out… there's nothing… . But as long as you have faith in the Lord, you are going to go ahead and take what He sends you. But there's times you really wonder.

Now compare Johnson's accounts with those of a second resident, Peter Rinehart. Like some other residents, Rinehart's story centers on lifelong equanimity and is conveyed in a dramatically different tone. He himself doesn't use the word *equanimity,* but the term suits the purpose of distinguishing the type of narrative he conveys from Myrtle Johnson's and others' accounts, which fall under the rubric "it's come to this."

A 77-year-old widowed white male, Rinehart was paralyzed from the waist down, the result of a fall from a roof, leaving him in chronic pain. The fall figures prominently in his story. But if it divides related biographical matters chronologically into before and after, especially his functional capacity, it does not shape the quality of his life in the nursing home, nor does it serve as a watershed for separating his life as a whole into parts.

Regularly referring to matters conveyed in Rinehart's lifestory, I encouraged him several times in his interviews to compare life now with what it was like in the past. Rinehart responded accordingly, retrospectively tying together now with then. But the ties were not embedded in an account with temporal scaffolding that gave them overall shape or form. Rinehart's accounts differed from the depressing public image of nursing home life, even while he repeatedly talked about how some saw nursing homes, knowingly flagging the big story in question. When Rinehart looked back, then and now were not evaluated in terms of better or worse or in terms of before and after. Rather, varied thens and nows were compartmentalized and constructed as different pockets of experience through time. If Rinehart's fall was a turning point, before and after that didn't extend to his life as a whole. While its consequences were still felt in the nursing home and he had hoped this might change, the fall was not a basis for his reckoning of life as a whole.

Rinehart was one of two male residents interviewed who had been itinerant travelers. He had worked in sales for the Oster Company and, according to Rinehart, was constantly on the move. The constructive tone of the two men's stories was organized against this background, in which coming-and-going was viewed as the normal state of daily affairs. Home was not so much a headquarters or base of operations as it was one more stop along the way. If anything, home was time-out from the routine matters of daily life. These men *went home* for vacation, they didn't leave it.

For residents like Rinehart, the overall meaning of life isn't puzzling because life's meaning is found in particulars, in its parts and occasions. Their narratives show that if life has a plotline, it doesn't move in a particular direction. It unfolds in moments along a purely temporal pathway. If life has a moral horizon, it's constructed in fits and starts, each of life's pockets having its own evaluative purview. If these stories center on anything it is on incidents along the road of experience, the nursing home being a kind of stopover along the way. For Rinehart, his current circumstance does matter, but it doesn't engulf his story in the way it does for Johnson and some others. He accepts the nursing home as a place offering care, security, and shelter for the weary, who might not otherwise be able to carry on.

Rinehart noted at various points in his interviews that the facility in which he resided wasn't home, but under the circumstances it was the next best thing to it. Care paraphernalia and sickness aside, for traveling men like Rinehart, the nursing home offered respite; it was a kind of hotel, having both the best and the worst qualities of such establishments. Residents more or less were fed, had beds to sleep in, and had their cares attended to, but understandably not to everyone's satisfaction. Rinehart took pride in the quality of his life and what he had accomplished, but his accomplishments were storied independently from his fall or his present circumstances. The following interview extract is telling.

> I see people that are worse off than I am. I feel sorry for them, but I'm not looking back with remorse. It's something I can't help. It happened [the disabling fall] and I have to live with it. Life's been happy and pretty good to me otherwise. I made a good living. You take the good with the bad.

When it first happened, I hoped that I would be able to get back to normal. Then I hoped to get... they got me in a wheelchair. I hoped to be able to stay in a wheelchair, maybe graduate to crutches and that. It never happened that way though. But it didn't make me despondent.

Gradually, I began to know that I would probably never walk again and I've been about the way I have been now for the last couple of years. They brought a specialist in from the University of Pittsburgh and he put a brain tap in the nerve center of my brain. But that didn't work.

I'm hoping to clear up the pain in my back so I can, if nothing else, sit up. But I read a lot and that takes time and they treat me good here. The aides come in and I kid with them and that. The rest of the time is about the same as an average day when you aren't working. Only instead of working now, I read. It's a long weekend, you might say.

CONCLUSION

I'll conclude with three important points, each of which has been touched upon. The first one, now clear enough, is that everyday biographical construction is both circumstantially and interpersonally sensitive. If stories of "poor dears" and the nursing home resident are recognizable in society at large, they do not overshadow their everyday constructions. Certainly, because ordinary biographical construction is part of society, it is affected by shared understandings. But, at the same time, narrative events provide for amazing diversity in story production.

The second point is explanatory and relates to how we view the way biographical construction operates in everyday life. The interplay of the biographically general and the biographically particular is complex and varied narrative terrain. Biographical construction should not be reduced to either the general or the particular. Big stories are not just agglomerations of little stories, just as little stories do not fully display what is more broadly shared. Neither should be overshadowed in research. Overshadowing individual accounts with shared stories risks driving everyday constructions into the mold of homogeneous narratives. Likewise, overshadowing big stories with individual accounts risks shortchanging the common challenges of biographical construction.

Finally, the moral contours of the concepts of play and interplay are notable. The concepts provide context for appreciating the complexity of everyday life. They are a way of bringing into view the individual accounts that creatively ramify or challenge what is experienced in common. While the concepts are not as analytically neat and efficient as, say, a vocabulary of causality, their moral bearings are richer and relate more suitably to active narrative agents of experience.

REFERENCES

Anderson, E. (1999). *Code of the street*. New York: W. W. Norton.

Bamberg, M. (2006). Stories: Big or small—why do we care? *Narrative Inquiry, 16*, 139–147.

Bauman, R. (1986). *Story, performance, and event: Contextual studies of oral narrative*. New York: Cambridge University Press.

Freeman, M. (2006). Life "on holiday"? In defense of big stories. *Narrative Inquiry, 16*, 131–138.

Georgakopoulou, A. (2006). Thinking big with small stories in narrative and identity analysis. *Narrative Inquiry, 16*, 122–130.

Goffman, E. (1961). On the characteristics of total institutions. In *Asylums: Essays on the social situation of mental patients and other inmates* (pp. 1–124). Garden City, NY: Doubleday.

Gubrium, J. (1993). *Speaking of life: Horizons of meaning for nursing home residents*. Hawthorne, NY: Aldine de Gruyter.

Gubrium, J., & Holstein, J. (2009). *Analyzing narrative reality*. Thousand Oaks, CA: Sage.

Hochschild, A. (1973). *The unexpected community*. Englewood Cliffs, NJ: Prentice-Hall.

Holstein, J., & Gubrium, J. (2000). *Constructing the life course*. Lanham, MD: Rowman & Littlefield.

Ochs, E., & Taylor, C. (1992). Family narrative as political activity. *Discourse and Society, 3*(3), 301–340.

Shaw, C. (1930). *The jack-roller: A delinquent boy's own story*. Chicago: University of Chicago Press.

Wieder, D. (1974). *Language and social reality*. The Hague, Netherlands: Mouton.

four

INVENTING YOURSELF: HOW OLDER ADULTS

DEAL WITH THE PRESSURE OF LATE-MODERN

IDENTITY CONSTRUCTION

Frits de Lange

To many older adults in late-modern society, the question "Who are you (now, still)?" is difficult to answer. With retirement from their jobs, they have lost their work identity; the key positions in society have been taken over by the next generation. Their societal role has come to an end; they are playing the "roleless role" (Burgess, 1960) of the aged. Later on, they may even be forced to develop the "institutional self" (Gubrium & Holstein, 2001) of a nursing home. Who are they? They are the ones who require care from others. Also, their private role-identity as a parent or partner is threatened. Children have their own lives; partners pass away. Being aged means having been somebody in earlier days, but also being nobody today. Who you are seems to be restricted to who you were; your identity seems to shrink to the story of your life in retrospection. Therefore, for older adults, a narrative identity often seems to be the only possible identity to have, and to keep.

In this chapter I would like to elaborate on why the development of a narrative identity for older adults is so important, as well as what older adults can do if they don't succeed in having one. The narrative paradigm has enormous potential in gerontology, but also comes up against some limitations. Often, older adults don't succeed in articulating their lifestory. The late-modern necessity of identity construction continues, however, to put pressure on their lives. Consequently, sometimes minor or major depression cannot be avoided. More common in later life is the experience of the meaninglessness of life. Nonetheless, many older adults seem to have found other ways of saving their endangered sense of self, even though they scarcely own the narrative power necessary to develop a coherent and purposeful lifestory.

THE BIRTH OF PERSONAL IDENTITY

"Personal identity" is a recent construction. To an individual in a holistic, premodern society, having a personal identity distinct from the community that one participated in did not make sense. Community and individuality mutually defined each other. In premodern Europe, the only personal identity that people had was an administrative identity. Starting in the fourteenth century, every newborn child was recorded in the parochial baptism register. Later on, weddings and funerals were also listed. After the French Revolution, the church records were handed over to the local government. Carrying one's identity in one's pocket or wearing it on one's skin was a later development, born by the administrative need for increasing state control. Historically, personal identity was a product of the political concentration of power in the nation state. In France, the *livret ouvrier* (worker booklet), the certificate that workers had to carry with them wherever they went, was introduced in 1781. In the twentieth century, the obligation became compulsory for everyone. Identity started as an administrative instrument of control, not as a philosophical idea (Kaufmann 2004b, p. 22).

In Western democracies, societal control has been interiorized and has become part of the internal self-government of individuals (Rose, 1990). Identity has become a psychological characteristic. In the work of Erik H. Erikson, who may be called the father of the *concept* of personal identity (Erikson, 1950), this concept seems to develop out of thin air. But his introduction of identity as a characteristic of the self is closely connected to a new phase in the history of modernity. Since World War II, Western societies have viewed a "decline of the institutions" (Dubet, 2002). Hierarchical institutional programs (such as education, religion, health care) in which universal values were collectively transferred to individuals have slowly lost their impact. New institutions (for example, the media) represent another kind of emerging social structure. They focus on personal subjectivity as the main instrument of control. In school, medicine, and finance, experts assist individuals in creating an inner-directed personality, instead of being only external authorities. Domination comes from within, less than from above. The area of "organized modernity" (Wagner, 1996) is replaced by a second modernity in which power shifts from collective institutions to the psyche of the individual. Discipline is disseminated and interiorized (Foucault, 1988a).

In this context, obtaining a personal identity becomes a precondition for leading a meaningful life. The new fear, articulated by popular existentialism in the 1950s, is being Nobody, falling into Nothing. Without the institutional support of a clear role identity, life loses structure and purpose. Erikson himself reflects in his own biography the late-modern quest for identity. Born in 1902 as a Jew with the name Erik Homberger, he was forced to invent a new self in the United States. In his theoretical work, Erikson follows Freud—who did not use the term *identity* in any sense other than a description of a logical relation—in his understanding of the mechanism of psychological identification. Through identification with their parents, children interiorize and appropriate important, primordial role models. Their identity is not a given, but a permanent process of ongoing identifications.

In Erikson's theory of identity, he takes over Freud's perspective. But he also suggests that identity is not just an ongoing story of identifications but represents its outcome as well. On the one hand, identity development is an open process that eventually, in the final and Erikson's eighth stage of adult life, leads to a balance of integrity and despair. At the same time, Erikson introduces a "final identity," "fixed at the end of adolescence" (Erikson 1968, p. 161). In his work, the perspective shifts back and forth between process and product. His seminal work expresses the search for a late-modern, substantial identity: unique, irreplaceable, and unchangeable as the *livret ouvrier* that workers once carried in their pocket.

IDENTITY AS A HOLISTIC DESIRE

Another aspect of Erikson's theory of identity is notable: its emphasis on crisis. Erikson had a clear view of the way life in Western society after the Second World War transformed itself into a "chronic identity affection" (Ehrenberg, 1995). This might clarify his (ambivalent) inclination to stabilize identity as a distinguishable, closed entity. The French sociologist Jean-Claude Kaufmann recognizes a primordial holistic desire in this temptation to understand personal identity in an essentialist or substantialist manner. Identity is the religion of free-floating individuals who are longing for secure "envelopes," no longer guaranteed by premodern communities and the institutional programs of first modernity (Kaufmann, 2004a). According to Kaufmann, the abstract individual, understood as a closed entity, is the provisional outcome of a long history of religious transformation. In religion, the idea of totality is fundamental: the religious myth articulates the faith in, and longing for, a holistic universe. In the first phase of modernity, science tried to take over this integrative function of religion with faith in Reason. In the twentieth century, however, the Enlightenment had to give up its holistic pretensions. Nothing and no one else other than the Individual seems to be in charge of taking over the task of guaranteeing ontological wholeness. Therefore, the individual has to be considered as an integrating micro-totality, creating from "the inside" the nomic order that is no longer offered externally.

Seen from this perspective, the construction of personal identity as a closed unity and totality fulfills not only a social and psychological function but also a metaphysical one: as a "protective cocoon" (Giddens, 1991, p. 126ff) it provides an ontological safe-haven in a desolate world. In the modern religion of the abstract individual, "having an identity" is synonymous with believing in a Self as a stable and identifiable unity. Being someone is to have meaning in life. "Narrative foreclosure" (Freeman, 2000; this volume), therefore, is not by definition a pathological phenomenon but one mode within the dialectics of openness and closure that characterizes every "normal" construction of identity. On the one hand, the synthesis of a personal identity is always provisional and incomplete, and constantly under the threat of falling apart in heterogeneity. Identity is an open process, permanently in crisis. On the other hand, however, its mechanism is fed by the holistic dream of unity and continuity. That is the reason why individuals like to represent themselves as being a fixed, rounded entity, a *homo clausus* (Elias, 1991). Perhaps they have to admit that their identity is a fiction. But "if men define situations as real, they are real in their consequences" (Thomas & Thomas, 1929, p. 572); the social world has been organized around this fiction. We cannot *not* believe in this representation of the Self. Identity is an anthropological concept that creates reality by the belief in its reality (Kaufmann 2004a, pp. 230–231). Identity construction is only thinkable as an imaginative process, constantly threatened in its holistic pretensions. However, for ontological reasons, fact and fiction, the individual and its identity, the social process and its imaginary representation are persistently mixed up.

THE PRESSURE OF INVENTING OURSELVES

So we may understand personal identity not as given but as the provisional result of constructed identifications (identity for me), intentionally to be confirmed by others (identity for others). In the remainder of this chapter,

I argue for understanding late-modern identity as a layered concept. Older adults in particular use different modes of identity construction, narrative identity being one of them. The compelling argument by sociologists such as Anthony Giddens (1991), Ulrich Beck (Beck & Beck-Gersheim, 2002), and Zygmunt Baumann (1995) may suggest that personal identity as a "self-reflexive project" (Giddens, 1991) is the only available option, but I have my doubts about that.

Their story goes like this: traditions and communities have lost their self-evident legitimacy, making people live under the pressure to invent lives on their own. The future can no longer be deduced from the past. This requires a constant attitude of reflexivity, an active and innovative self that is ready to create a coherent, purposeful identity in a constantly changing environment. Coherence of identity over time no longer consists in belonging to social group(s) but has to be personally constructed. Each transitional phase in the trajectory of life tends to become an identity crisis (Giddens, 1991).

By developing a narrative identity as late-modern individuals, we reflexively provide ourselves with a meaningful life. The self has a heroic job to do. It has "to bring together the different parts of ourselves and our lives into a purposeful and convincing whole," Dan McAdams writes (1993, p. 11). "We make ourselves through myth" (p. 13). Our world can no longer tell us who we are and how we should live; therefore, we must figure out our identity on our own.

After the individualization of the holistic ambition of totality, every single individual seems to be forced to create his or her own universe of meaning. Identity building is a synonym for meaning construction, a creation ex nihilo. The individual is the *principium*, the primordial beginning of its own world (Kaufmann, 2004a, p. 97). The pressure, hereby laid on the imaginative power of the auto-creative individual, is enormous. In the philosophy of Friedrich Nietzsche, this way of understanding personal autonomy finds its exemplary expression: "We... want to become who we are—the new, unique, incomparable ones, who give themselves their own laws, who create themselves!" (1882/1974, p. 335).

The power to create oneself out of nothing into a sovereign individual is the foundational myth on which modern culture is built. This narrative endows the culture of late-modern subjectivity with an enormous dynamic. Whoever starts creating him- or herself will never accomplish the job. Personal identity is an open, indeterminate process, a *creatio continua.* Self-actualization is permanent self-enhancement. Not everyone, however, is a Nietzsche. People who cannot cope with the pressure involved in the business of autobiographical construction will get into serious trouble.

The sociologist Alain Ehrenberg (1995) portrays the late-modern self as an "uncertain individual" who easily breaks down under the pressure of reflexive self-invention by fleeing into addiction or depression. He assumes a plain connection between the "depression pandemic" (Dehue, 2008) and late-modern identity pressure. Depression is the result of the breakdown of the identity machine. Somehow and somewhere, sand has been sprinkled in the engine of the self. Depression can be labeled as *la fatigue d'être soi*. One is tired of being oneself. Characteristic for late-modern depression is not the melancholia of earlier ages but the weakening and loss of the power of agency. Depression is the antonym of an enterprising spirit, the break-down of personal productivity (Dehue, 2008). Depression is the failure of the will that no longer has the power to will. The mission of self-creation is abandoned before it has even been taken up. Apathy, motionlessness, total asthenia, both mental and physical, is the essence of the late-modern depressive mood.

THE MYTH OF SELF-CREATION

The pressure to create oneself ex nihilo is a modern myth, in both senses of the word. On the one hand, it is the archetypical narrative of modernity, the religion to which we have to adhere in order to experience meaning. As the creation of meaning runs through the construction of identity, for older adults telling a coherent lifestory is an important instrument to save their threatened identity from despair. The better their story (see, for example, Randall & McKim, 2008), the more they are somebody, and the more their lives make sense. The development of narrative therapies and other methods of intervention, supporting older adults in the reconstruction of their lifestory, is of great help for their existential well-being.

On the other hand, narrative self-creation as the only means remaining for identity construction is a myth that distorts reality. There are other ways for late-modern individuals to construct their personal and social identity without much reflexive and/or narrative labor. It is important to see the scope and limits of the job done by narrative identity construction. But the construction of narrative identity requires an active subject, creating a coherent and enduring "self" in its imagination. Some older adults may lack the courage to take up that yoke and flee into depression. Others, however, discover alternative ways to create personal identity, ways "good enough" to keep their lives going without the escape into pathology. Different modes of personal identity can be distinguished that continue to exist next to one another (synchronically), though they have emerged diachronically, in the dynamics of subsequent historical constellations.

The work of the French sociologist Claude Dubar (2007) might be of great help here. In his typology of identities, he first distinguishes between two general forms of social identity: an identity of community and a societal identity. Both are *social* identities. Any kind of identity is simultaneously always identity for oneself and identity for others. Therefore, talking about premodern and modern identity as individual and collective identities is confusing. The first form of identity Dubar discerns, community identity— that is, Max Weber's (1920/2002) *Vergemeinschaftung*—is characteristic for holistic societies, in which no distinctive meaning is given to individuals. To be more precise, every individual has a social identity for him- or herself and for others. Psychologically, he or she surely is an I, and socially a Me. But in a holistic context it is by definition a We–I and a We–Me. There is no question of *personal* identity, in the sense of a distinctive identity, apart from that of the community. The meaning of an individual's life is defined by his or her contribution to the reproduction of the community, identical across the generations. Spatial, genealogical relationships determine one's individual identity. There is little openness for development: identity is given by heritage, gender, class, marriage. The place one occupies within the community and within the successive generations is expressed in one's name. Therefore, Dubar speaks of a "nominal self," characteristic for holistic societies. Until modern times, this type of identity dominated societies. Gender is the most important criterion for the distribution of power within such a holistic system. The anthropology of Claude Lévi-Strauss (1977) paradigmatically describes and analyzes this type of identity.

Modernity introduces a second, *societal* form of identity, namely, Weber's *Vergesellschaftung*. It presupposes a variable participation of individuals in different communities, with which they identify for a shorter or longer time. The biographical component in social identity, its time dimension, becomes more important than the spatial dimension. One can speak of *personal* identity in a more strict sense, distinctive—though not separated—from the identity within the community.

Within societal identity, several types of personal identity have developed in the course of modern history. We may call them, along with Dubar subsequently, reflexive identity, role (or status) identity, and narrative identity. Already within early Christianity the foundation was laid for a reflexive type of personal identity. *Reflexive* may be taken here with Dubar in a broad sense: it refers to a personal identification with an ideal, symbolic self, through introspection and dialogue. Michel Foucault (1988a) has described this type of identity in an exemplary way in his research on care for the self (*souci de soi*). The reflexive self becomes a project in time. Its power is not distributed by politics or economy but depends on the status one occupies within the symbolic order of a philosophical doctrine or a religious system. What counts is not whether one is rich or mighty, but whether one is a person of wisdom and virtue, or a saint.

Then, in the early Renaissance period, a different type of identity emerged at the European courts, coined "status identity" by Dubar. In the following centuries it slowly spread over the emerging bourgeois society and the newly constructed nation states. A person's social significance and personal identity were no longer attached to one's name and genealogy but to the role he or she played within the court hierarchy (early Renaissance) or the nation state (late nineteenth century). One's social role has become the essential identity marker, so we can also speak of *role identity*. Inner space is possible now between the self and its function within the fabric of society, a function that is not fixed once and for all: roles allow social mobility—upward, downward, and sideward. The determining mechanism for the distribution of power here is the expanding bureaucracy.

The last and fourth type of identity may be called "narrative identity." Dubar understands the term in a surprising and rather strict way. Its origins lie in early modernity. Max Weber's puritan, the hero of early capitalism, can count as its model. The puritan Calvinist wants to make a success story of his life for religious reasons. His lifestory has holistic importance: it reflects the glory of God (Weber, 2002). He presents his self as an entrepreneur, a *homo faber*, a self-made man. Perhaps John Bunyan's *Pilgrim's Progress* (1678) can be considered the archetypical model of modern narrative identity (De Lange, 2004). Telling the story of his life grants him continuity, coherence, and purpose—the major holistic guards against the loss of meaning. But the narrative can only do the job when it relies on the energy of a powerful will. The entrepreneur's personal identity is not determined by his name, nor is it given by the social role he plays. The degree to which his life makes sense depends on the choices he makes and the risks he takes throughout the total trajectory of his life course. The meaning of his life is given by the pilgrimage he undertakes. Who he is will be revealed after he has completed his earthly voyage.

A PLURALITY OF SELVES AND THE INTEGRATIVE ROLE OF NARRATIVE IDENTITY

Drawing on Dubar, I distinguish between a nominal, symbolic role and narrative self-identity (see Table 4.1). Dubar defends the thesis that personal identity in late modernity is in constant crisis, permanently threatened and in transition. He also suggests, in line with Giddens, Beck, and Baumann,

Table 4.1 Forms and types of personal identity*

Forms of identity	Identity types	Main characteristics	Exemplary research
Community identity	Nominal self	Name and place	Levi-Strauss
Societal identity	Symbolic self	Project and time	Foucault
	Role self	Role and institution	Elias
	Narrative self	Action and story	Weber

*After Dubar (2007).

that as the importance of reflexive and narrative identity increases, the more holistic communities and societal institutions come under pressure. He emphasizes, however, that all the mentioned types of identity still occur simultaneously in late-modern society. Personal identities often consist of composed amalgams of the four different identity types described previously (Dubar, 2007, p. 194ff). Even holistic survivals continue to be vitally present. Besides, though the role of institutions may have decreased and changed (they have become more flexible, aiming at personal "governmentality"), they continue to be vital structuring elements in society and in identity construction. Playing institutional roles is essential in the transmission of social memory and is still supportive for individual identities.

This layered, complex concept of identity can serve as the point of departure for the hypothesis that *the importance of developing a narrative identity for living a meaningful life increases as nominal, symbolic, and role identities are weakening.* Conversely, the stronger these types of personal identification fulfill their holistic function, the less integrative power is required by personal-narrative activity.

The thesis put forward here requires empirical support. Some preconditions, however, may be expressed in advance.

The first one is that a *nominal self* might be strong or weak. With the name someone carries, he or she is connected to earlier generations and to a family. By giving names to one's children, the identity of future generations is produced. During a lifetime, the meaning attached to the parental name can increase and/or decrease. But it can never be denied. Iván Böszörményi-Nagy (1920–2007), who developed a contextual approach to family therapy and individual psychotherapy, shows in his therapeutic work and theory how people are trans- and intergenerationally involved deeply in a network of invisible loyalties to their parents, grandparents, siblings, children, and grandchildren. Despite the individualization of society, the abstract individual is an illusion, not only synchronically, but also diachronically. In family and Christian names, a hidden, complex web of vertical and horizontal (dis) loyalties is revealed (Böszörményi-Nagy and Spark, 1984). Why do parents choose specific names for their children?

A stronger awareness of (affirmed) nominal identity often contributes to the construction of meaning in old age. Being able to say, "I have been a good (not only) Rockefeller, Kennedy (but also) Smith or De Lange," gives a comforting sense of continuity and purpose. Parents who name their child after a movie or pop star or a sports hero may transmit a much weaker nominal self to their child. But it will never be absent. A name represents a history and anchors a person in time and place; it is given by parents, not constructed by the child. The affirmed consciousness of being a link in the chain of generations may weaken the pressure on the imaginative power of self-creation. The beginning and end of one's autobiography are perhaps to be reconstructed, but not to be invented ex nihilo.

The second factor is that reflexivity leads to inner role distance. In late-modern society, no one coincides with his or her societal status. Role identities, however, continue to be important. The moment one engages personally with a role, "role distance" will shrink. In strong commitments, one will interiorize a role, will identify with it even physically. A happy, young father not only plays his role but also embodies it. He *is* father. Speaking in general about a process of "desinstitutionalization of society" is, therefore, inaccurate (Kaufmann, 2004a, in a critique of Dubet, 2002). It is not the impact of institutional roles that is decreasing, but their shape and character that are undergoing changes. There is a shift in the organization of societal order and political control away from collective, hierarchical institutions and toward subjective autonomy: late-modern institutions are focused on the production of "governmentality," an individuality that has acquired the mentality to govern itself (Foucault, 1988b; Rose, 1990). In second modernity, the life courses of individuals show a degree of flexibility and variability that requires a permanent reflective awareness of their social performances. It results in what one might call a "duplication of action schemes." There is a role to fulfill, but one fulfils it in an authentic, personal way. The institutional role identity becomes a personal "identity role" as well. In playing it, individuals acquire during the course of their lives an "identity salience," a reservoir of possible identity roles, to perform whenever the social need is felt by them (Kaufmann, 2004b, p. 74). Hazel Markus (1977) speaks of "self-schemata," or affective–cognitive structures modeled on accumulated individual experiences. An inner conflict might result when the expectations attached to formal institutionalized roles on the one hand, and the personal action repertoire in the form of self-schemes on the other hand come into competition. But normally, they run together smoothly, reinforcing each other.

For older adults, the repertoire of available institutional roles is decreasing radically. They are confronted with the need for inventing their lives anew. Many seniors in their "third age," according to the Dutch gerontologist Kees Knipscheer, experience their lives as "a second adolescence" (2005). While young people experiment dynamically with a broad spectrum of roles, in adult life and old age the repertoire is rather reduced and seems fixed. Retirement often implies the loss of occupational and professional roles, which are anchor places in society. Parental roles continue to exist but have lost their embeddedness in and connection with the educational system. However, older adults continue to behave according to patterned self-schemes that provide them with a satisfying personal identity. Many elderly people are involved in volunteer work, often organized informally. And seniors identify willingly and intensely with their role as grandparent. Sometimes, older adults even define their identity exclusively in terms of the informal care they give to their partner. This kind of strong personal role identity (or identity role) protects older adults from a loss of meaning and relieves, to a degree, the pressure on their narrative ability. They don't have to tell who they are; they simply show who they are.

To avoid the fatiguing labor of reflexive and narrative identity construction, older adults also may fall back on their accumulated *habits*. Habits are also identity roles that keep people going, but without the structured need of participants or a public. Narrative identity requires creative work, an enterprising self. As stated earlier, those who lack the power and energy to do this work may slip away into a depressive mood. And those who might have the energy but don't want to use it end up with a spiritual emptiness. This existential shallowness can be made bearable by lowering the expectations of life. Personal identity shrinks to only wanting to be what one is. This refusal of constructive identity work can be considered a desperate, though unconscious, act of resistance to late-modern self-creation, as well as a vital attempt to survive psychologically as a human being. One clings to the habitual course of life, still being the one that one has been before. Daily rhythms (breakfast, newspaper, meal rituals) are stretched out endlessly. One draws back from the social world into one's home or garden and watches television, because "one has to do at least something." Reflexivity is avoided. "It is as it is." "That's the way things go" (Kaufmann, 2004b, p. 229). The mental doubling required by living consciously one's roles is reduced to a minimum. One deliberately incarnates oneself in the pattern of daily, elementary acts. A certain serenity sets in. Though life expectations shorten, the experience of time lengthens. But one prefers boredom above the uncertainty of plans and projects. This description may be suited especially for lower middle-class retired couples. Among them, a large resistance to the effort of identity construction can be encountered (Kaufmann, 2004b, p. 237ff.).

Finally, the third factor to be considered here is that a strong *symbolic identity* may relieve the older adult from the demanding labor of maintaining identity. The symbolic power of nationalist, class, and confessional identities has significantly decreased in Western democracy. However, just as adolescents may strongly identify themselves with a pop group or artist, a sporting club or a fundamentalist movement, older adults may willingly identify with a spiritual world or a religious tradition. Whoever is a committed "child of God" appears less in need of autocreative energy and biographical reconstruction than someone poor in symbolic identifications. Accepting the fact of being a Muslim or a reborn Christian as one's one and only identity, and disregarding all other affiliations and group identities one has acquired in the course of one's life, not only simplifies one's existence but also gives it massive meaning—besides making it possibly intolerant and belligerent (Sen, 2006).

POSSIBLE SELVES AS NARRATIVE IDENTITIES, VERSION "LIGHT"

How can an experienced meaninglessness in old age be alleviated if older persons lack the energy, the will, or the power for intensive narrative identity construction? Interventions with life book methods (Noonan, this volume; Tromp, this volume; van den Brandt, this volume), however promising their results are, are not suitable for every older adult. Not everyone embodies an enterprising self and has the assembling imaginative power to compose a lifestory. Also, storytelling mostly requires special moments and occasions.

Helping to develop a "narrative identity, version light," may offer an alternative, especially for the oldest and most frail elderly (Smith & Freund, 2002). Not everyone is capable of narrating a Sunday version of his or her lifestory. But a daily "working self" (Markus & Nurius, 1986) that pragmatically responds to the concrete contexts in which some form of agency is required is usually available. The working self prefers to construct its identity not by openness but rather by fixation: "that's the way I am." This here-and-now-identity works with quick images, rather than with long stories.

Though this work identity has narrative structure, it requires only modest narrative power and energy. With imaginative, possible self-images, one is able to produce self-schemes that may guide—at least in the short term—future behavior. The inertia of coinciding with oneself, the refusal of mental doubling, is avoided. Possible selves are future representations of the selves that are hoped for or feared. By projecting possible selves in one's "little cinema," one is able to escape the stone-like, subhuman identity of "I am who I am": a self without a future, without projects and plans, waiting for its death (Kaufmann, 2004b). One gives oneself at least a tomorrow. The imagined self is a story, frozen in one positive or negative image: "I want to stay the lean and sportive man that I am now, and still a long distance runner at 70." "I would like to be always cheerful and laughing—which I am not at the moment." "I want to stay just as I am—someone who likes to help other people." "I would like to play the organ again, but I can't anymore." These are images that aim at an improvement, maintenance, or avoidance of some parts of one's actual self (Smith & Freund, 2002). The picture is not all-encompassing and does not stretch over a lifetime; it is limited in scope and scale. The job of creating images of possible selves is a modest endeavor, also in the sense that it does not allow too much freedom: accumulated biographical experiences and a set social context narrow the spectrum of available selves. It requires little psychic energy to lean on the amassed repertoire of identity roles, one's "identity salience." However, the mobilizing of one's possible selves requires at least some effort and some risk-taking, because the process can end up in disappointment. In developing possible selves, one accepts the invitation to work on oneself and strive, if not for a slight innovation of the actual self, at least for keeping it in shape. These possible selves provide persons with a dynamic motivational structure that helps them to confront the vicissitudes of life, although the fabric of images may have to be reset when what is strived for does not happen or what was feared actually occurs.

The imagination of possible selves may lose contact with reality by becoming too ambitious. Idealized selves are often only ephemeral, gratuitous, symbolic compensations for negative self-evaluations. Virtual identities that are transformed into work schemes for future selves are a minority. They may be called "possible selves" in the strong sense. Generally, however, much imaginary effort is not needed: possible selves may be composed of inner representations of established social roles in one's "little cinema." The narrative scenario thickens to one scene, shrinks to one image: "that's the way I would like to be." Or, conversely, "that's the me I never want to become." Possible selves also do not require much rational reflection. A working self's reflection is mostly repetitive, and seldom progressive. An open dialogue about possible self-images that one longs for or fears, however, will contribute to the externalization of personal identity, and liberate it from its isolation as an individual mental activity. A threatened personal identity is gifted with a rudimentary narrative plot, with a minimum of laborious imagination. As long as older persons say to themselves, "I want to stay healthy and carry on living as I am," or "I don't want to become grumpy" (Smith & Freund, 2002, p. 494), they keep unbroken their "capacity to keep a particular narrative going," the essential requirement in late-modern times for leading a meaningful life (Giddens, 1991, p. 54).

REFERENCES

Baumann, Z. (1995). *Life in fragments: Essays in postmodern morality.* Cambridge, UK: Basil Blackwell.

Beck, U., & Beck-Gernsheim, E. (2002). *Individualization: Institutionalized individualism and its social and political consequences.* London: Sage.

Böszörményi-Nagy, I., & Spark, G. (1984). *Invisible loyalties: Reciprocity in intergenerational family therapy.* New York: Brunner/Mazel.

Burgess, E. (1960). Aging in western culture. In E. Burgess (Ed.), *Aging in western societies* (pp. 3–28). Chicago: University of Chicago Press.

Dehue, T. (2008). *De depressie-epidemie: Over de plicht het lot in eigen hand te nemen* [The depression-pandemic: On the obligation to take fortune in one's own hand]. Amsterdam: Uitgeverij Augustus.

De Lange, F. (2004). Life as a pilgrimage: John Bunyan and the modern life course. In P. Holtrop, F. de Lange, & R. Roukema (Eds.), *Passion of Protestants* (pp. 95–126). Kampen, The Netherlands: Kok.

Dubar, C. (2007). *La crise des identités: L'interprétation d'une mutation* (3rd ed.). [The crisis of identities: The interpretation of a mutation]. Paris: Presses Universitaire de France.

Dubet, F. (2002). *Le déclin de l'institution.* [The decline of the institution]. Paris: Seuil.

Ehrenberg, A. (1995). *L'individu incertain.* [The uncertain individual]. Paris: Calman-Lévy.

Elias, N. (1991). *The society of individuals.* (M. Schroter, Ed.; E. Jephcott, Trans.). Oxford, UK: Blackwell. (Original work published 1987)

Erikson, E. (1950). *Childhood and society.* New York: W. W. Norton.

Erikson, E. (1968). *Identity: Youth and crisis.* New York: W. W. Norton.

Foucault, M. (1988a). *The care of the self. The history of sexuality, Vol. 3.* (R. Hurley, Trans.). New York: Vintage.

Foucault, M. (1988b). Technologies of the self. In L. Martin, H. Gutman, & P. Hutton (Eds.), *Technologies of the self: A seminar with Michel Foucault* (pp. 16–49). London: Tavistock.

Freeman, M. (2000). When the story's over: Narrative foreclosure and the possibility of self-renewal. In M. Andrews, S. Slater, C. Squire, & A. Treacher (Eds.), *Lines of narrative: Psychosocial perspectives* (pp. 81–91). London: Routledge.

Giddens, A. (1991). *Modernity and self-identity. Self and society in the late modern age.* Cambridge, UK: Polity Press.

Gubrium, J., & Holstein, J. (2001). *Institutional selves: Troubled identities in a postmodern world.* New York: Oxford University Press.

Kaufmann, J.-C. (2004a). *Ego: Pour une sociologie de l' individu.* [Ego: Toward a sociology of the individual]. Paris: Armand Collin.

Kaufmann, J.-C. (2004b). *L'invention de soi: Une théorie de l'identité.* [The invention of the self: A theory of identity]. Paris: Armand Collin.

Knipscheer, K. (2005). *De uitdaging van de tweede adolescentie.* [The challenge of the second adolescence]. Amsterdam: Free University.

Lévi-Strauss, C. (Ed.) (1977). *L'identité.* [Identity]. Paris: Grasset.

Markus, H. (1977). Self-schemata and processing information about self. *Journal of Personality and Social Psychology, 35*(2), 63–78.

Markus, H., & Nurius, P. (1986). Possible selves. *American Psychologist, 41*(9), 954–969.

McAdams, D. (1993). *The stories we live by: Personal myths and the making of the self.* New York,: William Morrow.

Nietzsche, F. (1974). *The gay science* (Vol. 4). (W. Kaufmann, Trans.). New York: Vintage. (Original work published 1882)

Randall, W., & McKim, A. (2008). *Reading our lives: The poetics of growing old.* New York: Oxford University Press.

Rose, N. (1990). *Governing the self: The shaping of the private self.* London: Routledge.

Sen, A. (2006), *Identity and violence: The illusion of destiny.* New York: W. W. Norton.

Smith, J., & Freund, A. (2002). The dynamics of possible selves in old age. *Journal of Gerontology, 57B*(6), 492–500.

Thomas, W., & Thomas, D. (1929). *The child in America: Behavior problems and programs* (2nd ed.). New York: A. A. Knopf.

Wagner P. (1996). *Liberté et discipline: Les deux crises de la modernité.* [Freedom and discipline: The two crises of modernity]. Paris: Métaillé.

Weber, M. (2002). *The Protestant ethic and the spirit of capitalism.* (P. Baehr and G. Wells, Trans.). London: Penguin. (Original work published 1920)

Five

IN WAVES OF TIME, SPACE, AND SELF: THE

DWELLING-PLACE OF AGE IN VIRGINIA

WOOLF'S *THE WAVES*

Rishi Goyal and Rita Charon

> *Now is life very solid or very shifting? I am haunted by the two*
> *contradictions. This has gone on forever; will last forever; goes down*
> *to the bottom of the World—this moment I stand on. Also it is*
> *transitory, flying, diaphanous. I shall pass like a cloud on the waves.*
> —Virginia Woolf, January 1929 (1977, p. 218)

The deepest fears and the broadest comforts of aging human beings emerge from the poles of the contradiction between the lasting and the fleeting. The contradiction is unseen in youth, as summer's sea-bathing lasts forever even though each wave disappears in its turn on the shore. Any adult knows what happens to endless summers. They shorten sequentially, perhaps abridged by responsibilities, sufferings, boredom, and the simple calculus that there are fewer and fewer of them in store. By the time of old age, the contradiction seems for some to shift dramatically toward the fleeting, the thoughtless sense of the great expanses of the life of youngsters eroded by pain in the hip, cataract-clouded vision, bills to be paid, houses to be cleaned, and the senior realization that, indeed, it will come to an obituated end.

One's experience of time is governed by one's position in it—how far into the river of it one has waded—or, more specifically, by the distance one finds oneself from either shore. The stages of life or the ages of human beings, the medieval *cursus aetatis*, has been an available trope for organizing the life course since antiquity—the proliferation of the image of the stairs with its parabolic course offers one example of its cultural penetration (Thane, 2000). Aristotle (1991) adopted a three-stage theory in *On Rhetoric,* while for Horace (1926) and Galen (1951) it was four; Saint Augustine (2002) argued in *On Genesis Against the Manichees* for a six-stage progress, as did Isidore of Seville (2006) in the *Etymologies.* Whether three, four, six, or seven, these stages of life stressed the correspondence of human time with geologic or religious phenomena—from the seasons according to Ovid's *Metamorphosis* (2005) to the planets in the heavens to the days of creation; and they all asserted the practical overlap of the last stage, old age, with death. For most pre-nineteenth century philosophers, writers, theologians, or physicians, old age was simply that period of life immediately prior to a physical leave-taking of this world; the appropriate behaviors for this stage then were resignation and acceptance. But with the end of the eighteenth and nineteenth centuries, whether because of the Enlightenment and the rise of scientific thinking, the secularization and de-Christianization of the world, urbanization, industrialization, the invention of retirement and pension funds, or real demographic shifts, the last stage of life was re-understood as a meaningful aspect of the earthly life and a distinct phase of life. With the lengthening of old age and its separation from death, old age emerged as an important aspect of the newly standardized life course. The notion that old age had a *duration* would have an immediate impact on thought in a variety of disciplines, including aesthetic theory, history, economics, and literature.

The person in old age will endure many temporal contradictions—not only the tension between the lasting and the fleeting, but also the value tension between well-used time and wasted time, the aspirational tension between completion and breakdown, and the acquisitory tension between desire and deprivation. A narrative gerontology suggests that there is some nourishment to be had from either narrative texts or the actions of engaging with them that alter these contradictions. In addition to the telling of one's lifestory and the reading of others' lifestories, we propose that specific novels might be mined for fresh ways of not solving but living with the contradictions. Although some novels might offer portraits of characters who "age well" that might inspire or console their readers, we have in mind novels whose creation and form lend some understanding to the very foreclosing (Freeman, this volume) or expanding tensions that are experienced by us as we traverse this newly discovered age of humankind.

It is not necessarily the stories told in the course of the novel—its so-called plot—that treat the contradiction between the fleeting and the lasting. Rather, the forms in which novels are told and received bestow narrative's gifts to all of us struggling to live within the grip of aging. The poetics of the novel grants its writers and readers access to a means of seeing whole a section of the random chaos of existence. By framing its domain, the novel canonizes a stretch of both time and place as its sphere of meaning-making. Russia at nineteenth-century war, the maturation of a pretty girl from Albany into the portraited lady of Europe, the coming of age of a German engineer by way of the tuberculosis sanatorium in the Alps: Leo Tolstoy (1869/2003), Henry James (1881/2003), and Thomas Mann (1924/1995) etched their scenes within times and settings narrow enough for visible detail and wide enough for contingent resonance. The narrative strategies adopted by novelists illuminate some of the escape hatches in the otherwise relentless trap of human time, by no means only the chronological ordering of events in time but all the narrative forces—imagery, allusion, characterization, conflict, narrative tension, point of view, narrating strategy, and desire—that animate every novel and let it tell its truth.

Most, perhaps almost all, works of fiction treat the passage of time. Indeed, as philosopher and literary scholar Georg Lukács writes, "We might almost say that the entire inner action of the novel is nothing but a struggle against the power of time" (1971, p. 122). What we today call narratology arose from the work of Russian formalists and linguists who studied the construction of folk tales to uncover the "rules" of storytelling (Propp, 1968; Shklovsky, 1929/1990). Their overriding concern was to describe the relations between story and discourse—that is, between the events being represented and the discursive acts that performed and then captured the accounts of them. By definition, these are temporal duties: how, most simply, to transpose an event from its occurrence in a "then" into a narrating "now" of telling. Gérard Genette's magisterial *Narrative Discourse* (1972/1979) brought into French structuralism the Russian scholars' concerns with temporal duplication, in text, of events of the so-called real world. (Genette's chapters are "Order," "Duration," "Frequency," "Mood," and "Voice," reserving three-fifths of the study for temporal concerns.) Tellingly, Genette chose Marcel Proust's *A la Recherche du Temps Perdu* [In search of lost time] (1913–1927/1999) as the text that he glossed in this authoritative study of the narrative process, in effect marking the narratological study of the novel as the narratological study of *time* in the novel. Such works as Henri Bergson's *Time and Free Will* (1910/1960) and Paul Ricoeur's *Time and Narrative* (1983/1984–1988) were profoundly influential in the thinking of literary scholars developing the then-young field of narratology.

The *sitedness* of the novel's action—unlike much poetry, for example, novels generally happen somewhere—adds a dimension to its temporal unfolding that a narrative gerontology might value. It is just of late that narratology has moved from a blinding concentration on temporality to recognize the weight of space in storytelling. Eminent narratologist Shlomith Rimmon-Kenan, author of two editions of *Narrative Fiction: Contemporary Poetics* (1983/2002), summarizes the work of such contemporary theorists as David Herman and Susan Stanford Friedman in inserting considerations of spatialization or spatial poetics into the narratological discourse: "Classical narratology has continued by and large to privilege time. Today, in what Herman (2002) calls postclassical narratology, this is no longer the case" (p. 231, n. 1).

Schools of thought have gathered around literary studies, anthropology, sociology, and phenomenology that privilege space. Such writers as Gaston Bachelard (1958/1994), Pierre Bourdieu (1977), Michel de Certeau (1980/1984), and Jean Baudrillard (1994) have given us some terms and concepts for mapping this domain within writing. Published originally in French from the late 1950s to the mid-1980s, these studies informed both the structuralist and the poststructuralist currents investigating the consequences of particular kinds of textual form in releasing meanings from literary works. The work of M.M. Bakhtin (1981) and A.J. Greimas (1987) before them, among others, opened up clearings where notions of the relativity of time and space in interpreting language and experience—be it in fiction, memoir, discourse, or life—were acknowledged. In turn, a generation of scholars, working within multiple humanities, social science, and cognitive science disciplines, continue to sharpen and expand our notions of the consequences, for interpretable meaning, of the spaces represented in our texts. Bachelard suggests in *The Poetics of Space* (1958/1994) that "space that has been seized upon by the imagination cannot remain indifferent space subject to the measures and estimates of the surveyor. It has been lived in, not in its positivity, but with all the partiality of the imagination" (p. xxxvi). Crossing the line from literary theory to visual aesthetics, the naming of a spatial poetics recognizes the obligatory sensory and envisionable nature of how our lives accrue meaning. Fundamental to the human ability to process whatever constitutes the actual is the skill to mentally represent where one is and has been, and that skill depends on a visual and dimensional responsiveness to the locations that contain and shape and surround the unfolding lives.

This liberating shift from an exclusive focus on time toward the "other" dimension of space makes room in the contemplation of novels and poems for acknowledging the physical, the indwelt, the surround.

Contemplating space permits one to distinguish the exterior from the interior—of houses, of shells, of cities, of bodies. Paying attention to the spaces in which events occur *grounds* them in the particularities of situations. It is not simply that scholars now notice more the setting of novels— Oxford South, iron cold New England, the plains of Willa Cather. It is instead, far more radically, that the shifts and pulses of space are accorded meaning and value. Readers now have permission to follow closely the opening and closing of doors and windows or to envision the dimensions of an overcoat. Ahead of his time, E.M. Forster (1927/1985) had this to say about space in *War and Peace* (Tolstoy, 1869/2003):

> Why is *War and Peace* not depressing? Probably because it has extended
> over space as well as over time, and the sense of space until it terrifies us is
> exhilarating, and leaves behind it an effect like music. After one has read *War
> and Peace* for a bit, great chords begin to sound, and we cannot say exactly
> what struck them. They come from the immense area of Russia.... Many
> novelists have the feeling for place.... Very few have the sense of space....
> Space is the lord of *War and Peace,* not time. (p. 39)

The study of aging might take the passage of time for granted, but it requires as well deep inspection of the problems and powers of space. If the "self" or the "soul" or the "personhood" is what declines, it is the dwelling it inhabits, very literally its body, that stands against evanescence and declares, absolutely and positively, that there is a "here" here. For the field of narrative gerontology and for narrative medicine in general, the shift toward recognition of a spatial poetics confers primacy on the space of concern to the clinician, that of the human body itself.

Virginia Woolf wrote *The Waves* (1931/2006) 10 years before she ended her life. Both the plot and the form of this experimental modernist novel repay close reading by the project of narrative gerontology. Like *The Years* (1937/1998), written in the same period, *The Waves* explores the possibilities of change and continuity in history through individual lives. Both novels flirt with formal structures based on historical reflexivity: *The Waves* (which is divided into sections based on the natural rhythms of the sun moving through the sky and the waves striking a beach) and *The Years* (structured as a series of chapters with year headings) are modeled on two opposing historical assumptions. *The Waves* borrows its structure both from Renaissance tropes of recurrence and from a cyclical epistemology of history (Vico's "*ricorsi,*" Croce, Spengler), while *The Years* projects history as a linear, eschatological movement: "It seems as if the two great conceptions of antiquity and Christianity, cyclic motion and eschatological direction, have exhausted the basic approaches to the understanding of history" (Lowith, 1949, p. 221).

But both works merge historical patterns and time with Woolf's most con-sistent principle of composition, the longevity of a human life. Both follow characters from childhood to old age (a span of approximately 60 years), directly linking historical movement and time with the human lifespan. While her early novels would often depict a day or a few days, these two novels of the 1930s, a historical period beset with the rising spectacle of fascism and a clearer view of the perils of imperialism, recognize meaning only in the whole of an imagined human life. As she wrote in her diary on October 16, 1935, "a kind of form is… imposing itself, corresponding to the dimensions of the human being" (1977, p. 347).

Virginia Woolf was interested in old age. All of her novels and essays engage strongly with the difficulty and importance of representing and imagining the obscure lives of the elderly. Throughout her fiction, she projects a variety of meanings in old age that is recognized differentially within individuals and across class and gender divisions. Beyond the focus on old age, many of Woolf's novels treat loss and mortality. Woolf scholar Gillian Beer (1989) comments that "all of Virginia Woolf's novels brood on death, and death, indeed is essential to their organization as well as their meaning… . Death was her special knowledge… but death was also the special knowledge of her entire generation, through the obliterative experi-ence of the First World War" (p. 185).

Starting with *A Room of One's Own* (2008/1929) and continuing to her death, Woolf's writing evinces a stronger, pressing concern with social poli-tics and history, with the real world, with what she would distinguish as "fact" and "vision." The two novels of this period, *The Waves* and *The Years,* take as their subject the human life course in its longevity (both redefine the historical novel as they follow characters and families from childhood to old age). By constructing old age as a biologically distinct period of life while standardizing human longevity into unique stages, the late nineteenth cen-tury gave a new impetus to the use of the human life course as a model or explanatory medium for historical processes. The metaphor of a human life divided into stages, available since antiquity (Cicero's *De Sinectute*, 1923) and regularly reaffirmed in the Renaissance, was given real explanatory power as science "proved" that different periods of life were underpinned by different biologies: the nineteenth century saw the birth of a science of childhood and of old age.

In *The Waves* and *The Years,* Woolf considers the biological meaning of stages of life while rethinking history as sociology. In these two novels, she develops age as a significant marker of difference by distinguishing between social age, chronological age, and historical age. In considering old age as a dynamic period that is sociologically, historically, and biologically mediated, in considering the human life in its totality or longevity, Woolf offers a more complete and open approach to studying the lifespan and old age in its totality.

Woolf's fiction is often motivated by what Mark Hussey in *The Singing of the Real World* (1986) calls the "fact of living through time" (p. 54). *The Waves* unfolds the life histories of six characters, in nine stages from the nursery to old age. The first three sections develop stages of education (nursery, boarding school, college); the next two turn on aspects of adulthood (marriage, parenthood); while the final four elaborate the characters' perceptions of time passing and their experience of getting older. Separating the "dramatic soliloquies" (presented in Roman type) of the narrative are brief poetic interludes (in italics) charting the course of the sun from its rise to its fall. In the earliest sections of the novel, the characters are caught in the ordering processes of church, education, and the playing fields; they alternate between individuation and reintegration. They come together, they separate, they come together, they separate. Bernard and Susan marry other people and have children; Louis and Rhoda become lovers; Neville is attracted to a seventh character, Percival, who is an absent/present figure in the text—he never speaks. Over the course of her many love affairs, Jinny lives in terror of physical deterioration. All of the characters acknowledge growing old: Neville, "Time passes, yes. And we grow old" (p. 129); Bernard, "I have lost my youth" (p. 143); Jinny, "How solitary, how shrunk, how aged! I am no longer young. I am no longer part of the procession" (p. 142).

The novel's underlying structural division, its juxtaposition of the cyclical rhythm of the natural order (poetic form) against a linear and irreversible movement (narrative), may be meant to highlight the question of pattern in human (individual, historical, cultural) time. While all of the characters age and proceed through life stages, only Bernard seems to develop and change. Rather than individuals living through time, the five other characters seem to represent positions against time. Susan embodies the natural rhythms of the animal and vegetable kingdoms, speaking self through fertility. Her tragedy is that once she has fulfilled her reproductive biological function, she grows dissatisfied and simply turns "grey before [her] time" (140), with no potential for a meaningful or productive old age. There is no place for an old woman in this natural order. Neville expands into the life of the mind, having lost his only love, Percival, to an early death. If Susan enacts the biological spring of fertility, Neville, the academic, lives out—or, rather, on—the ancestries of literature and culture that sustain or support persons toward their deaths.

Louis matures through neither biological nor cultural progenitors but through political and historical ones. Claiming his roots in colonial and working class Australia, Louis is awake not to the splendors of the Empire, but to the devastations and infamies it practiced on those it conquered. His civilization is the one in decline, recapitulating the individual life-that-ends-in-death with the grand cultural life-that-ends-in-death. Jinny represents the flesh-and-blood solutions to the facts of age. The woman of passion, of body, she exists only in the eyes of those who adore her. Woolf would have been terrified by the Kate-Moss-anorexic fashion models of these times or, indeed, the scarified, tattooed, pierced body artists who seem to declare the self on the visible canvas of the skin. In *The Waves,* Woolf depicts Jinny as the horror, the emptiness, the plight of the human who lives a life within only the shell of the body whose couturier or manicurist is the closest she might have to a confessor.

The only one of the six to die in the course of the novel, Rhoda is met as the existential truth-teller, the character who finds no solace in intimacy but rather can only declare self through isolation. Unlike the other characters, whose connections with those they love or at least desire expand their own purchase on the ground of existence, Rhoda cannot root herself in a life other than the present. She takes her life close to the end of the novel, apparently throwing herself off a precipice in Egypt while on a cultural pilgrimage, trying vainly to attach herself to a human effort at beauty or meaning and finding instead the absence of footholds and the inevitable fall into the abyss.

Bernard is the only character not fated to repeat only one experience of the world: for Louis, it is history and civilization; for Neville, literary culture from Catullus to Shakespeare; for Jinny, it is the pleasure of the body; for Susan, the generative capacity; and for Rhoda, a sense of alienation (even her suicide seems fated). These five characters exist in a static universe, repeating their same sense of experience at each stage of their lives. But Bernard seems different. Of all the characters, only Bernard embraces the possibility of change, particularly in old age: Jinny wards off "time's fangs" with "rouge, with powder, with flimsy pocket-handkerchiefs" (p. 168); and for a "middle-aged" Neville, "change is no longer possible" (p. 155).

In the final section (the longest), Bernard is an "elderly man, grey at the temples" (p. 176), who proposes to explain the meaning of his life, but has now become suspicious of all stories:

> I must tell you a story… stories of childhood, stories of school, love,
> marriage, death, and so on; and none of them are true. Yet like children we
> tell each other stories, and to decorate them we make up these ridiculous,

> flamboyant, beautiful phrases. How tired I am of stories… how I distrust
> neat designs of life that are drawn upon half-sheets of note-paper. (p. 176)

He wants to tell his lifestory because stories are the medium of meaning, but he distrusts "neat designs of life," distrusts stories as meaning. Yet he ultimately succumbs, beginning in the conventional sense: "In the beginning, there was… ." (p. 177). He tells the listener the "stories" of the other characters, each following one another amidst the pain of their individuation: "Louis was disgusted by the nature of human flesh; Rhoda by our cruelty; Susan could not share; Neville wanted order; Jinny love; and so on. We suffered terribly as we became separate bodies" (p. 179). Despite his expertise as storyteller, Bernard feels his narrative failure: "How impossible to order them rightly; to detach one separately, or to give the effect of the whole" (p. 190).

In old age, distinctions between individual characters seem to blur: "Am I all of them? Am I one and distinct? I do not know… . There is no division between me and them. As I talked I felt, 'I am you.' This difference we make so much of, this identity we feverishly cherish was overcome" (p. 214). In a letter to Goldsworthy Lowes Dickinson in October 1931 after finishing the novel, Woolf (1978) wrote: "The six characters were supposed to be one. I'm getting old myself—I shall be fifty next year; and I come to feel more and more how difficult it is to collect oneself into one Virginia" (p. 397). What appears to be at stake for Woolf, and for Bernard, is the integrity of the self over time.

As Bernard "sums up" his life he attempts to gather together all of the other characters or personalities into a collective mind and bind them there, but discontinuity and disillusion always seem to interrupt. The irrevocable deaths of Percival and Rhoda ("Into this crashed death," p. 195), the metaphysical fact of death calls forth from him "the contribution of maturity to childhood's intuitions—satiety and doom" but still also "how life is more obdurate than one had thought it" (p. 199). Even his "ageless" self no longer comes when he calls: "This self now as I leant over the gate looking down over fields rolling in waves of color beneath me made no answer… . His fist did not form. I waited. I listened. Nothing came, nothing… . This is more truly death than the death of friends, than the death of youth" (pp. 210–211).

The loss of the self (and the selves) in old age is experienced, paradoxically, as a greater embodiment: "There is the old brute, too, the savage, the hairy man who dabbles his fingers in ropes of entrails; and gobbles and belches;… well, he is here. He squats in me" (p. 215); and transparence: "I could worship my hand even, with its fan of bones laced by blue mysterious veins" (p. 216). All that remains are things, himself one of them: "Let me sit here for ever with bare things, this coffee-cup, this knife, this fork, things in themselves, myself being myself" (p. 219). He is "tired" in his old age, "spent" and "worn out" but he regains his sense of self: the "I, I, I" returns with the ticking of the clock and the rising of the sun (p. 218). "What is dawn in the city to an elderly man standing in the street looking up rather dizzily at the sky?" he asks himself. Whatever the exact answer, this elderly man flings himself forward, "unvanquished and unyielding" still, against death (p. 220).

To this temporal dimension of aging toward the inevitable end of life in death, we must now add a sensibility to the spatial poetics of the novel. *The Waves* is a visually rich text, filled with kinetic cinematic scenes and still-life tableaux. The plot itself revolves around the homes of these characters, from the tree houses and hideaways of their youth to the stately townhouses or threadbare garrets that they inhabit as they age. The underbrush through which the children crawl at the opening functions as an anchoring site for childhood attachment: "'Let us now crawl,'" said Bernard, "under the canopy of the currant leaves, and tell stories. Let us inhabit the underworld. Let us take possession of our secret territory.... Here, Jinny, if we curl up close, we can sit under the canopy of the currant leaves and watch the censers swing. This is our universe'" (p. 14)

The novel is governed by the master narrative of the sun rising and setting in relation to the sea and the shore. These cyclic spatial relation-ships—complexly worked out with angles of declension and maturations of shadows—stand for the very largest and most momentous movements in human beings' lives. In the wordless changes of the sun's topographical position vis-à-vis the beach, the stages of human lives are represented— dawning, promising, arriving, peaking, declining, setting. Cosmic, the move-ments contract and expand to represent both the progressions of state of each of these individual children as they age and the inexorably vectored mortal condition of the whole of the animal and vegetable kingdoms.

And yet the descriptions of the passage of the sun across the sky contain within them evocations of habitations, simultaneously shelter and address, as in an early interlude, as the sun is on the rise: "*Perhaps it was a snail shell, rising in the grass like a grey cathedral, a swelling building burnt with dark rings and shadowed green by the grass*" (p. 52). Unlike the military discipline of temporal ordering (once gone, never to return), the organic discipline of spatial ordering has give, grants metaphoric travel, allows for an Alice-in-Wonderland scale confusion that permits the snail shell to also be a grey cathedral, minute and massive all at once. A later interlude, now that the sun has sunk, also contains breathtaking evocations of the experience of being contained: "*Darkness washed down streets eddying round single figures, engulf- ing them… enveloping the solitary thorn tree and the empty snail shells at its foot*" (p. 174). The mood of isolation and decline is here countermanded by the images of the collectivizing of the darkness, the shared, if sad, plight of those single figures, engulfed here by the unifying waves of night, pledging us all to that sunken ship, at very least, together in it at last.

If one can argue that what "happens" in the novel is that time passes, one can argue as convincingly that what happens in the novel is that space is occupied. "*Space,*" writes de Certeau (1980/1984), "*is a practiced place*" that finds itself at the intersections of particular velocities, directions, and tem- poralities (p. 117). Washington Square in Greenwich Village in New York City is a place, marked by a memorial arch to the United States' first president, itself a replica of a memorial arch in Paris, doubling the memory implied in the stone. As I[1] walk through the square on a cool but sunny afternoon in October, returning overdue books to their shelves in New York University's Bobst Library so that others, too, can read the copy of *Practice of Everyday Life* (de Certeau, 1980/1984) that I've borrowed, I pass intense, silent, competitive money-on-the-table games of chess. I pass bell-bottomed, tie-dyed, acoustic-guitar-playing holdovers from more innocent times. I step smartly to avoid the dashing dachshunds and labradoodles on their way to the so-called run. I crane my neck to follow the full trajectory of the toddler strapped into her swing set chair, pushed gently but firmly by dad's hand on her little behind, arcing through space on the singing chains that free her, momentarily, from all the powers of the universe at that heart-stopping apogee of flight, that moment of heart-rending freedom from the forces that otherwise constrain and constrict and maintain her on earth. In my walk across the square, I transform the place into a space. Together with the kings and queens, the presidents and the generals, the cats and dogs, the fathers and daughters, I have not only lived through and walked through but created a *clearing* in this universe. I have cleared a space of meaning that, by walking through it mindfully and attentively, speaks to me of culture and belief and gains and losses. In that transit, I undergo myriad knowings—that the three-year-old will outgrow the swings, that the dogs will be put down, that this empire too will fall, that he not busy being born is busy dying. When I arrive at the circulation desk with my overdue de Certeau, I have altered whatever counts as my self by virtue of the cross- ing I have just accomplished, being now the person who has walked across the square on this October afternoon.

The salience of *The Waves* to the topic of aging is evident. It treats very literally the passage of time, the maturation of six characters, first met as school children, into their old age, one to her death. The fact of aging seems to be almost altogether uttered in the recognition—be it lament or triumph—that time passes. But as the sun rises and sets, the seashore remains, with its shells and caves and cathedrals revealed, illuminated, if then darkened. Woolf seems to give the reader of *The Waves* either a consolation prize or an ontological rescue raft in the notions of space. Space is no more constant than is time, yet its tactility, its physicality, its existence as *material* opposes the immateriality of time: currant bushes we can see and smell and crawl under. The world under the currant bushes is occupied by two people, Bernard and Jinny, whose mutual presence there *alters* the experience of having been there. Because two bodies nominate this clearing together, they are *included* in the space, each of them altered by the other's presence. As young children, Bernard and Jinny inhabited the currant bush cave, achieving a private vantage point from which they saw others pass, in which they remained unseen, and by virtue of which they become seers.

Much later in the novel, Jinny, now in her 30s, finds herself having had a series of lovers, having become a woman addicted to appearance, a woman who declares the self by virtue of others' response to her body. And yet, she remembers the currant bush practice. At a reunion of the six in their middle age, Jinny says, "Now let us talk, let us tell stories.... . Let us sit here under the cut flowers.... . (I am now past thirty, perilously, like a mountain goat leaping from crag to crag; I do not settle long anywhere; I do not attach myself to one person in particular)" (p. 126). Even though her mountain-goat existence refuses to give her settlement, her spatial practices—here, now, the cut flowers, but the same actions of sitting-under learned in childhood—endow her with a shared continuity and, maybe, a chance to cohere the "then" with the "now" in something other than savage cessation.

Unlike the experience one has of time as separating us from our former selves and, ultimately, separating each one of us from one another in our ultimate deaths, the spaces of our lives grant common ground onto which the intersubjective presence can be triangulated and, hence, acknowledged if not even enacted. As the reader moves through each of the six characters' accounts in *The Waves*, he or she experiences the crossings, the dwellings, the encampments made in the course of the lives of each of the six. Neville, referencing the "clock ticking on the mantelpiece," acknowledges that "[t]ime passes, yes. And we grow old" (p. 129). But he also tells us that time's meaning is not to be found in the staccato irrevocable tick-tock, but in the mood of communion: "Some spray in a hedge, though, or a sunset over a flat winter field, or again the way some old woman sits, arms akimbo, in an omnibus with a basket—those we point at for the other to look at. It is so vast an alleviation to be able to point for another to look at" (p. 130).

Sitting under the currant bushes or the cut flowers, sitting silently side by side on the bus, triangulated by pointing at the view they share and are thereby joined by, put into contact by a thing outside of them both—these are the methods of intersubjective connection. Unlike the temporal impressions of the unfolding of relationships in time, the before-and-after of the father pushing the infant on the swing and then, before he knows it, giving her away on her wedding day, a spatial poetics locates the intersubjective relation much more in the way the phenomenologist might, as the triangulating gaze on an alien point in space that locks the two who gaze (one from each skull) into relation through the very spatial link through the seen. Seeing what the other sees, one connects with the other "one-who-sees" through the agency of the seen. Our surrounding objects *link* us as common seers, perhaps thereby absolving the unforgiving isolation of each our separate eye sockets. No wonder we flock to the Metropolitan Museum of Art to gaze at the Cezanne seascapes or the Rembrandt portraits: we committed gazers are linked with all others who, in concert, gaze.

The death of Percival, whose voice is not heard in the text and yet whose presence and then absence governs the action, occasions Rhoda's reimaginings of her living: "Now that lightning has gashed the tree and the flowering branch has fallen and Percival, by his death, has made me this gift, let me see the thing. There is a square; there is an oblong… they make a perfect dwelling-place" (p. 118).

This realization, remember, is not enough to save Rhoda from her suicide. She is not able to inhabit these dwelling places she creates, and she flings herself from a cliff on a pilgrimage that was to have provided her with meaning. Spaces are not, by themselves, redemptive, although redemption, whatever that means, cannot come outside of space. In an essay on Djuna Barnes's modernist novel *Nightwood*, Brian Glavey (2009) suggests that "only once the text stands as a whole in the mind and the pattern of interior relations holding it together is apprehended spatially will its meaning be revealed" (p. 754). The best we might achieve in the way of redemption might well be this form of revelation.

In contrast, Susan creates a closed-off dwelling place, insulated, she thinks, from the shadows of time: "I am fenced in, planted here, like one of my own trees," she says. But there is desperation in the enclosure; she is "sick of natural happiness, and fruit growing, and children scattering the house with oats, guns, skulls, books won for prizes and other trophies"; she is sick, too, of her body and her "own craft, industry and cunning"; and she is sick most of all of "the unscrupulous ways of the mother who protects, who collects under her jealous eyes at one long table her own children, always her own" (p. 139).

The contradictions of aging, especially those between completion and breakdown or desire and deprivation, are perhaps not adjudicated so much in time as they might be in space. Susan sees the lie in her presumed solution to the problem of time—it just will not work to barricade her and her progeny against the shadow of time, trying through fruition to live forever. But here, perhaps, she might glimpse a release from the mother's unscrupulous cunning. The children will age out of their oats, no doubt, but perhaps that long table will persist, that gathering collectivity endowing them not with jaundiced jealousy but with a shared capacity to withstand the shadow.

By pairing the temporal interpretations of the lives of these characters with spatial beholdings of them within their dwellings, one might lengthen the shadows and deepen the *chiaroscuro* that represent their lives. We are left with more, simply put, than Bernard's hairy savage brute. We have more to go on than Neville's Shakespeare or Louis's empire. It may well be that Bernard, alone among the six characters, changes through time and that the rest of them are marooned in a stasis of repetition. And yet, perhaps, the others can be recognized as having *become* themselves not through temporal transformations but through their gifts of inhabiting fully the spaces they have created and discovered in life.

In reviewing and assessing our lives, as we tend to do as we age, we have the temporal "accomplishments" to inventory. We have, as well, these wordless and timeless spaces, inhabited and therefore created by us, that gather us in meaningful knots, that permit us to see ourselves *by virtue of the seeing of one another* throughout our lives. If the phenomenologist claims self-making in the triangulated or intentional gaze at alien objects, then we, too, ordinary souls trying for a self, seeking out intention, might rejoice in the capacity of our dwellings to reveal the self, to hold out in our cupped hands the "huge and very small" seen under the currant bushes. In our shells and nests, we rest from the glare of that sun on the sand and we find, within the cool shadows and glades, the means to behold and even accept these lives we so bravely face up to.

Gerontology has discovered the urgency of spaces—homes, material possessions, objects that contain and then can spill memory—in the ontology of aging. The work of such qualitative gerontologists as Graham Rowles

(1984), Mortimer Powell Lawton (1986), and Robert Rubenstein (Rubenstein & Parmalee, 1992) has explored the importance of spatial attachment and embodiment in the preservation of memory and the extension of self into the future. Habitual movement and practiced trajectories through space relinquish not only the sought (one finds the string by opening the drawer that one opens "by habit" when needing string), but also the meaning of the search. Without the temporal unfolding of storied narrative, the familiar object surrenders its significance like a " 'lightning rod for memory.' We see our past suddenly illuminated as a dazzlingly bright image, rather than an extended story… . The home thus becomes a 'total environment' of self-mirroring surfaces in which virtually every object serves to 'stiffen' identity" (Krasner, 2005, p. 214).

Contemporary geriatrics and gerontology are clueing in to space. The primacy of letting the elder return to his or her home instead of being remanded to a nursing home prevails, even though clinicians may not fully have assimilated the complex reasons for doing so. Research studies of clinical interventions for elderly patients are using as outcomes measure the "Life-Space Assessment" score that tabulates the elder's trajectories away from home, effectively tracking the radius of movement from the ground of home outward as a measure of the scope of the elder's social dwelling-space (Brown et al., 2009). The new focus on visual arts in geriatrics heralds this realization of the value of beholding as one comes to "terms" with the aging process. It is not simply just for fun that the Metropolitan Museum of Art sponsors art programs for senior citizens and even those with dementia. This growing practice instead, perhaps, hypothesizes that expanding an elderly person's self-experience with timeless non-narrative space— captured by the facility in simply standing in front of a painting and letting it work on one—might endow that old person with something otherwise unattainable: the Djuna Barnian or Woolfian practice to let "the text stand whole in the mind" so as to "apprehend spatially… its meaning… revealed" (Glavey, 2009, p. 754).

The impression is growing among those who care for the elderly that a life review, in search of meaning, brings not a cushion of consolation to the dying process but, more radically, a discovery of the point of having lived at all. The work of William Randall and Elizabeth McKim (2008) is illuminating most powerfully the advantages to the elderly and those who love them of building the capacity of "reading our lives," and thereby allowing ourselves to be legible to self and other. The twinned aspects of temporality and spatiality that this essay has tried to reveal in Woolf's magnificent, if challenging, novel are available to all of us and our patients as we review lives, gaze at their successive stages, and envision their successive shells and caves and cathedrals. Our efforts here to fortify a single-minded attention to passing time with a shared beholding of the dimensions of living might suggest to gerontology some new strategies for expanding a felt existence in a world one is preparing to depart.

NOTE

[1] One of the authors.

REFERENCES

Aristotle (1991). *On rhetoric: A theory of civic discourse.* (G. Kennedy, Trans.). New York: Oxford University Press.

Augustine (2002). On Genesis. In J. Rotelle (Ed.) and E. Hill (Trans.), *The works of Saint Augustine: A translation for the 21st century.* (Vol. 13, Pt. 1). Hyde Park, NY: New City Press.

Bachelard, G. (1994). *The poetics of space.* (M. Jolas, Trans.). Boston: Beacon Press. (Original work published 1958)

Bakhtin, M. (1981). *The dialogic imagination: Four essays.* (C. Emerson & M. Holquist, Trans.). Austin, TX: University of Texas Press.

Baudrillard, J. (1994). *Simulacra and simulation.* (S. Glaser, Trans.). Ann Arbor, MI: University of Michigan Press.

Beer, G. (1989). *Arguing with the past: Essays in narrative from Woolf to Sydney.* New York: Routledge.

Bergson, H. (1960). *Time and free will.* New York: Harper & Row. (Original work published 1910)

Bourdieu, P. (1977). *Outline of a theory of practice.* (R. Nice, Trans.). New York: Cambridge University Press.

Brown, C., Roth, D., Allman, R., Sawyer, P., Ritchie, C., & Roseman, J. (2009). Trajectories of life-space mobility after hospitalization. *Annals of Internal Medicine, 150,* 372–378.

Cicero (1923). *On old age* (De senectute), *on friendship, on divination.* (W. Falconer, Trans.). Cambridge, MA: Loeb Classical Library.

de Certeau, M. (1984). *The practice of everyday life.* (S. Rendall, Trans.). Berkeley: University of California Press. (Original work published 1980)

Forster, E. (1985). *Aspects of the novel.* San Diego: Harcourt. (Original work published 1927)

Galen (1951). *A translation of Galen's Hygiene* (De sanitate tuenda). (R. Green, Trans.). Springfield, IL: Thomas.

Genette, G. (1979). *Narrative discourse: An essay in method.* (J. Lewin, Trans.). Ithaca, NY: Cornell University Press. (Original work published 1972)

Glavey, B. (2009). Dazzling estrangement: modernism, queer ekphrasis, and the spatial form of *Nightwood. PMLA, 124,* 749–763.

Greimas, A. (1987). *On meaning: Selected writings in semiotic theory*. (P. Perron, F. Collins, Trans.). Minneapolis, MN: University of Minnesota Press.

Herman, D. (2002). *Story logic: Problems and possibilities of narrative*. Lincoln, NE: University of Nebraska Press.

Horace (1926). *Satires, epistles, the art of poetry*. (H. Fairclough, Trans.). Cambridge, MA: Loeb Classical Library.

Hussey, M. (1986). *The singing of the real world: The philosophy of Virginia Woolf's fiction*. Columbus, OH: Ohio University Press.

Isidore of Seville (2006). *The etymologies of Isidore of Seville*. (S. Barney, W. Lewis, J. Beach, & O. Berghof, Trans.). Cambridge, UK: Cambridge University Press.

James, H. (2003). *Portrait of a lady*. London: Penguin. (Original work published 1881)

Krasner, J. (2005). Accumulated lives: Metaphor, materiality, and the homes of the elderly. *Literature and Medicine, 24*, 209–230.

Lawton, M. (1986). *Environment and aging* (2nd ed.). Albany, NY: Center for the Study of Aging.

Lowith, K. (1949). *Meaning in history: The theological implications of the philosophy of history*. Chicago: University of Chicago Press.

Lukács, G. (1971). *The theory of the novel: A historico-philosophical essay on the forms of great epic literature*. (A. Bostock, Trans.). Cambridge, MA: MIT Press. (Original work published 1920)

Mann, T. (1995). *The magic mountain*. (J. Woods, Trans.). New York: A.A. Knopf. (Original work published 1924)

Ovid (2005). *Metamorphoses*. (C. Martin, Trans.). New York: Norton, 2005.

Propp, V. (1968). *Morphology of the folktale*. (2nd ed.; L. Scott, Trans.; rev. L. Wagner). Austin, TX: University of Texas Press.

Proust, M. (1999). *A la recherche du temps perdu* [In search of lost time]. Paris: Gallimard. (Original work published 1913–1927)

Randall, W. & McKim, A. (2008). *Reading our lives: The poetics of growing old*. New York: Oxford University Press.

Ricoeur, P. (1984–1988). *Time and narrative* (Vols. 1–3). (K. McLaughlin & D. Pellauer, Trans.). Chicago: University of Chicago Press. (Original work published 1983)

Rimmon-Kenan, S. (2002). *Narrative fiction: Contemporary poetics* (2nd ed.). London: Routledge. (Original work published 1983.)

Rowles, G. (1984). Aging in the rural environments. In I. Altman, M. Lawton, & J. Wohlwill (Eds.), *Elderly people and the environment* (pp. 129–157). New York: Plenum Press.

Rubenstein, R. & Parmalee, P. (1992). Attachment to place and the representation of the life course by the elderly. In I. Altman & S. Low (Eds.), *Place attachment* (pp. 134–163). New York: Plenum Press.

Shklovsky, V. (1990). *Theory of prose*. (B. Sher, Trans.). Elmwood Park, IL: Dalkey Archive Press. (Original work published 1929)

Thane, P. (2000). The history of aging in the West. In T. Cole, R. Kastenbaum, & R. Ray (Eds.), *Handbook of the humanities and aging* (pp. 3–24). New York: Springer.

Tolstoy, L. (2003). *War and peace*. (R. Edmunds, Trans.). London: Penguin. (Original work published 1869)

Woolf, V. (1977). *The diary of Virginia Woolf* (Vol. 3). A. O. Bell (Ed.). New York: Harcourt Brace Jovanovich.

Woolf, V. (1978). The letters of Virginia Woolf (Vol. 4, 1929–1931). N. Nicolson and J. Trautmann (Eds.). New York: Harcourt Brace Jovanovich.

Woolf, V. (1998). *The years*. London: Penguin. (Original work published 1937)

Woolf, V. (2006). *The waves*. Orlando, FL: Harvest Book/Harcourt. (Original work published 1931)

Woolf, V. (2008). *A room of one's own and three guineas*. (M. Shiach, Ed.). Oxford, UK: Oxford University Press. (Original work published 1929)

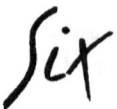

THE NARRATIVE FRAME IN DISCOURSE ON AGING:

UNDERSTANDING FACTS AND VALUES BEHIND

PUBLIC POLICY

Phillip G. Clark

Narrative approaches involving older adults are usually associated either with individuals and their lifestories or with research and interventions targeted on them. However, narrative understanding and methodology can also be applied to public policy as it responds to the issues associated with aging at the societal level. In this context, public policy can be defined as the "attempt to balance competing notions of the responsibility of individuals, families, and the state in developing programs to meet human needs" (Clark, 1993, p. 13). Such a balancing requires the development and assessment of various approaches to defining human needs, set against a backdrop of differing assumptions about the role of different players in the public policy arena in meeting them. In this sense, every policy position, statement, or recommendation is a story or substory within a larger narrative discourse or debate about a compelling public policy problem.

In particular, a public policy problem can be defined in terms of its empirical ("facts") and normative ("values") dimensions and the dynamic interrelationship between them. More importantly, the potential solutions to this problem are determined by its definition. A policy narrative creates a particular understanding and interpretation of a set of policy-relevant issues; interrogating or deconstructing the narrative affords us an opportunity to look below the surface to find the meaning underlying this policy discourse.

This chapter proposes an analytical framework based on the concept of *narrative frame* as a lens through which to examine public policy perspectives, positions, and proposals. In particular, this discussion focuses initially on an analysis of the interrelationships between facts and values. Subsequently, the narrative-frame approach is proposed as a structure for exploring the story and substories underlying any policy discourse about which there is open and ongoing discussion and debate. This framework serves as a tool to unravel the thematic threads used to weave together a policy narrative, as well as a method to reconnect them into a coherent storyline with texts, subtexts, and counterstories.

To explore the application of this framework and to illustrate its relevance to unpacking public policy discourse, the recent history and current debate on home care policy in Canada will be explored, especially from the perspectives of the federal government, national organizations, and the aging and disability communities themselves. Home care policy is an arena of rapidly growing relevance and urgency within Canada as the government, advocacy groups, and citizens debate its place within the larger discussion of health care renewal and reform. It is through applying this framework to the actual public reports, position papers, research findings, and recommendations on home care that the deeper meaning behind the public policy discussion becomes apparent and the application of the narrative-frame approach can be more fully understood.

DEVELOPING A NARRATIVE-FRAME APPROACH

Facts and Values

Any thorough examination of policy discourse requires an understanding of the role that values play in framing and addressing significant public policy problems. It is simply a myth that providing enough factual information alone about a complex social problem—empirically researched data—is ever sufficient to allow policy makers to make informed choices among alternative ways of defining and solving it. The reality is that every public policy problem consists of both an empirical description and a normative dimension—and a set of interrelationships between them (Potter, 1969). The values dimension represents cherished principles or beliefs that are affected in some way by the empirical state of affairs.

It is interesting and perhaps revealing that in the Canadian context, there is frequent and overt attention to values; the value-related Romanow

Commission report on the future of health care in Canada is titled "Building on Values," which suggests that values are the underpinning of the Canadian health care system, stated to be "equity, fairness, and solidarity" (Commission on the Future of Health Care in Canada, 2002, p. xvi). Research on uncovering various meanings in Canadian public policy statements emphasizes the power of expression used in policy discourse, drawing attention to the importance of analyzing patterns and uses of language to construct and deconstruct the world of public policy—"the meaning of words and the wording of meanings" (Iannantuono & Eyles, 1997, p. 1611). Of particular importance in this regard are words having "value valence," i.e., those with moral weight or ethical significance.

Reflecting on the power of ethics language used in policy discourse, Kenny (2004) notes, "The words used highlight some beliefs and values and obscure others. The framing of the discourse therefore influences the construction of meaning and the valuing of beliefs" (p. 5). For example, technical or scientific language can be used in empirical analyses to lend power and authority to official pronouncements or positions. In contrast, values may be more implicit in the type of language used in policy documents, and uncovering them may require more explicit interpretive analysis.

Various authors have drawn attention to the types of analysis needed to identify the values underlying particular public policy problems and options in light of relevant moral principles. For example, this process has been termed "public ethics" by Jonsen and Butler (1975), and Kelman and Warwick (1978) have developed a framework for analyzing the ethical dimensions of social interventions. In Canada, there is a pattern of using such approaches to understand values as drivers of health care policy development and implementation (Giacomini, Hurley, Gold, Smith, & Abelson, 2001, 2004).

Critical Narrativity

As discussed earlier, narrative approaches may also be developed to interrogate public policies and expose their underlying empirical and normative foundations. Conceptualizing the overall emergent policy discourse as a "story," the perspectives of different policy makers or advocacy groups on a particular issue can be read as subtexts to the main story or text (Levine & Murray, 2004). Biggs (2001) proposes the concept of "critical narrativity" to draw attention to the story underlying a particular way of framing a public policy problem, which invites the search for "counterstories" with different perspectives on the issue (Roe, 1994).

Similarly, Rein (1983) suggests the approach of developing a policy "frame," a way to understand how we see, what we say, and how we act in the world—integrating theory, facts, interests, and action within a policy framework. A policy frame is a way of viewing the world, "a way of inquiring, of making sense as well as masking sense of the world in which we live" (p. 99). This metaphor reinforces the point made earlier that language can both reveal and obscure important facts and values underlying policy discourse. For our use in this chapter, the concepts of narrativity and frame can be combined into the approach of narrative frame to capture both the sense of an emergent story and our own unique perspective on how it is developed and presented.

To illustrate the application of the narrative-frame approach, our analysis will now shift to an exploration of the emerging debate and discussion on home care policy in the Canadian context.

EMERGENCE OF THE DOMINANT NARRATIVE FRAME: HOME CARE DISCOURSE IN CANADA

Home care has emerged on the public policy stage in Canada as a major issue in the discourse on health care renewal (e.g., Health Council of Canada, 2008a, 2008b). Primary care and home care are paired as areas meriting attention and support as the government considers new emphases in responding to pressing health care needs now and into the future. Driven by the recognition of consumer preferences and fueled by growing awareness of the aging of the population, the increasing prevalence of chronic health conditions, and home care as an alternative to acute-care and institutional long-term care settings, governments are being pressed to develop both more effective primary health care delivery methods and more extended home care benefits (Canadian Home Care Association, 2008a, 2008b). How the voice of home care has emerged within the evolving story of health care in Canada is the focus of the discussion that follows.

Background to the Current Situation

Home care has been defined in Canada as "an array of services which enables clients, incapacitated in whole or in part, to live at home, often with the effect of preventing, delaying, or substituting for long-term care or acute care alternatives" (Health Canada, 1999a, p. 6). Its main functions have traditionally been to substitute for more costly acute-care services (e.g., hospitals) and long-term care in a nursing home and to support clients with health and functional deficits in maintaining their independence and preventing functional decline for as long as possible (Keefe, 2002; Shapiro, 2002). Home care is often linked to community care, which is a broader concept and encompasses a wider range of community-based services and supports.

Before 1970, home care programs tended to be local and community based, focused on acute-care needs and sponsored by hospitals or community health nursing agencies. Starting in the 1970s, some provinces expanded the objectives for home care services to include support for older adults and adults with disabilities (Health Canada, 1999a). The Canada Health Act includes home care services under the category of Extended Health Care Services, which are not insured or covered by restrictions on user fees or extra billing. Each province and territory has developed its own model of how to provide home care services, resulting in service inequities based on such factors as geographic location and user charges.

Emergence of Discourse at the Federal Level

The dominant public policy voice that has emerged in home care discussions, debates, and dialogues in Canada is that of the federal government. Based on a review of major written public documents, reports, and position papers by nonprofit professional associations, advocacy organizations, and policy research centers, this voice can be characterized as the primary narrative frame or "text" in this discussion. Direct quotations will be used to provide examples of the actual language employed in developing this emergent story.

Some national organizations in Canada call for the federal government's leadership in home care policy through statements that acknowledge its traditional role in creating a national health care system, moral authority that should now be extended into the home care arena (Canadian Association for Community Care and Canadian Home Care Association, ND; Canadian Home Care Association, 2004). Recognition of this presumed leadership is evidenced by the National Conference on Home Care, sponsored in 1998 by Health Canada to bring stakeholders together to foster dialogue on the complex issues associated with national approaches to home care (Health Canada, 1998). A strong consensus emerged that the federal government should assume a major leadership role by committing to the development of an integrated national home- and community-based care program.

A year later, Health Canada (1999b) sponsored a National Roundtable on Home and Community Care, in which participants cited the "values that Canadians consider important for the development of home care, including those related to protection, equity, fairness, support for independence, mobility, and valuing and respecting the needs and contributions of individuals, families and communities" (p. 2) as the basis for continuing to develop a national program. By describing these guidelines for policy development as "values," the power of normative language was invoked to lend moral weight to the growing momentum of a national home care program in Canada.

Romanow Commission Report

A major watershed in the emergent discourse on the future of health care in Canada, the Romanow Commission Report of 2002 devoted an entire chapter to home care, characterized as "the next essential service" in a revision of the Canada Health Act (Commission on the Future of Health Care in Canada, 2002). The Report cites empirical research by Hollander and Chappell (2002) suggesting that home care can both save money and improve quality of care and of life for those who might otherwise be institutionalized. It also suggests that priority be placed on determining the most important needs and developing a national foundation of services to be delivered uniformly across Canada only for the specific areas of mental health, post-acute care, and palliative care. "Textual commentaries" from nongovernmental groups in response to the Report's recommendations praised them as "good first steps" for their support of strengthening home care nationally, but they also pointed out that their focus was too narrow and short term (Canadian Association for Community Care, 2002; Canadian Home Care Association, 2002).

Early in 2003, the prime minister and provincial/territorial premiers from across Canada ("first ministers") agreed on a vision, principles, and an action plan for the renewal of the Canadian health care system, invoking Canadian values embodied in the five principles of the Canada Health Act (universality, accessibility, comprehensiveness, portability, and public administration). Once again, however, recommendations on home care coverage were limited to short-term, acute home care services and a compassionate care benefit for family caregivers (Health Canada, 2003). As if anticipating this restriction, the Canadian Home Care Association (2003) issued a position paper just prior to the First Ministers' Health Accord that called for the extension of publicly funded home care services as part of the Medicare envelope and a package of services to be included, again invoking the principles of the Canada Health Act. Its statement that "the challenge is one of determining which home care services should be defined as 'medically necessary health services' without compromising our social values or overextending scarce resources" (p. 11) recognized the potential conflict between important Canadian values and the financial reality of limited resources.

Also in 2003, a policy paper released by Hollander (2003) charged that both the Romanow Commission Report and the First Ministers Health Accord left a major gap in their policy recommendations by not addressing the home care needs of individuals with chronic health conditions. Empirical research is cited that home care should be included in a broader, integrated system of continuing care, because it is a cost-effective strategy in chronic care and an alternative to long-term care institutions. The paper accused policy makers of lacking the political will to shift the current policy to more adequately cover the costs of an integrated home care system, because of their fear of the possibility of dramatically rising costs.

Subsequently, in 2004, a new Ten-Year Plan to Strengthen Health Care was announced, based in part on the foundation laid previously by the first ministers in 2000 and 2003 (Health Canada, 2004). Recognizing the importance of the principles in the Canada Health Act, the plan restated the need for unified action in meeting national priorities for health care renewal. However, it did little to address the concerns of home care critics from the past by continuing to recognize needs only in the contexts of short-term post-acute care, short-term acute community mental health care, and palliative care at the end of life.

To monitor progress in achieving health care renewal, advocate for further changes where needed, and accelerate the rate of change in the health care system, the Health Council of Canada was formed and released its first report in January 2005 (Health Council of Canada, 2005). Noting that government recommendations and initiatives had previously emphasized short-term, acute, and palliative home care initiatives, it recommended that the government invest in home care services targeted on long-term and chronic-care needs to achieve their full potential. The factual foundation of governmental recommendations for the development of home care policy is disputed, with facts based on empirical research calling into question the assumptions made about the anticipated growth in costs associated with a comprehensive national home care program.

The next annual report from the Health Council of Canada (2006) also had a section focusing specifically on home care, observing that home care is undervalued and underfunded, leading to higher costs in other parts of the health care system. It recommended that home care services be expanded, especially for those with chronic illnesses. Subsequent reports in 2007 and 2008 (Health Council of Canada, 2007, 2008a, 2008b) emphasized the importance of holding the federal and provincial governments accountable for their earlier commitments to home care expansion. Both primary care and home care are considered the next major areas for investment and expansion, and calls have been made to proceed quickly to develop more unified and comprehensive models to meet growing health care needs in the future.

SUBTEXTS AND COUNTERSTORIES: AGING AND DISABILITY PERSPECTIVES

Using the metaphor of narrative frame, we find that subtexts or counter-stories may be proposed to either augment or challenge the dominant narrative or text by groups having an interest in the process and outcomes of public policy discourse. Here the term *subtext* refers to a perspective that is basically consistent with the overall empirical and normative dimensions of the text, whereas *counterstory* refers to a radically different perspective that may call into question the fundamental ordering of facts and values in the prevailing dominant text. In the case of the Canadian home care policy narrative, these are provided respectively by the aging and the disability communities.

Aging Community Subtext

The voice of the gerontological community in the public discourse on home care in Canada is remarkably soft, perhaps because those groups advocating for the interests of older adults and their families assume that they are already a major target group for home care policy reform. The perception is that expressions such as "those with chronic illnesses" or "those with long-term care needs" are primarily identified with older adults. In addition, population aging is often mentioned as a critical factor in fueling the demand for home care services.

An exception to this observation is the Canadian Association on Gerontology's official statement, published as an editorial in the *Canadian Journal on Aging* in 1999: "Home care is not currently available to Canadians on a universal basis; it falls outside of the realm of Medicare... . Yet, for many, home care is considered a necessary part of an appropriate and integrated health care system" (p. i). The research on cost-effectiveness, funding levels, and needs of informal caregivers is considered, and the statement concludes with the recommendation that "federal, provincial, and territorial governments move without delay to ensure a universally accessible, comprehensive home care program for Canadians" with adequate funding, national standards, and appropriate services (p. ii).

Similar statements have been released by the National Advisory Council on Aging (NACA), which was created in Canada in 1980 to assist and advise the minister of health on issues related to the aging of the Canadian population and the quality of life of older adults. In 2000 it adopted an official statement on home care, suggesting that "[we have] come to the conclusion that while some progress has been made on the road to universal home care, the subject needs to remain at the forefront of discussions on how to revitalize the health care system. Governments must take action without delay" (National Advisory Council on Aging, 2000, p. 1). The NACA statement goes on to restate its strong historical support for home care services: "Home care prevents and delays institutionalization and promotes the social integration of seniors. It responds to the changing health needs of older Canadians in a flexible, holistic manner and provides support to their informal caregivers" (p. 5). Citing evidence of continued unmet needs for home care services and popular support for the development of a national home care system, the report asserts that "the federal government has a responsibility to act as a role model for other jurisdictions and other employers. This is an opportunity to use moral suasion as another method for advancing home care" (p. 14). Importantly, the term "moral suasion" explicitly incorporates value-laden language to advance a public policy agenda—a point previously addressed in this discussion.

Again, in advance of the Romanow Commission Report in 2002, NACA issued further recommendations on the future of health care in Canada that included the statement that "maintaining and expanding the provision of home care is critical to a reformed health care system" (National Advisory Council on Aging, 2002, p. 3). Asserting that home care prevents and delays institutionalization and improves the quality of life of older adults by allowing them to remain in the community, NACA recommended that "a national, publicly-insured home care program be established... that provides, at a minimum, a 'core' set of services for everyone" (p. 9).

Disability Community Counterstory

Counterstories offer a fundamentally different way of framing a policy debate from the dominant textual and subtextual analyses. In the home care policy discourse in Canada, the disability community represents adults of all ages with cognitive, physical, or developmental disabilities. It places the discussion of home care services within a larger framework of discourse on community supports, where it is overtly based on an explicit set of articulated values and principles.

For example, a policy paper on informal and formal caregivers of persons with disabilities in Canada begins with a strong ideological statement regarding the deficit model of disability and its implications, including the exclusion and marginalization of persons with disabilities (Roeher Institute, 2003). There is a perceived lack of accessible, affordable in-home supports and services for informal caregivers. The creation of communities that are more inclusive, including improvements to home care through changes in the Canada Health Act and provincial care policies, is considered to be an appropriate solution to this problem.

Another policy paper on improving access to community supports (Roeher Institute, 2002) adds a statement based on values language and the rights of persons with disabilities: "[The] provision of disability supports in Canada should be strengthened through: a guiding vision of the full citizenship of people with disabilities and improved access, enhanced portability, more consumer control and greater responsiveness to individual needs" (p. 1). Subsequently in this report, there is stronger support for the inclusive community and the principles and values it embodies—equality, respect for diversity, fairness, individual dignity and responsibility, and mutual aid and responsibility—as well as the rejection of objectification, marginalization, and exclusion of persons based on gender, level of ability, race, age, and sexual orientation. It is clear that home care issues are conceptualized within the alternative, ideologically driven counterstory of supports provided within an inclusive community.

REVISITING THE NARRATIVE FRAME IN PUBLIC POLICY ANALYSIS

This discussion has been based on the proposed conceptual approach of narrative frame, suggesting that there can be a dominant narrative and subnarratives, a primary text and subtexts, and stories and counterstories that shape the policy discourse on such a topic as home care. Overall, the narrative frame draws our attention to the empirical and normative dimensions characterizing policy discourse. Thus, deconstructing the emerging discourse on home care policy requires an analysis of facts and values in policy statements and positions regarding programs and services for populations of older adults and adults with disabilities. An examination of the evolving primary text or story of home care policy, along with the consideration of subtexts and counterstories, can help to reveal the underlying assumptions, structures, and tensions in this unfolding public policy debate.

Employing the concept of narrative frame to analyze this emergent discourse from the federal perspective, one can observe a distinct tension between the value and the factual components: the ethical imperative of the Canada Health Act, with its collectivist principles, runs counter to the potential empirical reality of concerns over the uncontrolled costs and consequences of home care policies. Given the perceived uncertainty over the impacts and associated costs of expanded public policy in an area of increasing service demand, government is reluctant to exercise the political will and moral leadership that is expected of it.

Further examination of this tension between facts and values reveals that the factual information is viewed through a conservative lens; namely, empirical research suggesting overall cost savings in the health care system with an expansion of home care services is discounted. The interpretation of facts viewed from a conservative perspective is more compelling than the assertion of important social values. Though values may have the power of historical significance and moral argument, it seems that they cannot trump the interpretation of data, no matter how accurate or scientific. Values may be invoked to rally political support, but they cannot overcome (assumed) economic realities.

Similarly, the subtexts and counterstories provided by other groups and constituencies can either expand and enrich the dominant story line or confront and call into question the emerging discourse based on different ideological interests, emphases, and agendas. By comparing and contrasting the aging and disability community responses to the dominant federal voice in home care, we have extended the use of narrative-frame analysis to include different values and voices, differing lenses for interpreting empirical research, and alternative priorities in a public policy debate.

Overall, a narrative-frame analysis of significant public policy issues reveals the underlying textural contours of policy discourse and draws attention to the importance of deconstructing policy positions and perspectives to reveal their prevailing assumptions about facts and their ideological structures of values. The metaphor of "policy as story" invites research into the history of the development of the storyline, the evolution of the plotline of the story, and the search for other voices that may either enrich or call into question the emerging direction of policy discourse. It is clear that the application of narrative methods in public policy analysis is an important tool in investigating and intervening with issues involving older adults (see also Ubels, this volume).

NOTE

This chapter is based, in part, on an earlier and more extensive discussion of home care policy in Canada, published by the author as "Understanding the Aging and Disability Perspectives on Home Care: Uncovering Facts and Values in Public Policy Narratives and Discourse," in the *Canadian Journal on Aging*, 26 (Suppl. 1), 47–62. The original research was part of a Major Collaborative Research Initiatives program funded by grant No. G124130363 from the Social Sciences and Humanities Research Council of Canada.

REFERENCES

Biggs, S. (2001). Toward critical narrativity: Stories of aging in contemporary social policy. *Journal of Aging Studies, 15*, 303–316.

Canadian Association for Community Care. (2002). CACC welcomes Romanow report as a good beginning (November 28, 2002 press release). Toronto: Author. Retrieved January 19, 2004, from http://www.cacc-acssc.com/english/newsroom/20021128.cfm

Canadian Association for Community Care and Canadian Home Care Association. (n.d.). Sustaining Canada's health care system: The role of home and community care. Toronto: Author. Retrieved January 19, 2004, from http://www.cacc-acssc.com/english/pdf/brief.pdf

Canadian Association on Gerontology. (1999). Editorial: Canadian Association on Gerontology policy statement on home care in Canada. *Canadian Journal on Aging, 18*(3), i–iii.

Canadian Home Care Association. (2002). *Romanow recommendations—A foundation for strengthening home care* (November 28, 2002, press release). Ottawa: Author. Retrieved January 19, 2004, from http://www.cdnhomecare.ca/chca_admin/documents/nov_28_02_e_romanow_media_release.pdf

Canadian Home Care Association. (2003). *Expanding the Medicare envelope: Publicly funded home care services.* Ottawa: Author. Retrieved January 19, 2004, from http://www.cdnhomecare.ca/chca_admin/documents/expanding_medicare_jan_03.pdf

Canadian Home Care Association. (2004). *Home care: A national health priority: Visionary leadership can make it happen.* Ottawa: Author. Retrieved March 15, 2005, from http://www.cdnhomecare.ca/chca_admin/documents/home_care_a_national_health_priority_june_2004.pdf

Canadian Home Care Association. (2008a). *Canadians want more home and community-based health care services.* Ottawa: Author. Retrieved April 10, 2009, from http://www.cdnhomecare.ca

Canadian Home Care Association. (2008b). *Home care and primary health care: A solid basis for the future.* Ottawa: Author. Retrieved April 10, 2009, from http://www.cdnhomecare.ca

Clark, P. (1993). Public policy in the United States and Canada: Individualism, familial obligation, and collective responsibility in the care of the elderly. In J. Hendricks & C. Rosenthal (Eds.), *The remainder of their days: Domestic policy and older families in the United States and Canada* (pp. 13–48). New York: Garland.

Commission on the Future of Health Care in Canada. (2002). *Building on values: The future of health care in Canada* (Romanow Commission Report). Ottawa: Government of Canada. Retrieved February 12, 2003, from http://www.hc-sc.ca/english/care/romanow/hcc0086.html

Giacomini, M., Hurley, J., Gold, I., Smith, P., & Abelson, J. (2001). *"Values" in Canadian health policy analysis: What are we talking about?* Ottawa: Canadian Health Services Research Foundation. Retrieved January 12, 2005, from http://www.chsrf.ca/final_research/ogc/pdf/giacomini_e.pdf

Giacomini, M., Hurley, J., Gold, I., Smith, P., & Abelson, J. (2004). The policy analysis of "values talk": Lessons from Canadian health reform. *Health Policy, 67*, 15–24.

Health Canada. (1998). *Proceedings of the National Conference on Home Care.* Ottawa: Author. Retrieved August 9, 2004, from http://www.hc-sc.gc.ca/hcs-sss/finance/htf-fass/reference/conf/home-domicile2_e.html

Health Canada. (1999a). *Home care in Canada 1999: An overview.* Ottawa: Author. Retrieved April 19, 2004, from http://www.hc-sc.gc.ca/hcs-sss/pubs/care-soins/1999-home-domicile/index_e.html

Health Canada. (1999b). *Report on the National Roundtable on Home and Community Care.* Ottawa,: Author. Retrieved August 9, 2004, from http://www.hc-sc.go.ca/homecare/english/rt1.html

Health Canada. (2003). *2003 first ministers' accord on health care renewal.* Ottawa: Author. Retrieved April 19, 2005, from http://hc-sc.gc.ca/hcs-sss/delivery-prestation/fptcollab/2003accord/index_e.html

Health Canada. (2004). *First ministers' meeting on the future of health care 2004: A 10-year plan to strengthen health care.* Ottawa: Author. Retrieved April 19, 2005, from http://www.hc-sc.gc.ca/hcs-sss/delivery-prestation/fptcollab/2004-fmm-rpm/index_e.html

Health Council of Canada. (2005). *Health care renewal in Canada: Accelerating change.* Toronto: Author. Retrieved February 12, 2005, from http://www.healthcouncilcanada.ca/docs/rpts/2005/Accelerating_Change_HCC_2005.pdf

Health Council of Canada. (2006). Home care. Excerpt from *Health care renewal in Canada: Clearing the road to quality.* Toronto: Author. Retrieved July 20, 2006, from http://www.healthcouncilcanada.ca/docs/rpts/2006/EX_Home_EN.pdf

Health Council of Canada. (2007). *Health care renewal in Canada: Measuring up?* Toronto: Author. Retrieved April 10, 2009, from http://www.healthcouncilcanada.ca

Health Council of Canada. (2008a). *Fixing the foundation: An update on primary health care and home care renewal in Canada.* Toronto: Author. Retrieved April 10, 2009, from http://www.healthcouncilcanada.ca

Health Council of Canada. (2008b). *Rekindling reform: Health care renewal in Canada, 2003–2008.* Toronto: Author. Retrieved April 10, 2009, from http://www.healthcouncilcanada.ca

Hollander, M. (2003). *Unfinished business: The case for chronic home care services.* Victoria, Canada: Hollander Analytical Services Ltd. Retrieved January 12, 2005, from http://www.hollanderanalytical.com/main.html

Hollander, M., & Chappell, N. (2002). *Final report of the national evaluation of the cost-effectiveness of home care* (synthesis report). Victoria, Canada: Hollander Analytical Services Ltd. Retrieved January 12, 2005, from http://www.homecarestudy.com

Iannantuono, A., & Eyles, J. (1997). Meanings in policy: A textual analysis of Canada's "Achieving Health for All" document. *Social Science and Medicine, 44,* 1611–1621.

Jonsen, A., & Butler, L. (1975). Public ethics and policy making. *Hastings Center Report, 5*(4), 19–31.

Keefe, J. (2002). Home and community care. In M. Stephenson & E. Sawyer (Eds.), *Continuing the care: The issues and challenges for long-term care* (pp. 109–141). Ottawa: CHA Press.

Kelman, H., & Warwick, D. (1978). The ethics of social intervention: Goals, means, and consequences. In G. Bermant, H. C. Kelman, & D. Warwick (Eds.), *The ethics of social intervention* (pp. 3–33). Washington, DC: Hemisphere.

Kenny, N. (2004). *What's fair? Ethical decision-making in an aging society.* Research Report F/44. Ottawa: Canadian Policy Research Networks. Retrieved July 26, 2006, from http://www.cprn.org/en/doc.cfm?doc=776

Levine, C., & Murray, T. (2004). Caregiving as a family affair: A new perspective on cultural diversity. In C. Levine & T. Murray (Eds.), *The cultures of caregiving: Conflict and common ground among families, health professionals, and policy makers* (pp. 1–12). Baltimore: Johns Hopkins University Press.

National Advisory Council on Aging. (2000). *The NACA position on home care.* Ottawa: Author. Retrieved January 12, 2005, from http://dsp-psd.pwgsc.gc.ca/Collection/H71-2-2-20-2000E.pdf

National Advisory Council on Aging. (2002). *Waiting for Romanow: Recommendations on the future of health care in Canada.* Ottawa: Author. Retrieved July 28, 2009, from http://dsp-psd.pwgsc.gc.ca/collection_2007/naca-ccnta/H39-639-2002E/pdf

Potter, R. (1969). *War and moral discourse.* Richmond, VA: John Knox Press.

Rein, M. (1983). Value-critical policy analysis. In D. Callahan & B. Jennings (Eds.), *Ethics, the social sciences, and policy analysis* (pp. 83–111). New York: Plenum Press.

Roe, E. (1994). *Narrative policy analysis.* Durham, NC: Duke University Press.

Roeher Institute. (2002). *Moving in unison into action: Towards a policy strategy for improving access to disability support.* North York, Canada: Author.

Roeher Institute (2003). Caregivers of persons with disabilities in Canada… and policy implications. North York, Canada: Author.

Shapiro, E. (2002). *Health Transition Fund Synthesis series: Home care.* Ottawa: Health Canada Publications. Retrieved July 20, 2006, from http://www.hc-sc.gc.ca/hcs-sss/pubs/care-soins/2002-htf-fass-home-domicile/index_e.html

Part 2 Investigations

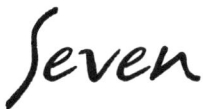

THE POWER OF STORIES LEFT UNTOLD:

NARRATIVES OF NAZI FOLLOWERS

Stephan Marks

We humans have been storytelling creatures since the earliest times. Telling stories about our world, our relationships, and our selves is fundamental to how we make meaning. But what about the stories we do *not* tell? What meaning can we make when fundamental stories are barred from being told? If narratives about our past help us understand where we are going, then where are we going if we cannot listen to the stories of where we have come from? Who are we without them? When it comes to listening to the stories of our elders, how can we honor their dignity, how can we care for them, if their narrations are about not-caring, about contempt, betrayal, perfidy, violence, and murder? These are some of my questions as I reflect on the research that my colleagues and I have been conducting in recent years and that I will be referring to throughout this chapter. But let me start with a few personal remarks, plus a rough outline of the ways in which, since 1945, Germany has dealt with its Nazi past.

SOCIETAL STORIES ABOUT
GERMANY'S NAZI PAST

I grew up in a small village in southern Germany in the 1950s. My country and its past felt dark, depressing, evil. It was a burden that no one would talk about. A number of men from the village were known to have "fallen" or "stayed in the war," and there were rumors about a neighbor (he often wore a long, dark, leather coat) who had been member of the SS—whatever that was. It sounded like something frightening and demonic. In high school, during the early 1960s, history classes started with the Ice Age and ceased with the German unification in 1871. One day, a new pupil named Jacob joined our class. I remember how we all stood frozen and aghast the moment he stated his religious affiliation with the one word, "Jewish." Without having any real knowledge of National Socialism and its crimes, we knew with every atom of our bodies that something egregious had just happened. A few weeks later, Jacob left the school after being isolated and bullied by his classmates—us. In the late 1960s, our history classes still starting with the Ice Age, I recall this one day when, quite abruptly while on a school outing, we were guided through what had been a Gestapo torture chamber. I was deeply shocked to see the large hooks on the walls. At that time, many of my generation—the first post-Nazi generation—attempted to ask our parents, "What did *you* do during the Nazi years? What did *you* know?" Very few of us got answers. Instead, our questions were warded off with anger and rage. Typically, family relations in post-Nazi Germany were frozen beneath the ice of denial.

During the first two decades after World War II, the topic of National Socialism and its crimes was widely taboo in West German society. (Things were somewhat different in East Germany, or the GDR). As Arthur Koestler observed in 1953, "Whenever Auschwitz or Belsen (site of the concentration camp Bergen-Belsen) is mentioned, Germans, even many obliging and intelligent ones, react with ironclad silence and piqued face, like a Victorian lady in whose presence the offensive word 'sex' is mentioned. One doesn't talk about such things, period" (as cited in Volker, 1995). This was the first pattern of Germans dealing with their Nazi past: by *not* dealing with it, by "silence"—as various researchers have characterized those years (see Arnim, 1989; Mitscherlich, 2000; Heimannsberg & Schmidt, 1992; Bar-On, 1996). By the term *pattern* here, I mean "paradigm" or "societal narrative." I mean the larger story that German society put together about its Nazi past: in other words, German discourse on the matter, its (provisional) effort to make sense of it. In this case, the larger narrative was: "Let's not talk about those things; let's work instead. With our industriousness we'll prove to the world that—except for Hitler and a few Nazi leaders who were solely responsible for 'all of that'—we're good people after all." This attitude changed, however, as a consequence of the famous Frankfurt lawsuits from 1963 to 1968 against Auschwitz perpetrators, of the student revolt of the years around 1968, and ultimately of the film series *Holocaust*, which was broadcast on

German TV in 1979 (Chomsky, 1978). Since then, Germans' ways of dealing with the past have been dominated by two other paradigms.

A growing number of historians have researched the Nazi past, bringing to light the facts, the data, the names, and the numbers of National Socialism and its crimes. Except for a few notorious deniers, German public opinion has accepted the fact that the Holocaust did indeed happen. This knowledge is present in literature, films, television, and the media. It is also an essential part of the curriculum in schools, not just in history classes but in civic education, in religious studies, and in German classes, too. We can summarize this paradigm under the heading "facts." In this case, the larger story is: "By being well informed about all the facts, the data, names, and numbers of National Socialism and the Holocaust, we can prove—to ourselves as well as to the world—how much we have learned about our past."

In recent decades, numerous concentration camps and former synagogues have been restored and made into places of information and remembrance. Memorial sites such as the *Denkmal für die ermordeten Juden Europas* (The Holocaust Memorial) in Berlin and a commemoration day, January 27, have been established to honor the victims of the Holocaust and to acknowledge their suffering. Survivors are invited to share their stories in schools, at conferences, and on public TV. We can call this paradigm "commemoration." Here, the larger story is: "By giving so much attention to the victims of the Holocaust, we can prove that we have become good people, true democrats."

The flip side of these two stories (facts and commemoration) goes like this: "Let's not talk about the millions of ordinary men and women who agreed with and actively supported Hitler and the Third Reich—the Nazi followers, bystanders, and perpetrators as they are commonly named. 'Those old Nazis' will become extinct eventually anyway, so let's talk about the victims instead."

THE MISSING STORIES

Clearly, both facts and commemoration are essential. However, National Socialism and the Holocaust are still frequently regarded as the work of Adolf Hitler and a core group of a few hundred thousand Nazi leaders and SS perpetrators, with the majority of the non-Jewish population regarding themselves as not involved ("unpolitical"), as resistance fighters, or, at worst, as passive "bystanders." This trivializing of the Nazi years was challenged with the *Wehrmachts-Ausstellung* (Wehrmacht Exhibition; Heer & Naumann, 1995), an exhibition that, from 1995 on, documented some of the crimes of the German Wehrmacht in Eastern Europe, where more than 15 million civilians were killed. This exhibition was highly disputed, however, for it tried to call attention to the almost unimaginable war crimes committed by (a not yet defined number of) members of the army. The Wehrmacht consisted of more than 17 million soldiers, more than 12 million of whom returned from the war.

Also, the notion of "unpolitical" noninvolvement has to be questioned. After all, the Nazi Party (NSDAP) received some 44% of the vote in the 1933 elections, and by 1945, 7.5 million Germans had become party members. So, where have they all gone? Many of those former members of the Wehrmacht and the party are still alive today. In 2005, more than three million Germans, born in 1925 or earlier, were still living: almost one million men and more than two million women. What are *their* stories about the Nazi years?

Interestingly, although the situation is slowly changing, this question has, until recently, hardly been asked. Instead, public discourse in Germany has been dominated by facts and commemoration, with the following consequences. The "need to remember" is regularly stressed, for instance, by politicians during the various commemorative events. In a speech to the Israeli parliament (the Knesset) in 2000, former federal president Johannes Rau insisted that "there is no life without remembrance. Therefore, we need to pass on the memory to the youth." Similarly, Wolfgang Thierse, former president of the German parliament, stressed the importance of remembrance in a lecture he delivered in Freiburg in 2007. In all such statements, however, it is solely the memories of Holocaust survivors (a small minority in Germany at present) that are thought of, *not* those of former followers, bystanders, and perpetrators, who remain a considerable part of the German population. In discussion with him, I asked Thierse about this: "How are we dealing with the memories of those citizens who were excited about Hitler and the Third Reich, and may still be today—many of them claiming they didn't notice when their Jewish neighbors were taken away to be transported to Auschwitz? Instead, they remember their fascination with Hitler and the Nazi movement. What are the effects of their stories, of their memories, on their grandchildren, for example?" It was impossible to make myself understood. The man seemed to have no idea what I was talking about. Instead he repeated his emphasis on the importance of—only the victim's—memories.

While undoubtedly important to commemorate the victims, to honor their narratives, and to have knowledge of the facts about National Socialism and the Holocaust, the stories of Nazi followers are widely regarded as improper, as off-limits. Thus, a core component of German history remains missing. In the following statement, a high school student addresses this taboo in German society today:

> There was this history teacher who always told us about the victims, for hours and hours, about the Jews, the communists, the gypsies, the Russians— nothing but victims. I never really believed him. One day, one of my classmates asked him: "What was so great then? Why did so many scream 'Hurray' and 'Heil Hitler'? Why were they all so excited? There must have been something else?" At that, the teacher looked quite silly and started to blame the student for being a neo-Nazi, accusing him of having no respect for the victims. But we wouldn't let go. At last, someone had vocalized this question. We wanted to know what really happened then. After all, we had seen it in the films that he had shown us: the laughing children, the shining eyes of the women. Hundreds of thousands in the streets, and they were all cheering. Where did their excitement come from? (Sichrovsky, 1987, pp. 41–42)

THE EFFECTS OF A TABOO

What are the effects of such a taboo on the narratives of seniors who had been Nazi followers? In a project founded in 1998 (Marks, 2007) and entitled *Geschichte und Erinnerung* (History and Memory), an interdisciplinary team of us at the University of Education in Freiburg set out to analyze such narratives. Our team consisted of 10 professionals from a range of fields in the social sciences, including history, psychology, psychoanalysis, education, social work, and social education. All of us were born in the years after 1945, making us members of the first post-WWII generation.

We conducted interviews with 43 senior citizens (born in 1925 or before) who had agreed with, and actively supported, Hitler and the Third Reich, as members either of Hitler Youth organizations (HJ, BDM), of the SA, SS, NSDAP, or Wehrmacht, or of other Nazi organizations. For purposes of comparison, 11 interviews were conducted by students (i.e., members of the second post-WWII generation), and 12 intergenerational sharing groups were organized. Overall, we were interested in the narratives, not so much of prominent Nazi leaders or of "extraordinary" mass murderers, but of ordinary people. The interviews were analyzed in relation to the following questions: What motivated the interviewees to agree with and actively support Hitler and National Socialism? In what ways is the experience of the Nazi years still present, cognitively and emotionally, in interviewees' lives today? What happens when people who were actively involved in the Nazi movement and members of subsequent generations communicate with one another about National Socialism (Marks, 2001)?

As it turned out, our interviewees were strongly affected by the taboo. One of our very first interviews began as follows. The interviewer had made an appointment with an elderly woman by telephone. As soon as he rang the doorbell, the door was flung open: "It's about time!" she exclaimed. "For 50 years we were not allowed to speak." What ensued was like opening a can of worms. The interviewer was barraged with rapid-fire words: "I was born into history, lived with history, and always lived *in* history, in the middle of it—very close, as close as could be. That's one thing, and the other is that 98% of my generation were involved in those years—somewhere, somehow, whether passively, actively, or as resistance," etc., etc. She continued in this manner for more than two hours, leaving the interviewer in such a state of confusion that he had a minor car accident on his return.

Altogether, these interviews were not a pleasant experience for us. Regularly, whether during the interviews or afterward, we felt confused, sickened, emptied, abused, depressed, knocked down, or overrun. Often we felt shame, as if something evil had been stuffed into us. And some of us suffered nightmares during the nights that followed. After a seven-hour interview with a former SS officer, one interviewer dreamed that someone broke into her home and besmirched the walls and the furniture with blood. Two of the eleven student interviewers were left with crying fits, while another fell into a state of fascination, as if he had been infected by the interviewee's fascination with Hitler himself. As a result, we discontinued working with student interviewers, for it would have been irresponsible to expose young people to such harmful situations. Instead, we continued with interviewers who were well experienced. With peer counseling and supervision (individual and team), we tried both to cushion and to analyze the harmful effects of the interviews (Marks & Moennich-Marks, 2002). In what follows, I will try to present some of our findings in relation to two questions.

INDIVIDUAL STORIES, SOCIETAL STORIES

What is the interplay between the stories of individuals and those of the society they live in—in this case, between the narratives of individual Nazi followers and the larger narratives of post-WWII Germany as regards National Socialism? On the basis of interviews we conducted, I came to two conclusions. First, the dominating larger stories of post-WWII Germany served as a cover-up, keeping individuals' stories from being brought to the surface, expressed, and thus worked through. In terms of William Randall's (2007) metaphor of memory as a *compost heap*, the individual's experiences seemed to be sealed beneath a thick plastic wrap, which kept them from being aired and ultimately being turned into humus—into fertile, life-giving soil in which something new could grow. On top of the plastic wrap were interviewees' declarations in keeping with the larger, politically correct story of present-day Germany. In many cases, however, these declarations seemed disconnected from their experiences of the Nazi years. Those stories were sealed off, were taboo. This may be why in many of these interviews we felt like we were opening a can of worms. It may also be why many interviewees' voices sounded young and energetic as soon as they spoke about the Nazi years, whereas their voices when recounting the years before and after were rather depressed. And it may be why most texts were rather confusing to listen to and seemed self-contradictory. In other words, while interviewees were well-informed about National Socialism and WWII (many of them proudly pointing to their bookshelves loaded with numerous volumes dealing with those years), their individual experiences during the Nazi years seemed to have been little reflected on and integrated into their lifestory as a whole (see Coleman, 1999). For instance, an interviewee might call Hitler a "criminal" and the Holocaust a "mistake," yet a few minutes later speak with excitement and shining eyes about his "encounter" with "HIM."

Second, the cover-up function of the larger stories may at the same time have been a lifesaver, allowing millions of Nazi followers to survive their immeasurable guilt and shame. Here a comparison can be made with veterans of the Vietnam War. During the 1960s, numerous young U.S. citizens volunteered or were drafted to fight in Vietnam. At the time, according to the larger story of American public opinion, it felt right to "fight against communism, for freedom and democracy." Yet when many of them became involved in war crimes, public opinion shifted. Many a veteran who returned from the jungle and landed in his hometown was accused of being a baby-killer. The congruence between individuals' stories and the larger story had gotten lost. Veterans were left alone with their shame and guilt about the crimes in which they had been involved. In the years that followed, in fact, more Vietnam vets lost their lives through suicide than had been killed in combat.

This example helps to illustrate how crucial the interplay is between individuals' stories and larger stories. Compared to WWII and the Holocaust, of course, the crimes committed by American soldiers in Vietnam were minor. How is it, then, that millions of Nazi followers and perpetrators did *not* commit suicide when the war was over? Veterans of the Wehrmacht, who returned from WWII in 1945 or from prison camp in the years that followed, came back to a defeated, destroyed, and traumatized country. However, they were not accused as killers—not yet. They were shielded by the prevailing larger stories, shielded by public opinion. With silence, with the projection of collective guilt onto Hitler and a small number of Nazi leaders and hard-core perpetrators, and with public opinion focused on facts and commemoration, they were granted protection.

In 1967, psychoanalysts Alexander and Margarethe Mitscherlich suspected that, through silencing, the German population prevented itself from a collective depression (Mitscherlich & Mitscherlich, 1975). Based on today's information about the extent of German war crimes and the participation of ordinary Nazi followers, I would go even further, in fact, and say that the silence of the 1950s and 1960s prevented a mass suicide. So maybe, in some ways, it was unavoidable? But is it unavoidable still?

WHY BOTHER?

Why rock the boat? Why stir up those old, unpleasant stories? Why not wait until the present generation of German seniors has died out? Why should we listen to the stories of Nazi followers after all these years? I suggest four reasons why we should.

First, the amount of research done on National Socialism and its crimes has been remarkable, as are all the efforts to convey the facts, names, and numbers in the German media, in schools, and so forth. Also, it is indispensable to commemorate the victims and honor their suffering. However, this is not enough. Learning *about* history is not the same as learning *from* history. Knowing facts about crimes that were committed by others does not necessarily change oneself—for example, today's students. Being confronted with other people's suffering does not necessarily initiate moral growth. In fact, it may lead to saturation or aversion instead. Learning *from* history involves facing the motives of those who agreed with, and actively supported, Hitler and the Nazi movement—that is, the motives of our parents, our grandparents, or our ancestors. For this learning to occur, we have to hear the stories of the men and women who were involved. We have to listen to their answers to the question posed by the high school student: "What was so great then? Why did you scream 'Hurray' and 'Heil Hitler'? Why were you so excited? Where did your excitement come from?" This is the homework that we, non-Jewish Germans, still have to do. Nothing can replace this. Why, after all, should other people trust us Germans? Because we are such industrious folks? Because we are so well informed about the Holocaust? Because we commemorate the Jews so often?

Second, without the stories of the bystanders and perpetrators, the stories of the Holocaust cannot be complete. In his psychotherapeutic work with Holocaust survivors, psychoanalyst Dori Laub, professor of Psychiatry at Yale University School of Medicine and Education, and co-founder of the

Fortunoff Video Archive for Holocaust Testimonies, made a remarkable observation. Survivors felt there was no longer a "thou," because in the concentration camps

> the executioner does not heed the victim's plea for life and relentlessly proceeds with execution. Human responsiveness came to be nonexistent in the death camps.... The natural outcome is a lonesomeness in one's internal world representation: "In the Lager... everyone is desperately and ferociously alone" (Jean Améry). This despair to communicate with others diminished the victims' ability to be in contact and in tune with themselves, to be able to register, to reflect to themselves about their own experience. (Laub, 2000)

The stories of Holocaust survivors need to be matched, therefore, by the stories of the bystanders and perpetrators. The victims' accounts of their experience will never fade as long as they encounter silence on the part of non-Jewish Germans. They must be responded to with the others' stories: "Yes, this is what happened."

The third reason for listening to Nazi followers' stories is that offering senior citizens opportunities to tell their stories about their participation in National Socialism is not a "betrayal" of the victims of the Holocaust, as we secretly feared before we started our interviews in 1998. Rather, listening may be a way to support them in their efforts to restore their mental health (Radebold, 2005) and, ultimately, their sense of human dignity. Having lost that sense in their past is what made National Socialism possible in the first place (Marks, 2007). So far, German society is not very open to listening to such narrations. Quite often, one can hear such comments as, "Why bother? Them old Nazis will die out soon anyway." As psychoanalyst Tilman Moser (1996) has observed, nursing home care for seniors in Germany is often impeded by the latent hostility harbored toward them because of their involvement in National Socialism. This may be one of the reasons why, compared to all other European nations, Japan, and the United States, the quality of German senior citizens' homes has been identified as the poorest (Hildebrandt, 2005).

Finally, having suffered tremendously from the silence and emotional coldness of the post-Nazi years, I can well understand the resentment against former Nazi followers. However, tit-for-tat is harmful to all. Listening may well be an act that restores the listener's dignity as well.

REFERENCES

Arnim, G. (1989). *Das grosse Schweigen. Von der Schwierigkeit, mit dem Schatten der Vergangenheit zu leben* [The great silence: About the difficulty of living with the shadow of the past]. Munich: Knaur.

Bar-On, D. (1996). *Die Last des Schweigens. Gespräche mit Kindern von Nazi-Tätern* [Legacy of silence: Encounters with children of the Third Reich]. Reinbek, Germany: Rororo.

Chomsky, M. (Director). (1978). *Holocaust. Die Geschichte der Familie Weiss* [Holocaust: The history of the Weiss family]. [Television series]. New York: NBC.

Coleman, P. (1999). Creating a life story: The task of reconciliation. *The Gerontologist, 39*(2): 133–139.

Heer, H., & Naumann, K. (Eds.). (1995). *Vernichtungskrieg. Verbrechen der Wehrmacht 1941 bis 1944* [War of extermination: Crimes of the Wehrmacht 1941 to 1944]. Hamburg: Hamburger Edition.

Heimannsberg, B., & Schmidt, C. (Eds.). (1992). *Das kollektive Schweigen. Nationalsozialistische Vergangenheit und gebrochene Identität in der Psychotherapie* [The collective silence: National-Socialistic past and broken identity in psychotherapy]. Cologne: EHP.

Hildebrandt, A. (2005, December 23). Der Mann mit den zwei Gesichtern [The man with two faces]. *Badische Zeitung*, p. 3.

Laub, D. (2000). Not knowing is an active process of destruction: Why the testimonial procedure is of so much importance. *Trauma Research Newsletter* 1, Hamburger Institute for Social Research, July 2000. Retrieved from www.traumaresearch.net/focus1/laub.htm.

Marks, S. (2001). Research project "History and Memory." In M. Kiegelmann (Ed.). *Qualitative research in psychology* (pp. 150–154). Tübingen, Germany: Ingeborg Huber.

Marks, S. (2007). *Warum folgten sie Hitler? Die Psychologie des Nationalsozialismus* [Why did they follow Hitler? The psychology of National Socialism]. Düsseldorf: Patmos.

Marks, S. & Moennich-Marks, H. (2002). The researcher is the instrument. In M. Kiegelmann (Ed.). *The role of the researcher in qualitative psychology* (pp. 131–138). Tübingen, Germany: Ingeborg Huber.

Mitscherlich, A., & Mitscherlich, M. (1975). *The inability to mourn: Principles of collective behavior* (B. Placzek, Trans.). New York: Grove Press.

Mitscherlich, M. (2000). Schweigen, Wegdenken oder Trauer um die Opfer unserer politischen Vergangenheit [Silence, thinking away, or mourning for the victims of our political past]. *Psyche, 53*, 234–241.

Moser, T. (1996). *Dämonische Figuren. Die Wiederkehr des Dritten Reiches in der Psychotherapie* [Demonic figures: The return of the Third Reich in psychotherapy]. Frankfurt: Suhrkamp.

Radebold, H. (2005). *Die dunklen Schatten unserer Vergangenheit. Ältere Menschen in Beratung, Psychotherapie, Seelsorge und Pflege* [The dark shadows of our past: Senior citizens in counseling, psychotherapy, pastoral care and nursing]. Stuttgart: Klett-Cotta.

Randall, W. (2007). From computer to compost: Rethinking our metaphors for memory. *Theory & Psychology, 17*(5), 611–633.

Sichrovsky, P. (1987). *Schuldig geboren. Kinder aus Nazifamilien* [Born guilty: Children from Nazi families]. Cologne: Kiepenheuer & Witsch.

Volker, U. (1995, April 21). Weggesehen, weggehoert [Looking away, hearing away]. *Die Zeit*, p. 17.

Eight

YOUNG BODIES, OLD BODIES, AND STORIES

OF THE ATHLETIC SELF

Cassandra Phoenix

Bodies are realized and created in the stories that they tell. According to medical sociologist Arthur Frank (1995), when people tell stories about their bodies, the actual body gives the story a particular shape and direction. Such sentiments have been echoed more recently by myself and my colleague, Andrew Sparkes, in arguing that the kind of body one has and is, and the stories one learns to tell about one's self and one's body, is important for the way in which order is imposed on one's experiences and sense is made of actions in one's life (see Phoenix & Sparkes, 2009). Likewise, Randall and McKim (2008) have noted the relationship between the body, storytelling, and meaning-making. Our storytelling, they propose, is always relevant and connected to what our body itself is telling us. In this sense, our physical being is central to our being-in-the-world, and given meaning through the stories that we tell. Drawing attention to the implications of this relation-ship for one's sense of identity, they suggest the following:

> Our body is not merely the housing of our life; it is the setting of our story, the main (though ever moving) environment in which that story unfolds.... . What is more, this character-cum-setting is continually changing, and sooner or later such changes impel us to rethink our identity: "Who am I, now that I am no longer youthful or able?" Changing bodies means changing stories (pp. 119–120).

If meaning-making is inseparable from storytelling, and if storytelling is always connected to the body, making sense of the physical changes brought about by the aging process calls for new and different stories to be told. Given the salience of the body in shaping the stories that we tell, experiences of aging might be understood more fully, therefore, when considered in relation to the type of body they are spoken from (active, inactive, young, old, and so forth). Indeed, Smith (2007) has argued that narrative researchers should resist being content with theories and conceptual considerations *on* and *about* the body. They should also seriously consider generating stories *from* and *with* the bodies of people at different stages of the life course so that a more comprehensive insight might be developed into how aging bodies become known and connected through narrative (see also Goyal & Charon, this volume).

Drawing upon life history data from a group of young, competitive athletes ranging in age from 19 to 27 and a group of mature, natural (i.e., "drug-free")[1] competitive bodybuilders from ages 54 to 73, this chapter examines stories told about and through the aging, athletic body (the athletes' names have been changed for the sake of anonymity). I explore the ways in which such stories come into being and the consequences they have for those who embody them. In addition, I consider the extent to which the athletes' ontological narratives or personal stories (Somers, 1994) are connected to and shaped by broader meta-narratives circulating within society regarding the aging body. Prior to discussing this in more detail, however, I reflect on why the athletic body should matter to those interested in narrative gerontology.

Athletic populations are inclined to inhabit and engage with the world via particular kinds of "high-performance" bodies that have particular characteristics. They tend to be highly disciplined and shaped by various regimes and technologies designed to ensure corporal control and predictable performance outcomes (Sparkes, 2004). Moreover, while the body is immediately relevant to the identity that any individual attempts to promote, it holds particular significance to the young athlete whose self-identity is constructed and maintained around possessing an able, pain-free, physically fit, and performing body. Experienced and expected physical changes associated with the aging process, however, can disrupt the meaning of the physical body and subsequently call into question who the athletes think they are, think they were, and think they can become in the future. Like others who depend on characteristics of youth for their livelihood, this scenario can arise long before athletes reach middle age. The consequence of this, suggests Neikrug (2003), is that concerns about the aging process may be more intense and immediate than those of people who inhabit different kinds of bodies in their youth. With all of this in mind, I now turn to the project that explored these issues in greater depth.

YOUNG ATHLETIC BODIES AND STORIES OF SELF-AGING IN CONTEXT

Given the salience of the body in the construction and maintenance of an athletic identity, combined with the seemingly premature arrival of "old age" within the subculture of sport, previous research that I have been involved in has explored stories of self-aging told by a group of young athletes (see Phoenix & Sparkes, 2006a, 2006b, 2007; Phoenix, Smith, & Sparkes, 2007). Their typical response to the notion of growing older is shown in the following comments from two of the participants. When asked, "Do you consider yourself to be an athlete now?" 21-year-old Laura replied, "Yes, I do." When asked, "and in the future?" her response was "Urgh," followed by a seven-second silence, and then: "I just think that it's all going to go. Everything. Like, who I am, and everything that I enjoy now, my whole life that I've built up for myself, my interests, the things that I'm interested in, I just relate it to being young and healthy and fit... . Then, when I'm older, it's like a different life and I won't have this one anymore. I'll have to give it up." Twenty-three-year-old Nick had this for an answer: "I think, for an athlete, having had what's sort of thought of as an athletic shape, for them just starting to sag and lose that shape as they get older, is a lot more depressing than someone who hasn't had that athletic figure in their early life."

As illustrated by Laura and Nick, one way in which the athletes gave meaning to their aging process was by considering the type of body they inhabited at present in relation to the type of body they envisaged becoming in the future. The stories they told about their bodies relative to these different periods of the life course signaled a sense of inevitable physical deterioration and decrepitude. In other words, a structural analysis (Lieblich, Tuval-Maschiah, & Zilber, 1998) of the data revealed that the stories told about growing old by the young athletes were indicative of a *tragic* plotline— or what cultural studies scholar, Margaret Morganroth Gullette, in *Aged by Culture,* refers to as the "narrative of decline" (2004, p. 17).

Indeed, employing multiple forms of analysis with this data—the benefits of which I have discussed elsewhere (see Phoenix, Smith, & Sparkes, 2010)—resulted in rich and increasingly nuanced insights into the young athletes' experiences and expectations of the (aging) body across the life course.

For example, in addition to identifying a narrative of decline via structural analysis, I examined the means by which cultural context was produced in the lives of the young athletes—where, when, and by whom—and how it was salient in their stories of self-aging (see Phoenix & Sparkes, 2008). This analytical procedure, advocated by Holstein and Gubrium (2004), revealed the ways in which people, places, and time periods (the *who*, *where*, and *when*) embedded within the participants' everyday living helped to support the narrative of decline by cultivating and sustaining assumptions that the body would physically deteriorate over time. In part, this was achieved via the association of three distinct selves that were (perceived to be) character-istic of certain periods throughout the life course. The centrality of these selves to the young athletes' stories of self-aging illustrated how qualifiers of aging for youth, midlife, and old age not only referred to a fixed biological chronology but were also shaped by cultural pressures and expectations spanning the whole life (Gullette, 2004). These selves were identified as a sporting self (present/youth), a settled self (midlife), and a reflective self (old age) (Phoenix & Sparkes, 2008). They were given meaning by the parti-cipants in terms of three individual plotlines: do it now (sporting self), have it now (settled self), and remember it now (reflective self).

Do it now involved making the most of the present (i.e., university years), enjoying a lack of responsibility to anyone or anything other than them-selves, and subsequently having an ability to dedicate their time, their energy, and their bodies to sport performance. This plotline was instigated and supported by a sporting self, which was developed by the means of a youth-ful, performing body and dominated the young athletes' identity hierarchy. Moreover, focusing on the ways in which these selves were constructed and maintained through their cultural context, the analysis illustrated how sporting selves existed and moved alongside other similar bodies (who) within the social contexts of university sport, the university campus, and nightclubs (where)—places and spaces suited and often restricted to bodies within the youthful stages of the life course (when). It seemed, therefore, that the sporting self's reliance on social contexts tailored toward physical prowess, and indeed youth, made sustaining it especially difficult, and its dominance unlikely at other points in time (e.g., old age).

In contrast to the plotline of do it now and the associated sporting self, the young athletes' expectations of life as an older person were understood via the plotline of *remember it now*. This plotline was indicative of the past being perceived as more valuable than the present and future. In old age (when), a reflective self was expected to shift to the foreground of their iden-tity hierarchy as a result of the anticipated loss and the absence of others such as friends and partners (who). In contrast to the embodiment of the sporting self, the reflective self was perceived to be motionless, experiencing the passing of time from a wheelchair or bed (where). This was illustrated in the following comments, once again from Nick, aged 23:

> I think your body in old age, it's almost like growing old has really taken its toll. You're sort of bed bound, wheelchair bound, possibly slightly crippled. I think with old age, it's really just a time for reflection and looking back on your life and reminiscing. But then it can also be seen as painful and a time when you think…"I'd rather be dead," if you know what I mean. You may be thinking "why is my life still stringing on? Why am I still going?"

What this can show is that, via the absence or presence of specific forms of social context, the foregrounding of particular selves within one's lifestory can be ordered by, positioned in, and indeed restricted to certain periods of the life course. Furthermore, the interpretation of these selves by the young athletes—whether they were perceived as being unbeatable, welcomed, or feared—illustrated the ways in which social contexts are tied to the development and maintenance of certain selves across the life course. It also illuminates how social context and self can shape and be shaped by what Henning Eichberg (2000, p. 91) describes as the "life curve mode" (Fig. 8.1).

The inverted "U" of the life curve model locates the meta-narrative of decline in a broader context. According to Eichberg (2000), it depicts the expectations and associated emotions we have of life, while simultaneously forming the foundation for practical decisions regarding our life management. As illustrated in Figure 8.1, the life curve portrays an upward tendency at the beginning of our life, followed by a "peak" or zenith. Soon after this point, following a period of stagnation, the way leads downward as the body weakens and becomes less productive. Elsewhere I have illustrated how this model was inscribed into and projected by the bodies of young athletes through the stories they told about the life course (see Phoenix & Sparkes, 2008). The "upward tendency" of the life curve model resonated with the aspirations of the participants' sporting self as it strove to invest in experiences

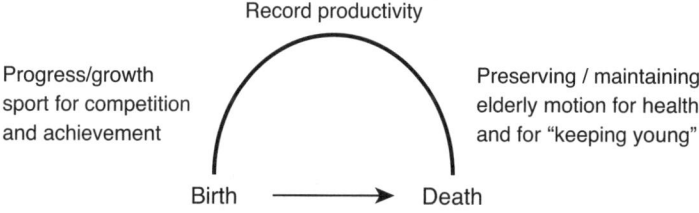

Figure 8.1 The life curve.

and memories that would be subsequently drawn upon during the latter half of life as a reflective self. Specifically, the participants believed that the notion of investment during youth (as a sporting self) was important, given the lack of meaning and purpose that they currently associated with life in old age. Indeed, with no future trajectory, and virtually no other function besides reflection, reminiscence, and soon death, old age was viewed by many of the participants as a period that held little or no meaning.

Analyses of the young athletes' stories of self-aging also illustrated how the foregrounding of different selves throughout the life course could have implications for the ways in which biographical time was experienced (see Phoenix et al., 2007). As a reflective self, it was expected that time would feel static and empty, with a sense of the *past being in the present*. This scenario bears similarity to McCullough's (1993) notion of "arrested aging," whereby individuals demonstrate an inability to respond to the passing of time and, instead, become imprisoned in a past (i.e., a youthful, sporting self), which is believed to contain all that really mattered. In this sense, the later chapters of life are believed to be already known in that they are assumed to hold no meaning. As such, with the future believed to be a foregone conclusion of meaningless existence, the young athletes appeared destined to live out a story with a pre-scripted ending. This sense of "narrative foreclosure" (Freeman, this volume) was a pertinent issue in relation to the stories that the participants told about their aging, athletic bodies.

YOUNG ATHLETIC BODIES AND NARRATIVE FORECLOSURE

According to psychologist Mark Freeman (2000), with pre-scripted narratives of decline well in place, there often appears little choice but to resign oneself to a "narrative fate" with regard to the aging process (p. 81). Freeman asserts that individuals can experience a sense of narrative foreclosure in that the types of stories they can tell about their aging bodies are severely limited. In this sense, the story of one's aging athletic body is thought to go this way, not that. As a result, one's ability to perceive and live one's life meaningfully and productively in all stages of the life course is believed to be severely restricted. More recently, Randall and McKim (2008) have considered narrative foreclosure in relation to aging, proposing that it can lead to a "shutting down" of stories despite one's life continuing to unfold. Consequently, one may "give in to getting—as opposed to growing—old" (p. 7) and potentially overlook opportunities to age in a way that is rich in meaning and wisdom. In this sense, narrative foreclosure denotes a loss of imagination, a failure to continue working on, expanding, and finding meaning in one's stories. Randall and McKim argue that the propensity to close one's story down and commit to a fate of narrative foreclosure may be further exacerbated when one's self-image is tied too tightly to one's body image. Alas, this is especially relevant for athletic populations whose image and identity are closely aligned to a youthful, powerful, agile, fast, and strong, performing body.

The stories told about a foreclosed identity, however, do not just spring from the minds of individuals. Rather, as Zilber, Tuval-Mashiach, and Lieblich (2008) point out, echoing numerous other narrative scholars, stories are always constructed intersubjectively: "People construct stories in relation to their social sphere and their position in it and in light of the 'social stock of stories' and local social conventions available to them" (p. 1048). One's lifestory is never solely an expression of a unique and private self. In other words, ontological narratives (our personal stories) are shaped by institutionally based public narratives, which in turn are informed by broad societally based meta-narratives.

Viewed in this manner, the life curve model and indeed the concept of narrative foreclosure are eminently social phenomena. Both of them con-nect to the reification of cultural storylines and the tendency, for many, to internalize these storylines in a manner that severely constricts their own field of narrative expression. Indeed, the analyses signaled that, for the young athletes, narrative foreclosure was in part a result of their internalization of cultural storylines regarding when "peak athletic performance" *should* be achieved, when one *should* be married, when one *should* have children, retire from work, and so forth. As such, the life curve helped to shape their onto-logical narratives associated with feeling "on time" or "off time" according to the social clocks regulating cultural expectations across the life course (see De Vries, Blando, Southard, & Bubeck, 2001). Thus, telling stories about a (feared and restricted) future was not just a personal story unique to the individual. These stories also reflected the current inadequacy of public and meta-narratives to provide young athletes who invest highly in a particular type of performing body with varied and accessible resources needed for constructing alternative storylines about the aging process.

If narratives of aging are socially situated as opposed to being located simply in the minds of individuals, then *where* and *how* did the young athletes come to know aging? *Why* were they able to form such powerful beliefs regarding life stages that they had yet to encounter first hand?

How did meta- and public narratives associated with aging infiltrate the participants' ontological narratives? Understanding the answers to questions such as these is important if we are to gain a purchase on how we might offer a means of resistance against the prevailing narrative of decline. Focusing on the concept of *narrative mapping* has been a useful starting point in this process.

NARRATIVE MAPS OF AGING

In defining a narrative map, Pollner and Stein (1996) propose that when seeking to grasp an unfamiliar world beyond the horizon of the here and now, newcomers may seek knowledgeable or experienced others for orientation, information, and advice regarding the psychosocial and physical landscape that presumably awaits them in the future. In this sense, narrative maps can contribute to socialization and social reproduction by confirming cultural stereotypes and forms of embodiment or, alternatively, by acting to challenge and problematize these stereotypes.

Relationships between young and older adults can therefore be significant in providing narrative maps that describe for newcomers the people, practices, and problems they are likely to encounter as they age. For example, in *re*-presenting their experiences of the aging body and of inhabiting/living through different kinds of bodies, older people can provide younger people with *pre*-presentations of what is to come as they age and how they might experience different forms of embodiment. In earlier publications, I have illustrated this by identifying three prevailing sources of narrative maps of aging from which the young athletes drew when storying their own aging process (see Phoenix & Sparkes, 2006a, 2006b, 2007). These sources were older family members, older teammates, and parts of the curriculum covered in the Bachelor of Science degree program (sport and exercise sciences) in which all of them were currently enrolled at university. The narrative maps of aging projected from these sources were consequential for how young athletes perceived their aging bodies because they shaped a number of *possible selves*.

According to Markus and Nurius (1986), possible selves include the selves that we would ideally like to become in the future (i.e., *preferred selves*), and the selves that we are frightened of becoming in the future (i.e., *feared selves*). Some of my earlier research illustrated how the narrative maps of aging utilized by the young athletes to make sense of their own aging continually emphasized inevitable physical decline and deterioration (see Phoenix & Sparkes, 2006a, 2006b, 2007). This was illustrated in the following comments from Vicky (age 19), as she explained where she gathered her information from regarding the aging process:

> I look at my parents, who I would describe as being middle-aged. I see what life is like for them, and I guess it will be similar for me. Perhaps the biggest difference that I notice with my mum is that she has gained more weight over the last few years, and now she's getting more wrinkly (laughs), though don't tell her I said that. Dad is still pretty fit, but his knees give him trouble if he overdoes it. But that's what growing old is; your body is starting to fail. My grandparents are both still quite independent and that's how I would like to be, but I worry about how much longer that will last. Last year my Nan was taken ill and it made me realize how fragile she is now. It's all quite depressing really, isn't it? I mean things are basically going to get worse from here.

These comments show how older family members acted as narrative resources, which Vicky drew from in order to develop some understanding of the unfamiliar world that she believed awaited her in the future. The stories that she told were characterized by a series of embodied events displayed by family members. These events included weight gain, sagging skin, illness, physical dependence, and impaired mobility. In this sense, the narrative maps of aging that she used facilitated and strengthened a number of feared selves she anticipated in the future. These were linked to the loss of bodily predictability relative to athletic performance and the loss of a youthful appearance. Similar narratives were also projected by older teammates, plus the content of the Bachelor of Science curriculum in which they were currently enrolled. As a consequence, the young athletes' perceptions of growing old were instilled with a sense of fear and trepidation. This scenario was heightened by the somewhat limited information projected through the narrative maps of aging.

Given all of the points raised thus far, the following could be surmised: older adults are important in the process of projecting narrative maps of aging to younger people; and young athletes place great emphasis on the athletic body in terms of who they think they are at present, and who they think they can become in the future. Related to both of these points, it would seem that the bodies of older adults are a key site for projecting messages about aging. It could be interesting, therefore, to flip the coin and examine the stories told by older athletic bodies regarding how they view the passage of time. Of course, this is not to champion the aging athletic body over other types of bodies moving through the life course. Nor is it to align the older athletic body with notions of personal responsibility and successful aging (see Dionigi, 2008, for an overview of relevant debates regarding this issue).

Rather, my intention here is to offer insight into some *alternative storylines* about the aging body—that is, storylines offering an additional version of growing old, aside from those that do little other than reinforce inevitable physical deterioration and subsequent loss of athletic identity. Having gained some insight into young athletes' perceptions of self-aging, stories of self-aging as told by older athletes themselves would seem a logical extension in further developing an understanding of aging bodies and stories of the athletic self.

OLDER ATHLETIC BODIES AND THE REOPENING OF A FORECLOSED NARRATIVE?

Recently, I undertook some research with older adults who appear to resist stories of inevitable, age-associated physical decline through their involvement in natural bodybuilding. There were 10 participants in total: 8 males and 2 females, ranging in age from 53 to 73. These individuals assert that their method of developing a symmetrical, proportioned, and muscular physique is more focused on a healthy lifestyle than on other forms of bodybuilding.[1] Using lifestory interviews and a range of visual methods, including auto-photography (see Phoenix, 2009; in press) and researcher-created images, one of my purposes was to explore how these individuals story their aging process and, in doing so, give meaning to their aging bodies.

The analyses of these spoken and visual narratives illustrated disparities between common assumptions regarding the aging body reflected in the narrative of decline (i.e., physical deterioration, lack of future trajectory) and the participants' actual experiences of embodied aging. For example, one salient storyline that emerged from the analyses was that of *lifelong learning*. This storyline opposed notions of a "finished personality," "certain stagnation," and "the way leading downward," as depicted in the life curve (Eichberg, 2000, p. 91), by emphasizing a sense of *ongoing accumulation of knowledge* over time. This was relative to their involvement in natural bodybuilding, as shown in the following comments from Carol, age 56:

> I think I'm learning more now than when I was younger. I'm learning because of dieting for contests and things. I understand more about how my body works and what foods to eat, the right foods to eat. I know what will make me fat. I know what foods I fancy and what I shouldn't eat, the so-called healthy foods. I know things that I could get away with before, but try not to eat so much of now.... So yes, I'm still on a learning curve. You know that you've got things wrong at times, but you learn as you go along. I'm still learning. I'm still learning new training methods, and I think I'm working with my body better as time goes on.

The participants described how their involvement in natural bodybuilding enabled physical training, dieting, and competition to be experienced. In turn, this provided them with a sense of progress through facilitating learning and an accumulation of embodied knowledge over time.

A second storyline that emerged as being salient to the mature body-builders reflected their *experiences of competition.* Competing in natural bodybuilding contests offered a sense of purpose toward which the partici-pants' disciplined lifestyles were directed. It also provided them with an opportunity to perform on stage with and through their aging, trained bodies. The strict preparatory procedures (dieting, gym training, and so forth) that were followed prior to the event, along with competition day itself, supported different forms of embodiment that are perhaps less typically associated with aging. This issue was highlighted in Bill's rich description of what com-peting in natural bodybuilding competitions involved:

> It's hard to describe to people who are not involved, the buzz and the excitement and the adrenaline rush you get when you're at these competitions. The really hard training is done between four and eight months before the competition, when you're going to the gym and you're really pushing things as hard as you can. Coming near the competition, those last four months, you start to train smarter, your rest periods are cut down, you're maybe going to use less weight but you're going to be resting less between your sets, and you're starting to think more about your diet. You're cutting out a lot of the food which is not doing you much good—the junk food, as they call it. You start to eat a bit cleaner and then again as the competition gets nearer, that diet becomes even more important. You eat really clean: chicken, fish, rice, sweet potatoes, rice, eggs, oatmeal. Your food supplements are very important. The last couple of weeks before [the competition], you're not eating any junk food at all. That's when you can really feel things happening to your body.... On the day itself, it's a lovely feeling. To go up there and stand on the stage doing my compulsory poses and my routine, well, it's a feeling that I would not have believed all those years ago. I didn't think it was possible to feel the way I feel about what I do now.

Echoing many of the other participants, Bill's experiences of preparing for and participating in bodybuilding competitions contrasted with those more usually associated with older exercisers. The meaning of exercise in old age, as signaled in the life curve model, is associated with the idea of preserving motion, and of general health and well-being (Eichberg, 2000). In the latter half of one's life, it is generally understood or presumed that less intense leisure pursuits will be undertaken. Lawn-bowling, walking, gentle swim-ming, and so forth are the types of activities deemed especially suited to the aging body. However, within the literature on sport and health sciences, and on sociology, so Rylee Dionigi (2008) and Emmanuelle Tulle (2008) have argued, these stereotypical assumptions regarding "appropriate" exercise habits of older adults can further reinforce the narrative of decline and construct older people as a homogenous population who are not interested in being competitive, achieving personal bests, or being able to exercise at physically intense levels. As a reflexive body project, Bill was acutely aware of these cultural expectations placed upon his aging body and explained how he had negotiated them:

> When you were younger, you just think in your mind that, when you're old, you have to sit in a chair, once you reach a certain age, you just sit in a chair, do a nice gentle walk, or you go down to the pub and sit. You think that you can't go to a gym and train because your body couldn't cope with it. But what I've found is that by keeping my body doing it [lifting weights] all those years, my body is accustomed to it and doesn't know anything else.

For all of the participants, living through an aging athletic body in such a way that could challenge cultural expectations about growing older was a positive experience. Their stories depicted notions of purposefulness as opposed to stagnation, and progress as opposed to decline and deterioration. Thus, while powerful and potentially oppressive, on this occasion, the narrative of decline appeared vulnerable and subject to subtle contestation. The stories told by the mature natural bodybuilders showed that a gap can exist between what the master narrative (i.e., narrative of decline) demands of certain people (i.e., older adults) and what some of those people actually do or are. This, of course, contrasts with the young athletes' perceptions of their future and beliefs about aging. In this instance, stories of the athletic self can act as a counterstory.

For philosopher Hilde Nelson (2001), *counterstories* are the stories that people tell and live that offer resistance to dominant cultural narratives. It is in their telling and living, suggests Andrews (2004), that people can become aware of new possibilities. Becoming aware of new possibilities, however, is not restricted only to individuals telling counterstories. Rather, as I illustrated earlier in this chapter, older adults—as projectors of narrative maps of aging—can influence the types of stories that younger generations tell about their aging bodies. Living and telling counterstories through one's aging, athletic body, such as that witnessed with the mature natural bodybuilders, might be a fruitful way of directing young people toward alternative storylines about aging. In doing so, it might challenge the unreflexive social reproduction of storylines about growing old and loosen the hold of

narrative foreclosure. The value of this process is apparent when the dominant storyline—such as the narrative of decline—can be harmful and
oppressive for individuals as they attempt to give meaning to their life as
a whole.

REFLECTIVE COMMENTS

In this chapter, I have highlighted the ways in which a population of young
athletes gave meaning to the notion of self-aging by drawing upon narrative
maps that portrayed information about growing old. These maps were
intertwined with the life curve model. I proposed that the narrative resources
currently available to young athletes can potentially restrict their ability to
construct meaningful stories about their aging bodies and ultimately lead to
a sense of narrative foreclosure. As a means of reopening a foreclosed narrative, I then suggested that alternative and varied storylines relating to aging
should be offered and that the stories told by mature natural bodybuilders
may be suited to this task. The stories that these older adults told about their
bodies seemed to have the potential to act as counterstories to the narrative
of decline by foregrounding purposefulness and progress.

All of this, however, is not to celebrate the athletic body over and above
other types of bodies as they age. As I indicated in the previous section, this
strategy can be problematic if and when the ability to be physically active in
older age becomes a marker of successful aging. To champion the aging,
athletic body in such a manner could, as Nelson (2001) warns, simply replace
one oppressive master narrative with another. That is, what of those who do
not have the ability, financial resources, or indeed desire to engage in serious
physical leisure in later life? These questions require a degree of critical
awareness when discussing, for example, the potential of older athletic
bodies for challenging the narrative of decline.

That noted, I would argue that these issues should not steer narrative
gerontologists away from the stories told by athletic bodies across the life
course. It is my belief that they have much to offer our understanding of the
intricate relationships between the body, narrative, and growing old. They
can also provide insight into the role of intergenerational relationships and
the transmission of stories between different aged bodies within a specific
context (i.e., physical culture). Of course, there is still much to be learned
regarding whether or not providing additional and alternative storylines
about the aging process has any bearing on how young people anticipate
their own aging bodies. But that, as they say, is another story.

NOTE

¹ Natural bodybuilders are routinely tested for illegal substances (via urine samples and/or polygraph tests) and are banned from future contests for any violations. They assert that their method of developing a symmetrical, proportioned, and muscular physique is more focused on a healthy lifestyle and competition than are other forms of bodybuilding. What qualifies as illegal substances are those prohibited by regulatory bodies, not only those that are illegal under the laws of the relevant jurisdiction. For example, anabolic steroids, prohormones, and diuretics are generally banned in natural organizations. Natural bodybuilders must have been "drug free" for a set period of time (from 5 years to "life," depending on the organization) in order to align themselves with natural bodybuilding federations.

REFERENCES

Andrews, M. (2004). Opening to the original contributions, counter-narratives and the power to oppose. In M. Bamberg & M. Andrews (Eds.), *Considering counter-narratives, narrating, resisting, making sense* (pp. 1–6). Philadelphia: John Benjamins.

De Vries, B., Blando, J., Southard, P., & Bubeck, C. (2001). The times of our lives. In G. Kenyon, P. Clark, & B. de Vries (Eds.), *Narrative gerontology: Theory, research and practice* (pp. 137–158). New York: Springer.

Dionigi, R. (2008). *Competing for life: Older people, sport and ageing.* Saarbrüken, Germany: VDM.

Eichberg, H. (2000). Life cycle sports: On movement culture and ageing. In J. Hansen & N. Nielsen (Eds.), *Sports, body and health.* Odense, Denmark: Odense University Press.

Frank, A. (1995). *The wounded storyteller: Body, illness, and ethics.* Chicago: University of Chicago Press.

Freeman, M. (2000). When the story's over: Narrative foreclosure and the possibility of self-renewal. In M. Andrews, S. Sclatter, C. Squire, & A. Treader (Eds.), *Lines of narrative* (pp. 81–91). London: Routledge.

Gullette, M. (2004). *Aged by culture.* Chicago: University of Chicago Press.

Holstein, J., & Gubrium, J. (2004). Context: Working it up, down and across. In C. Seale, G. Gobo, J. Gubrium, & D. Silverman (Eds.), *Qualitative research practice* (pp. 297–331). London: Sage.

Lieblich, A., Tuval-Mashiach, R., & Zilber, T. (1998). *Narrative research: Reading, analysis, and interpretation.* London: Sage.

Markus, H., & Nurius, P. (1986). Possible selves. *American Psychologist, 41*(9), 954–969.

McCullough, L. (1993). Arrested aging: The power of the past to make us aged and old. In T. Cole, W. Achenbaum, P. Jakobi, & R. Kastenbaum (Eds.). *Voices and visions of aging: Toward a critical gerontology* (pp. 184–204). New York: Springer.

Neikrug, S. (2003). Worrying about frightening old age. *Aging & Mental Health, 7,* 326–333.

Nelson, H. (2001). *Damaged identities, narrative repair.* Ithaca, NY: Cornell University Press.

Phoenix, C. (2009). Auto-photography in auto-biographical research: Exploring the life of a mature bodybuilder. In A. Sparkes (Ed.), *Auto/Biography yearbook 2008*. Nottingham, UK: Russell Press.

Phoenix, C. (in press). Auto-photography in aging studies: Exploring issues of identity construction in mature bodybuilders. *Journal of Aging Studies*.

Phoenix, C., Smith, B., & Sparkes, A. (2007). Experiences and expectations of bio-graphical time among young athletes: A life course perspective. *Time and Society*, *16*(2/3), 231–252.

Phoenix, C., Smith, B., & Sparkes, A. (2010). Narrative analysis in aging studies: A typology for consideration. *Journal of Aging Studies 24*, 1–11.

Phoenix, C., & Sparkes, A. (2006a). Young athletic bodies and narrative maps of aging. *Journal of Aging Studies*, *20*, 107–121.

Phoenix, C., & Sparkes, A. (2006b). Keeping it in the family: Narrative maps of ageing and young athletes' perceptions of their futures. *Ageing and Society*, *26*, 631–648.

Phoenix, C., & Sparkes, A. (2007). Sporting bodies, ageing, narrative mapping and young team athletes: An analysis of possible selves. *Sport, Education and Society*, *12*(1), 1–17.

Phoenix, C., & Sparkes, A. (2008). Athletic bodies and aging in context: The narra-tive construction of experienced and anticipated selves in time. *Journal of Aging Studies*, *22*, 211–221.

Phoenix, C., & Sparkes, A. (2009). Being Fred: Big stories, small stories and the accomplishment of a positive ageing identity. *Qualitative Research*, *9*(2), 83–99.

Pollner, M., & Stein, S. (1996). Narrative mapping of social worlds: The voice of experience in Alcoholics Anonymous. *Symbolic Interaction*, *19*(3), 203–223.

Randall, W., & McKim, A. (2008). *Reading our lives: The poetics of growing old*. New York: Oxford University Press.

Smith, B. (2007). The state of the art in narrative inquiry. *Narrative Inquiry*, *17*(2), 391–398.

Somers, M. (1994). The narrative constitution of identity: A relational and network approach. *Theory and Society*, *23*, 605–649.

Sparkes, A. (2004). Bodies, narratives, selves and autobiography: The example of Lance Armstrong. *Journal of Sport & Social Issues*, *28*(4), 397–428.

Tulle, E. (2008). *Ageing, the body and social change: Running in later life*. Basingstoke, UK: Palgrave.

Zilber, T., Tuval-Mashiach, R., & Lieblich, A. (2008). The embedded narrative: Navigating through multiple contexts. *Qualitative Inquiry*, *14*(6), 1047–1069.

Nine

THE RAGING GRANNIES: NARRATIVE

CONSTRUCTION OF GENDER AND AGING

Linda Caissie

People naturally tell stories to explain experiences or events to others. Increasingly, social scientists are exploring the meaning and value of story-telling, and narrative in general, in understanding human behavior (Kenyon, 1996). However, there has been very little study of the role of narrative in social movements, despite the abundance of stories that can be found within such movements and among activists themselves (Davis, 2002). My aim in this chapter is to try and fill some of this gap by discussing how the Raging Grannies, a group of older women activists, challenge the social construction of age and gender through their collective stories and provide a powerful "counterstory" to dominant narratives of both (Gimlin, 2007; Gullette, 2004; Nelson, 2001). What is unique about the Raging Grannies is that they call into question not only stereotypes of women activists but also negative images of older women generally in a society that places so much value on youth.

Many older women (i.e., 55 and over) who spent their earlier years in solitary work and/or in nurturing husbands and children are now discover-ing the external world of activism, politics, and social causes because of less pressure to conform to societal expectations (Heilbrun, 1988; Steinem, 1994). Even during the first and second waves of feminism, there were many exam-ples of older women being involved in activism. According to Steinem (1994), the nineteenth-century wave was started by older women who had been through the experience of getting married, giving birth, and becoming the legal property of their husbands—or, alternatively, the experience of not getting married and of being treated as spinsters, which limited their freedom. Even during the second wave of feminism, many early activists of the 1960s were organized by women who had experienced the civil rights movement or by homemakers who had discovered that raising children and doing housework did not occupy all their talents. Many older women were also holding press conferences and giving speeches on social issues. At the time of the second wave, most women in their teens and 20s had not yet experienced one or more of the major life-changing events of a woman's life: getting married and discovering that marriage is not an egalitarian institution (yet can be a violent one); entering the paid labor force and experiencing its limits, from the corporate "glass ceiling" to the "sticky floor" of the pink-collar ghetto; having children and finding out who takes care of them and who does not; and finally, aging itself, still the most impoverishing event for many women. Yet, as Steinem (1994) points out, the academic literature, including the literature on feminist theory, fails to recognize older women involved in activism. Further, many feminist groups still judge older women by age instead of individuality, and are concerned more about attracting younger women than about including older ones, even though the "older years can provide role models of energized, effective, and political older women" (p. 250).

WHO ARE THE RAGING GRANNIES?

According to Acker and Brightwell (2004), the Raging Grannies are a group of older women who have ideas about what is wrong with society and how to make it right. They began in Victoria, British Columbia, Canada, in 1987 and eventually spread across the country, with some "gaggles"—or chapters—forming in the United States, England, and Australia, as well (Acker & Brightwell, 2004; Roy, 2004). The Grannies are made up of mainly Caucasian, middle-class, educated older women, approximately 52 to 67 years of age, and represent a variety of backgrounds—teachers, nurses, artists, homemakers—and statuses: married, widowed, or never married. The first gaggle, in 1987, was formed to protest the U.S. Navy nuclear warships in the water surrounding Victoria. After not being taken seriously because they were regarded as old women, they decided "to break the stereotype of nice but negligible grandmothers by becoming outrageous" (Acker & Brightwell, 2004, p. xi) in order to gain attention and to challenge the status quo.

The Grannies use creative street theater as their method of protest (Acker & Brightwell, 2004; Roy, 2004). They dress in colorful, outrageous clothing as a spoof of older-women stereotypes. They also employ a number of props, such as flowers, umbrellas with holes (to represent acid rain), laundry baskets of women's undergarments (to represent their "briefs"), and banners, so as to draw attention to their message in a peaceful yet effective manner. The Grannies are most noted for their use of humor through cheeky satirical songs to express their social and political views. They have also attended presentations, conferences, speeches, and hearings uninvited, as a method of action. Despite their street theater, Grannies do not wish to be known as entertainers; they wish only to "make waves and make people listen" (Acker & Brightwell, 2004, p. 13), and to challenge the view of aging women.

METHODS

The main goal of my study was to gather and interpret narratives of older women involved with the Raging Grannies. Guiding me was the perspective of a feminist gerontology. According to Ray (2004), in feminist-inspired research and practice, dialogue, exchange, conversation, engagement, and response are placed at the forefront. In addition, feminist researchers recognize the importance of women's stories (Reinharz, 1994) and the fact that women narrate and interpret their lifestories differently from men (Kealey-McRae, 1994). The aim of feminist gerontology is to improve the negative images of older women by challenging negative stereotypes of them and emphasizing women's development over the entire life course. Furthermore, it provides the necessary insight to examine ageism and age relations more deeply (Calasanti, 2004; Ray, 2004).

One criticism of feminist literature has been its lack of recognition of older women. Instead, it has often focused on issues surrounding younger women and middle-aged women, such as reproductive rights and childcare; issues pertaining to older women have been neglected. Nonetheless, feminist gerontologists believe that feminism has played a vital role in contributing to the study of women and aging (Garner, 1999; O'Beirne, 1999). While feminism continues to seek social change and individual empowerment as mechanisms for enhancing women's lives, feminist gerontology acknowledges the dual importance of social action and individual empowerment as tools to enhance the lives of *older* women. In addition, feminist gerontology recognizes that older women not only connect with one another by telling stories about their lives but also validate their current worth through collective problem-solving and through using the skills and strengths they identify in sharing their stories. One manner in which older women can develop new roles, empower themselves, and identify their strengths is through activism (Garner, 1999).

In my study, I employed an interpretive paradigm, which is rooted in the belief that a researcher can gain an understanding about persons and their lives from everyday conversations and observations (Sanker & Gubrium, 1994). I therefore used qualitative methods to gather my data "to understand social life by taking into account the meaning, the interpretive process of social actors, and the cultural, social, and situational contexts in which these processes occur" (Jaffe & Miller, 1994, p. 52). In searching for meaning, the focus of interpretive research is on the taken-for-granted and common-sense understandings that people have about their lives. As well, interpretive researchers presume that social phenomena are best understood from the participants' own perspectives and so encourage them to speak in their own voices (Babbie, 2001; Lincoln & Guba, 1985).

My primary method of gathering these women's narratives was via in-depth active interviews (Holstein & Gubrium, 1995). Twenty-one Raging Grannies agreed to participate in the study. The questions I asked were open-ended in nature to allow them the freedom to refuse to respond, if they wished, yet at the same time enable me to probe beyond their answers (Berg, 1995; Reinharz, 1992). Open-ended questions permit an interviewer to understand and capture the world as seen by the participants themselves without predetermining their reality through the prior selection of questionnaire categories (Patton, 2002). In-depth, active interviews are used to collect detailed, information-rich narratives focused on the collaboration between interviewer and participant (Holstein & Gubrium, 1995). Active interviews also benefit participants by permitting them to share their stories in their own voices, an opportunity that is important to provide insofar as storytelling can be rich in personal meanings (Kenyon, 1996). In addition, open-ended interviewing offers researchers access to participants' ideas, thoughts, and memories using participants' own words rather than those of the researcher (Reinharz, 1992).

DISCUSSION

Throughout their stories of involvement in the Raging Grannies, it was evident that the women I interviewed resisted traditional gender roles and challenged the stereotypes of older women. While some older women conform to societal expectations, others challenge these prescribed gender roles. The following is a discussion of the Grannies' *counternarratives* in relation to a range of broad themes: defining one's self; reclaiming "old"; reclaiming public space; the strength of a women's community; and the power of humor and music. As explained by Perkins-Young (2006, p. 4), a counternarrative "demonstrates how the narrator does not think, feel, or behave the way the dominant structure says she is supposed to" (see also Nelson, 2001; Personal Narratives Group, 1989).

Defining One's Self

Gender is not a one-time identity that is acquired through socialization and remains unchanged throughout one's life. Consequently, past the age of 50, many women (and men) have the opportunity to resist traditional gender roles because they no longer have the social expectations of their youth—for example, the focus on finding a spouse, getting married, having children, and establishing a career. Older women have greater opportunities for developing identities other than wife, mother, or paid worker and for taking on new roles and activities that they may not have had time for when younger. They may now have choices and new opportunities to continue learning and growing through their continuing abilities and expanding interests (Arber, Davidson, & Ginn, 2003; Calasanti & Slevin, 2001; Morell, 2003; Silver, 2003).

During the interviews, I asked participants to tell me about themselves. The Grannies provided a variety of stories that indicated how they defined themselves, and in so doing, revealed that they shared similar social identities and values. They would first describe themselves, however, as "an activist," "a feminist," "a rabble-rouser," "a retired professor," or "an educator" before mentioning, for instance, that they were married or had grandchildren. They did not define themselves immediately in terms of traditional gender roles. It was not until much later in the interviews, in fact, that I realized some of them were indeed married or had grandchildren. The Grannies would actually stress their abilities and interests, for instance, their involvement in activism, their love for music or street theater, and their interest in social justice. Explained Granny Edith, "I'm an activist and feminist . . . have been a feminist since the 60s . . . read all those feminist writers. . . . My parents were even shocked over my feminist views." She also defined herself as a wise older woman: "I became a crone at 55 years old when I entered my third stage of life . . . and I am a hard worker and have a good attitude." Granny Dorothy, too, defined herself as an activist and feminist:

> I am an activist and feminist and I have been since I was about 25. . . . Yes,
> I would describe myself as a feminist. . . . It didn't come when I was a lot
> younger like some are more active in their teens and that sort of stuff but

certainly women's issues and gender analysis and that sort of thing has
always been fairly significant to me.

I also asked participants to describe the Raging Grannies group itself. Once
again, they would use images of older women that run counter to societal
expectations. As Granny Anne put it,

> It is a group of older ladies who care passionately about society, want to see
> injustices corrected; wherever possible, and are quite willing to make their
> point out in public; and we don't care if we look ridiculous but we would
> like you to listen and would like to get out there and be part of life so that
> people will listen.

Reclaiming "Old"

Gail Wilson (2002) discusses how older men and women are seen as "old"
before they are characterized in any other way, and how other attributes and
characteristics take second place to age. Being old becomes a person's main
social identity, something Wilson attributes to society's ageist attitudes
toward older adults in general. Nevertheless, she argues, there is a positive
side to ageism. Older adults have the opportunity to turn these negatives to
their benefit. For instance, "when you reach a certain age, if they don't like
what you say, they think you're a bit batty anyway, so you get away with it"
(p. 9). According to Calasanti and Slevin (2001), many older women are
reclaiming *old* by using the term in a positive way. Even researchers can be
guilty of using it in a negative way, especially when their research is focused
on such aspects of aging as disability and illness. Some researchers argue,
however, that *old* is only negative if we define it that way. By using *old age* in
positive ways, we are saying that there is nothing wrong with being old.

Based on my background in the sociology of aging, I assumed that being
older would be a topic the Grannies would be interested in speaking about.
I was mistaken. I was told on a number of occasions that being old was not
an issue. "One's attitude and spirit was what mattered," said Granny Lois.
They are not marginalized just because they are older women, as Granny
Margaret made clear: "I don't feel marginalized as an old woman because I
am not going to let people push me around. It's all in how you stand, present
yourself, and I present myself with confidence."

Age also gives a group of older women more of an advantage when
demonstrating. When describing the advantages of being older, Granny
Mary remarked that "older women as a group are more powerful." What
makes these older women more powerful? Some of the Grannies indicated
that, compared to a younger person, they can get away with more during

a protest. Said Granny Anne, "It is unlikely that . . . people would get violent with older women, so perhaps in a way we are cheating, you know, having the advantages of protest without the disadvantages." Granny Faith made a similar statement in discussing the advantages of being part of a group of older women: "We are old, so why would someone want to gather up a bunch of old women and put them in jail? So I guess in a way it is safer the way we are doing it now than when we were young." Like other Grannies, Granny Katherine spoke about the reluctance of the police to arrest old women: "The police won't hurt the Grannies because we are old ladies with silly hats on."

Many of the Grannies spoke about how as older women they have more freedom because they no longer have to follow the same societal expectations placed on women in general. They no longer have the obligations of family, work, body image, and so on. To quote Granny Beth, "There is a certain freedom in being in a group of older women doing things. A lot of the baggage of being younger is gone, so that you don't feel restricted. Older women as a group are more powerful, so that is sort of fun."

Likewise, Granny Dorothy, when speaking of the advantages of being with a group of older women, stated that older age means having more freedom to do what one pleases and being less self-conscious:

> I think . . . one of the things that we forgot when we were younger is that
> "oh, I am doing this for somebody else, I am doing this for the cause." You
> know, wait a minute, we are part of that cause too, and it's important that we
> look after ourselves as well. So I think that maybe that is a function of age
> in that somehow we have permission to look after ourselves and to do the
> things that we wish, and to see the activism in what we do as self-nurturing
> as well. This is where the age factor comes in, where we have worked so hard
> on so many things that it's time to have a little bit of fun also. There is also
> an internal getting away with it. There's an internal freedom that somehow
> what people think of you doesn't matter quite as much anymore.

When I first envisioned the Raging Grannies, I wondered if their persona was not reinforcing stereotypical images of older women. Also, through this persona, were they hiding their aging bodies? As a group of older women, could they be heard without wearing costumes? Many of the Grannies did admit that they could not protest without wearing their costumes, but it was not because they were old. Rather, the costumes gave them more self-confidence to be out in public and acted almost as a shield of protection. According to Biggs (1997), the use of persona is a coping strategy for maintaining an acceptable identity: "[T]he personae is simply a device through which an active agent looks out at and negotiates with the world, to protest and to deceive" (p. 559). The Raging Grannies are certainly not attempting to present a more youthful public image. On the contrary, said Granny Faith, "They are putting age out there."

More importantly, they are "making fun of the stereotypes with their costumes—it is all tongue in cheek," claimed Granny Katherine. The costume serves to grab people's attention in order to get their message out. It is one of the Grannies' symbolic tools of protest, and it is something they are enjoying as a way of expressing their creative side. Granny Faith made this comment when asked if their image reinforces traditional stereotypes:

> I don't think anyone has a stereotype of a granny looking like a Raging Granny. No, you deconstruct the stereotype when you do that. I don't think anyone sees us as grandmothers or the grandmotherly type. Reinforcing the stereotype is not what we are doing; it's not what we look like. I find there isn't a lot out there for older women like me, and older women are invisible in this culture and to put on weird costumes and sing as an older woman is quite strange and disruptive. We get looks because we are old; we are putting age out there.

Similarly, Granny Ingrid felt that their image was not reinforcing a stereotype:

> Oh, I don't think so. No, in fact it's almost breaking the stereotype. I mean are these older women sitting on the shelf? I don't think so. I think that is part of the reason why it's fun, we are changing the idea of what an older women should be.

Reclaiming Public Space

Traditionally, women's proper place has been in the home and men's place, in the public sphere. For over a century, women have been discouraged from entering many areas of public life (Day, 2001). The home is another place where power relations between women and men can be constructed (Browne, 1998; Massey, 1994). The phrase "a woman's place is in the home" is grounded in the gendered division of labor, which assigns women to the domestic sphere, where they are confined more often than men to domestic obligations and family commitments. Massey (1994) claims that the attempt to confine women to the private sphere has been both a spatial control and a societal control on identity. The identity of "woman" and of the "home place" are intimately entwined: "home is where the heart is and where the woman is also" (p. 180).

One method of resisting and redefining gender roles is by reclaiming public space (Day, 2001; Koskela, 1997; Massey, 1994). Doing so allows women to fill their space with whatever persons, objects, activities, or thoughts they may choose. Wearing (1998) suggests that women create their own spaces for spirituality, literature, support groups, and storytelling; for controlling financial and workplace stress; and for mental and physical pleasure—all on their own terms. Some feminist writers have argued that women have a history of using public spaces for social activism, where they have relied on noninstitutionalized or unconventional strategies to confront power structures (Boulding, 2000; Kuumba, 1991). Through their activism, the Raging Grannies are certainly reclaiming public space. They often march on the Parliament buildings in Ottawa, chanting, singing, and holding banners against a number of government policies, even putting on a skit in which they openly mock people in positions of power, i.e., politicians. They are also known for crashing political events, once considered the domain of white, middle-class men. The Grannies are not only reclaiming public space as older women but also refusing to be confined to their rocking chairs. As Granny Josephine explained, "We are not going to be relegated to wearing shawls and sitting in rocking chairs, in fact, we are going to get out there and take action." Granny Anne described her experience of being out in public, protesting, as follows:

> It's fun shaking people! Fairly enjoyable, perhaps it shouldn't be so enjoyable, although it's fun. It's an important part of who I am, who I was, and who I want to be. So I would say that it is . . . very important for me. I don't think I ever had a voice until I came here. I feel a freedom with the Raging Grannies to do anything that is me, and that is marvelous, right?

Granny Geraldine shared similar thoughts: "The Grannies is an opportunity to be my weird self. I can't talk about what I believe in many other places. Not that I couldn't do activism, but nobody would hear it. The Grannies give you a chance to be seen."

The Raging Grannies reclaim public space by expressing their anger and political concerns in spaces once dominated by men.

The Strength of a Women's Community

Another space where women provide counterstories or "progress narratives" of aging (Gullette, 2004), by challenging the social construction of age and gender alike, is in a women's community. Throughout the Grannies' narratives of being involved in a group of women, they often describe their community as having no hierarchical structure, but rather practicing collective decision-making in accordance with reciprocity and mutual respect. Their community involves social support through which their values and beliefs are reinforced with like-minded people working together for a common goal. The sharing of similar stories also assists in sustaining and strengthening a group member's commitment to change (Polletta, 2002). The Grannies often described being involved with a group of women as "the feeling of belonging to something bigger than oneself" (Granny Dorothy). Asked to describe what it was like to be involved with such a group, Granny Josephine answered,

> Activism is more fun with women. It's interesting and lively and motivating and I think there is a really nice feeling of camaraderie between us. The camaraderie and the idea of the local action [are] very satisfying. It inspires me. They are so strong and they have such power and will to continue, which energizes me.

Some of the feminist literature stresses the importance of women creating all-women environments, free from masculine values. Woman-centered culture is often focused on responsibility, connection, community, negotiation, and nurturance, in contrast to male culture, which is focused on self-interest, combat, and hierarchy. The Grannies I interviewed noted that, if men were allowed to join, they would attempt to dominate the group and allow the women little freedom to speak their minds. As Granny Ingrid pointed out, "Men discuss in a different way and they interact by taking authority. They don't have nearly as much empathy for people in the community as women do—they are just used to taking charge."

Boulding (2000) argues that women have a greater understanding of such social issues as violence, child poverty, and unemployment, because often they have been affected by these issues directly. The Grannies frequently mentioned that women had more empathy because of their nurturing side. As soon as my interview with Granny Beth began, she went into detail as to why the Raging Grannies should remain a women-only group, and why it was only "natural" for women to be organizers:

> Women are the ones who should be involved in activism because of their nurturing side. Women have always been doing this kind of work—just look at the volunteering in churches and hospitals. So if you want something done, ask a woman. Women get things done because as a group we communicate and delegate instead of fighting. A group of women are more powerful than a group of men because they are better at understanding both sides of an issue. If men were involved with the Raging Grannies, they would just take over and would try to dominant the group. Women also have fun together. We can laugh together and laugh at ourselves, while men take themselves way too seriously.

Interestingly, what caught my attention when the Grannies described their community were the stereotypical characteristics associated with feminine and masculine traits. By the same token, one must remember that the Grannies are inevitably influenced by the values and beliefs from their generation regarding gender roles (Rose, 2001). Some of the Grannies discussed how, in their generation, roles between men and women were much more defined than they are today. Granny Louise and Granny Helen explained, for instance, how women were more tied to the home and family, with men more tied to the workforce. Granny Helen also remarked that women of her generation were socialized to be more passive and quiet. I recall the interview with Granny Beth, who went on at length about how women have been always involved in caring work because of their "nurturing side," emphasizing stereotypical feminine traits. Nevertheless, being involved with a group of women gave the Grannies social support, collective action, camaraderie, and, no doubt, strength in numbers. Granny Ingrid noted the following when describing the advantages of being in such a group:

> The beauty of being with the Grannies is that there is safety in numbers. You can be more effective in a group of women than [as] one woman writing letters to the editor or writing petitions. It's like the next step from the individual is action in a group, and it's something about being older and wearing funny hats that diffuses hostility, for the most part. The people you are singing to may not always like the message you are singing, but they sort of forgive you because you are old and you look so funny with your hat; it's gestures crossed with humor, where there may be hostile actions otherwise.

Granny Lois also made an important statement regarding the exceptionality of a group consisting of older women:

> The very fact that [we are] a group of women in itself is a revolutionary thing because women as groups haven't done things like individual women who were tremendous, like Marion Parent who was the union leader or Emma Goldman. I mean these are extraordinary women, but they were individual people. But for a group of older women to get together and say "here we are" is exceptional.

The Power of Humor and Music

Women have a history of using nonviolent, creative methods of protest, including song, dance, poetry, humor, play, and symbolic imagery (Boulding, 2000; Kuumba, 1991). As discussed earlier, the Raging Grannies use street theater, cheeky songs, humor, play, and symbolic imagery as their principal methods. Kuumba (1991) has described some women involved in social protest using the only tools available to them: waving kitchen utensils or banging on pots and pans. The Grannies will also use props that are symbolic of who they are: umbrellas, spoons, pots, pans, mops, and even their own flag, namely the Canadian flag, except that the maple leaf is replaced by the picture of a Raging Granny. According to Kuumba (1991), the names that women pick for their groups are often symbolic and project a relevant image to which the public can relate. For example, using the term *mother* in the names of some groups projects a certain public image that could very well be used to the group's advantage. For the women I interviewed, the term *Raging Granny* had been carefully chosen. The women who began the first group were angry that the politicians and the public were not listening to older women and they blamed the ageist attitudes of society. *Granny* portrays the image of a "little old lady," yet rage (which represents their anger toward injustice) contradicts the stereotype of the "sweet little old lady."

Street (2003) claims that protest music can also be a means of resistance and empowerment for the group. Similarly to street theater, music can be used to have the message heard by the masses and challenge those in power without appearing threatening. Furthermore, compared with speeches, protest songs may reach more people and spread the group's message more effectively. Whereas a speech may be heard only once, songs are learned and repeated indefinitely. The songs, therefore, can perpetually promote and reinforce the messages of the group. While protest songs may not usually offer solutions to the perceived problem but are used mainly to criticize, educate, and evoke some sort of emotion, they are a vehicle to have the group's voice heard and to gain sympathy from its audience (Knupp, 1981).

Another effective tactic used by the Raging Grannies is humor, through their intentionally outrageous costumes and props and their satirical songs. The Grannies I interviewed repeatedly used humor and laughter to challenge power and express their desire to see change. Other women's groups, according to some feminist scholars, use humor especially during actions related to the women's movement (Barreca, 1991; Crawford, 2003; Gillooly, 1991; Gouin, 2004; Robinson & Smith-Lovin, 2001). Traditionally, feminists evolved a distinctive humor as a powerful tool of political activism. Furthermore, women sharing humor and laughter can create solidarity through a shared sense of reality. As with protest music, humor can also define group identities. The use of humor and laughter can help create and affirm the group's own meanings. Developing a sense of identity and solidarity is the first step toward political and social change.

According to Crawford (2003), humor can be a way of challenging those in power, expressing opposition, and proposing change. Humor that involves mimicking politicians, religious leaders, or the rich and famous vents feelings, questions the justice of the hierarchy, and temporarily reverses the power. Humor and laughter can function as a socially acceptable release for anxiety, especially if the group is conveying a message that some may find controversial. Making light of a situation can ease a situation that is uncomfortable while, at the same time, getting one's message across. Furthermore, women who use supposedly inappropriate humor are actually deconstructing traditional gender roles (Robinson & Smith-Lovin, 2001). Although the literature on women and humor tends not to address older women, the Raging Grannies are also resisting traditional gender roles through their use of humor, especially since some of their lyrics may be regarded by the general public as inappropriate for little old ladies. As Granny Edith observed, "We grab attention because people can't believe the audacity of older women doing this and their blatant disregard for everything other people think that is normal—their crazy hats, in-your-face mocking lyrics. . . . We sound so defiant. . . . We go against the grain."

CONCLUSION

Many older adults regard old age as an opportunity for continued development, given the knowledge of accumulated experiences that comes with their mature years (Auger & Tedford-Little, 2002; Friedan, 1993; Hatcher, 1994; Kaufman, 1986). For many, old age is the culminating chapter of a lifetime's work. Perhaps one's political philosophy becomes modified, yet one's basic belief remains the same. Attitudes and behaviors based on a sense of civic duty that began early in life will often continue, therefore, into later life, because one has developed the necessary skills for working toward social change (Burr, Caro, & Moorhead, 2002).

In the view of some researchers, moreover, now that the women's movement is maturing, so are the younger feminist activists who bring their common life experiences with them into their mature years (Liss, Crawford, & Popp, 2004; Polleta & Jasper, 2001; Reinharz, 1997). Older activists can carry their acquired skills and knowledge into old age to continue working for social change. In addition, older women can use the past as source material from which to challenge stereotypical views of older women (Biggs, 1997). With the knowledge they have gathered through their life experiences, they now have the tools to form collective action, as well as to empower themselves through the creation of spaces where relationships are built on feelings of trust, reciprocity, and commonality and are developed through continued interaction and a sense of belonging, acceptance, affirmation, and mutual aid (Browne, 1998; Cox & Parsons, 1996; MacRae, 1990; Narushima, 2004). Thus, the Raging Grannies have provided the space and the environment where these older women have the opportunity to not only seek social justice but also assist in challenging the conventional image of older women as weak, passive, and dependent and in transforming it into one in which they are strong, political, and independent.

Activism has provided these women a tool of empowerment by taking control through the selection of their own symbols, situations, and people and by challenging prevailing master narratives (Benford, 2002; Brown, 2002; Gullette, 2004). As Granny Katherine expressed it, activism is "giving the Raging Grannies the opportunity to come together as a community to educate and make a better world." Moreover, activism gives them freedom from the expectations of their youth. In the words of Granny Beth, "There is a freedom being with other older women. There's a freedom away from younger expectations."

The Raging Grannies remind me of a group of older women called the Hen Co-op, who write about challenging the traditional views of growing old and write poetry as well. Like the Grannies, the Hen Co-op (1993) comes from a generation that was socialized to put their own needs aside in order to attend to others. Some had had demanding jobs both outside and inside their homes, which left them little time for self-nurturing. However, they had reached a period in their lives when their work obligations were reduced. Now they had found the time to connect with other older women and reinvent themselves. They decided to grow old disgracefully:

> We use "growing old disgracefully" as a challenge to the image of "growing old gracefully," which implies that we are to be silent, invisible, compliant and selflessly available for the needs of others. In other words, to age gracefully is to continue to be the passive, obedient, unobtrusively good girls we were socialized to be. Well, we're not prepared to do that; we're going to make up for lost time. (1993, p. 106)

The Raging Grannies provide other older women with stories of empowerment by offering counterstories (Nelson, 2001) that challenge the "narrative of decline" (Gullette, 2004). For these women are not passively *getting* old but actively *growing* old (Randall & McKim, 2008). By reading the Raging Grannies' stories, younger women can draw upon the "narrative maps" (Phoenix & Sparkes, 2006; Pollner & Stein, 1996; Phoenix, this volume) that the Grannies provide as they formulate their own maps of aging and redefine their own aging selves.

REFERENCES

Acker, A., & Brightwell, B. (2004). *Off our rockers and into trouble: The Raging Grannies.* Victoria, Canada: TouchWood Editions.

Arber, S., Davidson, K., & Ginn, J. (2003). Changing approaches to gender and later life. In S. Arber, S. Davidson, & J. Ginn (Eds.), *Gender and ageing: Changing roles and relationships* (pp. 1–14). Maidenhead, UK: Open University Press.

Auger, J., & Tedford-Litle, D. (2002). *From the inside looking out: Competing ideas about growing old.* Halifax, Canada: Fernwood.

Babbie, E. (2001). *The practice of social research* (9th ed.). Belmont, CA: Wadsworth/ Thomson Learning.

Barreca, R. (1991). *They used to call me Snow White but I drifted: Women's strategic use of humor.* New York: Penguin.

Benford, R. (2002). Controlling narratives and narratives as control within social movements. In J. Davis (Ed.), *Stories of change: Narrative and social movements* (pp. 53–78). Albany, NY: State University of New York Press.

Berg, B. (1995). *Qualitative research methods for the social sciences* (2nd ed.). Boston: Allyn & Bacon.

Biggs, S. (1997). Choosing not to be old? Masks, bodies and identity management in later life. *Ageing and Society, 17,* 553–570.

Boulding, E. (2000). *Cultures of peace: The hidden side of history.* Syracuse, NY: Syracuse University Press.

Brown, M. (2002). Moving toward the light: Self, other, and the politics of experience in New Age narratives. In J. Davis (Ed.), *Stories of change: Narrative and social movements* (pp. 101–122). Albany, NY: State University of New York Press.

Browne, C. (1998). *Women, feminism, and aging.* New York: Springer.

Burr, J., Caro, F., & Moorhead, J. (2002). Productive aging and civic participation. *Journal of Aging Studies, 16,* 87–105.

Calasanti, T. (2004). New directions in feminist gerontology: An introduction. *Journal of Aging Studies, 18,* 1–8.

Calasanti, T., & Slevin, K. (2001). *Gender, social inequalities, and aging.* Walnut Creek, CA: Altamira Press.

Cox, E., & Parsons, R. (1996). Empowerment-oriented social work practice: Impact on late life relationships of women. *Journal of Women & Aging, 8*(3/4), 129–143.

Crawford, M. (2003). Gender and humour in social context. *Journal of Pragmatics, 35,* 1413–1430.

Davis, J. (2002). Narrative and social movements: The power of stories. In J. Davis (Ed.), *Stories of change: Narrative and social movements* (pp. 3–30). Albany, NY: State University of New York Press.

Day, K. (2001). The ethic-of-care and women's experiences of public space. *Journal of Environmental Psychology, 20,* 103–124.

Friedan, B. (1993). *The fountain of age.* New York: Simon & Schuster.

Garner, J. (1999). Feminism and feminist gerontology. In J. Garner (Ed.), *Fundamentals of feminist gerontology* (pp. 3–12). New York: The Haworth Press.

Gillooly, E. (1991). Women and humor. *Feminist Studies, 17*(3): 472–492.

Gimlin, D. (2007). Constructions of ageing and narrative resistance in a commercial slimming group. *Ageing & Society, 27,* 407–424.

Gouin, R. (2004). "What's so funny?": Humour in women's accounts of their involvement in social action. *Qualitative Research, 4*(1), 25–44.

Gullette, M. (2004). *Aged by culture.* Chicago: University of Chicago Press.

Hatcher, S. (1994). Personal rights of passage: Stories of college youth. In A. Lieblich & R. Josselson (Eds.), *Exploring identity and gender: The narrative study of lives* (pp. 169–194). Thousand Oaks, CA: Sage.

Heilbrun, C. (1988). *Writing a woman's life.* New York: W. W. Norton.

Hen Co-op. (1993). *Growing old disgracefully: New ideas for getting the most out of life.* London: Piatkus.

Holstein, J., & Gubrium, J. (1995). *The active interview.* Thousand Oaks, CA: Sage.

Jaffe, D., & Miller, E. (1994). Problematizing meaning. In A. Sankar & J. F. Gubrium (Eds.), *Qualitative methods in aging research* (pp. 51–66). Thousand Oaks, CA: Sage.

Kaufman, S. (1986). *The ageless self: Sources of meaning in late life.* Madison, WI: University of Wisconsin Press.

Kealey McRae, S. (1994). A woman's story· E pluribus unum. In A. Lieblich & R. Josselson (Eds.), *Exploring identity and gender: The narrative study of lives* (pp. 195–229). Thousand Oaks, CA: Sage.

Kenyon, G. (1996). The meaning/value of personal storytelling. In J. Birren, G. Kenyon, J.-E. Ruth, J. Schroots, & T. Svensson (Eds.), *Aging and biography: Explorations in adult development* (pp. 21–38). New York: Springer.

Knupp, R. (1981). A time for every purpose under heaven: Rhetorical dimensions of protest music. *Southern Communication Journal, 46*(4), 377–389.

Koskela, H. (1997). "Bold walk and breakings": Women's spatial confidence versus fear of violence. *Gender, place, and culture, 4*(3), 301–319.

Kuumba, M. (2001). *Gender and social movements.* Walnut Creek, CA: Altamira Press.

Lincoln, Y., & Guba, E. (1985). *Naturalistic inquiry.* Beverly Hills, CA: Sage.

Liss, M., Crawford, M., & Popp, D. (2004). Predictors and correlates of collective action. *Sex Roles, 50*(11/12), 771–779.

MacRae, H. (1990). Older women and identity in later life. *Canadian Journal of Aging, 9*(3), 248–267.

Massey, D. (1994). *Space, place, and gender.* Minneapolis: University of Minnesota Press.

Morell, C. (2003). Empowerment and long-living women: Return to the rejected body. *Journal of Aging Studies, 17,* 69–85.

Narushima, M. (2004). A gaggle of Raging Grannies: The empowerment of older Canadian women through social activism. *International Journal of Lifelong Education, 23*(1), 23–42.

Nelson, H. (2001). *Damaged identities: Narrative repair.* Ithaca, NY: Cornell University Press.

O'Beirne, N. (1999). Growing older, getting better: Than what? In J. Onyx, R. Leonard, & R. Reed (Eds.), *Revisioning aging* (pp. 8–12). New York: Peter Lang.

Patton, M. (2002). *Qualitative research and evaluation methods* (3rd ed.). Thousand Oaks, CA: Sage.

Perkins-Young, P. (2006). *How late middle-aged women define contributions in counter-narrative and narratives of acceptance.* [Doctoral dissertation]. Fielding Graduate University. UMI Microfilm #3205511.

Personal Narratives Group (Ed.). (1989). *Interpreting women's lives: Feminist theory and personal narratives.* Bloomington, IN: Indiana University Press.

Phoenix, C., & Sparkes, A. (2006). Keeping it in the family: Narrative maps of ageing and young athletes' perceptions of their futures. *Ageing & Society, 26*, 631–648.

Polletta, F. (2002). Plotting protest: Mobilizing stories in the 1960 student sit-ins. In J. Davis (Ed.), *Stories of change: Narrative and social movements* (pp. 31–52). Albany, NY: State University of New York Press.

Polletta, F., & Jasper, J. (2001). Collective identity and social movements. *Annual Review of Sociology, 27*, 283–305.

Pollner, M., & Stein, S. (1996). Narrative mapping of social worlds: The voice of experience in Alcoholics Anonymous. *Symbolic Interaction, 19*, 203–223.

Randall, W., & McKim, A. (2008). *Reading our lives: The poetics of growing old.* New York: Oxford University Press.

Ray, R. (2004). Toward the croning of feminist gerontology. *Journal of Aging Studies, 18*, 109–121.

Reinharz, S. (1992). *Feminist methods in social research.* New York: Oxford University Press.

Reinharz, S. (1994). Feminist biography: The pains, the joys, the dilemmas. In A. Lieblich & R. Josselson (Eds.), *Exploring identity and gender: The narrative study of lives,* (pp. 39–82). Thousand Oaks, CA: Sage.

Reinharz, S. (1997). Friends or foe: Gerontological and feminist theory. In M. Pearsall, (Ed.), *The other within us: Feminist explorations of women and ageing* (pp. 73–94). Oxford, UK: Westview Press.

Robinson, D., & Smith-Lovin, L. (2001). Getting a laugh: Gender, status, and humor in task discussion. *Social Forces, 80*(1), 123–158.

Rose, S. (2001). New age women. *Women's Studies, 30*, 329–350.

Roy, C. (2004). *The Raging Grannies: Wild hats, cheeky songs, and witty actions for a better world.* Montreal, Canada: Black Rose Books.

Sankar, A., & Gubrium, J. (1994). Introduction. In J. Gubrium & A. Sankar (Eds.), *Qualitative methods in aging research* (pp. vii–xvii). Thousand Oaks, CA: Sage.

Silver, C. (2003). Gendered identities in old age: Toward (de)gendering? *Journal of Aging Studies, 17*, 379–397.

Steinem, G. (1994). *Moving beyond words.* New York: Simon & Schuster.

Street, J. (2003). "Fight the power": The politics of music and the music of politics. *Government and Opposition, 38*(1), 113–130.

Wearing, B. (1998). *Leisure and feminist theory.* London: Sage.

Wilson, G. (2002). "I'm the eyes and she's the arms": Changes in gender roles in advanced old age. In S. Arber & J. Ginn (Eds.), *Connecting gender and ageing: A sociological approach* (pp. 98–113). Buckingham, UK: Open University Press.

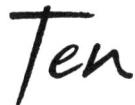
Ten

NARRATIVE AND GENDER DIFFERENCES: HOW MEN AND WOMEN INTERPRET THEIR LIVES

Patricia O'Neill, James E. Birren, and Cheryl Svensson

Gender role stereotypes have long been the premise on which male and female differences have been evaluated, and this chapter will discuss some of the research that has focused on these differences. This will be followed by an analysis of qualitative data from guided autobiographies to investigate the validity of gender stereotypes when men and women tell their own stories.

NARRATIVE, GENDER, AND AGE

Guided autobiography is a form of narrative life review that consists of theme-based autobiographical writing and the sharing of one's stories (Birren, 2006; Birren & Cochran, 2001; Birren & Deutchman, 1991). A narrative tells a person's story within a context, and context has unlimited forms—for example, race and ethnicity, socioeconomic background, geography, the culture and times in which one has lived, or the age, gender, and family of the storyteller (Ray, 1999/2000). Context depends not only on who the storyteller is but also on the audience, including those who analyze the stories, all of whom come from their own backgrounds and points of view (Ochberg, 1994).

The stories we tell reflect our personalities, and many believe that telling them helps to form our identities. How we organize the plots of our lives, how our audience responds, how we reorganize our stories to achieve an end that supports our self-esteem or self-concept—all of this happens repeatedly with ever-changing results throughout our lives (Ochberg, 1994; Ray, 2000). In the process, we may gain clarity and meaning from accumulated life experiences, resolve issues, and learn to accept ourselves and others (Birren, 2006).

In this investigation, we are particularly interested in how people interpret their lives within the context of gender and age. Men and women will certainly tell their stories differently. Women are more likely to express their emotions and be more verbal than men. Men may be more factual or chronological. In both cases, there is an expectation that traditional gender role ideologies will be represented (Ray, 1999/2000, 2000).

Likewise, as people age, their personalities change, so individuals of different ages will tend to tell their stories from different perspectives. Neugarten (1965/1996a), for example, observed that middle-aged storytellers see themselves as risk-takers, feeling empowered and using their narratives to problem-solve. Ray found that between ages 46 and 59, individuals are predisposed to restructuring and re-evaluating their identities, whereas older adults revert to more conventional behavior. Older adults, then, may take a broader perspective, exercise more caution in storytelling, emphasize the positive rather than the negative events in their lives, and distance themselves from both (Ray, 2000).

Neugarten posits that beginning in our 50s, our "inner life," or what she calls "interiority," becomes more important. We become more preoccupied with fulfilling our personal needs, less focused on others, more reflective, and concerned with controlling rather than responding to our environment (Neugarten, 1972/1996c).

Whatever age or gender, stories tend to reflect what is important to us, how we see ourselves in the greater scheme of things, how we think and what we feel about the events and outcomes of our personal histories (Kenyon, 2003). Accordingly, examining guided autobiographies should add to the literature on age and gender roles in a unique and effective way, as we explore what individuals say about their lives in their own words and how they interpret the causes of the outcomes of their lives.

HISTORICAL DIFFERENCES IN GENDER NORMS AND IDENTITY STATUS

Gender role expectations have historically been different for women and men. The female identity is inseparable from the ability to bear children and the need to nurture. Women are viewed as accommodators, destined to serve others, and fulfillment is dependent on their status as wife and mother. Identity formation is postponed to allow them to focus on interpersonal relationships (Anthis, Dunkel, & Anderson, 2003).

This interpersonal or relational aspect of women's identity is supported by several studies on social role theory which suggest that gender differences are learned through socialization of sex role expectations (Archer, 1996). According to social role theory, it is the mutual exchange of feelings and experiences that fosters closeness among women. Women desire greater intimacy than men. They are more "communal," more tender-hearted, more trusting and anxious than men, and more vulnerable in relationships. Women are expected to be compliant, responsible, reserved, and self-sacrificing (Archer, 1996). Social role theorists believe that whatever power women achieve is derived from respect and good will, earned from exhibiting gender-acceptable behavior (Barry & Beitel, 2006).

Gender role ideologies are also expected to manifest in personality traits. Women are believed to exhibit "expressive traits" such as gentility, affability, submissiveness, dependence, cooperation, and deference to and consideration of others. They are expected to be emotional, sensitive, warm, caring, and tactful, and to be promoters of harmony. In repeated tests during the 1980s, using the Bern Sex Role Inventory (BSRI), the most frequently identified expressive traits included being understanding, sympathetic, and loyal (Moore, 2007; Mueller & Dato-On, 2008).

In contrast, the same applications of the BSRI typically resulted in men being described as analytical, decisive, and assertive, and as demonstrating leadership abilities. These traits, identified as "agentic" and "instrumental," also include domination and control (Moore, 2007). Additionally, where women have historically been depicted as "interpersonal" and "relational," men have been defined as "intrapersonal," or occupational, as withholding personal thoughts and exercising emotional control, for fear of appearing vulnerable. Toughness, achievement, and stature are all qualities for which men have traditionally been socialized and by which they define themselves (Anthis, et al., 2003; Archer, 1996; Blazina, Pisecco, Cordova, & Settle, 2007; Brahnam, Margavio, Hignite, Barrier, & Chin, 2005).

Traditional gender role ideologies portray men as providers and decision-makers. They are seen as competent, ambitious, aggressive, independent, objective, and confident (Barry & Beitel, 2006; Mueller & Dato-On, 2008). Studies by social role theorists have found that men's relationships are based more on shared activities than on emotions. Traditional men do not depend on others, nor do they disclose intimacies about themselves or speak about personal matters. In contrast to women, most of the men in one study, for instance, could not even name their best friend (Archer, 1996).

The cumulative effect of traditional gender role ideologies for both sexes has been the creation and internalization of a rigid, interrelated belief system in which females are encouraged to become dependent and in need of protection, care, and support. Males, by contrast, are expected to be powerful, yet emotionally constricted (Snyder, 1997).

GENDER IDENTITY CROSSOVER

There is a considerable body of research suggesting that as men and women enter middle age, gender stereotypes weaken and individuals either become more androgynous or exchange traditional gender role ideologies for those of the opposite sex. Pioneering work in this regard was conducted by Bernice Neugarten and David Guttman in the 1960s, who used the "Thematic Apperception Test" (TAT), a construct based on a drawing that subjects aged 40–70 were asked to evaluate. Simplified, younger respondents identified the old man in the drawing as the authority figure and the old woman as submissive. Older respondents perceived the reverse. From this, the authors suggest that, as we age, women are more likely to integrate agentic qualities and men, communal traits (Neugarten, 1968).

Theories hypothesizing why this happens are largely advanced by Jung (as cited in Harker & Solomon, 1996) and Guttman (as cited in Harker & Solomon, 1996, and in Neugarten, 1979/1996b), both of whose views originate with the separation of powers among young couples raising children. According to Jung, childrearing and work form the fulcrum upon which society is balanced. Social mores designating women as caregivers and men as providers become self-fulfilling as women nurture children and men go out into the world to achieve. Activities and goals beyond the scope of these assigned roles are forfeited, and urges are suppressed until middle age, when one's direction becomes less focused on the needs of society and more focused on individuation or the integration of self. Moving from the same core belief, Guttman differs only to the extent that he views release from childrearing as a time when both men and women revert to their natural androgynous states.

Today there does not appear to be any real consensus as to whether androgyny, gender role reversal, or neither occurs, or whether this is unique to middle age, old age, or both. Further, the demarcation between middle and old age, if there is such a thing, is its own controversy (Lachman, 2004; Neugarten, 1987/1996d; Strough, Leszczynski, Neely, Flinn, & Margrett, 2007).

Of course, there are many influences that could account for the diversity of opinion. James, Lewkowicz, Libhaber, and Lachman (1995) reached inconsistent results when they tested using the TAT and self-reporting, subsequently arguing that crossover is both more complex than previously believed and more individual, related neither to parenting nor to age. The culture one grows up in, the relationship between one's own parents (e.g., weak father, strong mother), the degree to which one is dependent on one's spouse, or whether or not one's spouse is ill, are among the many potential restraints on midlife change (Huyck, 1999). There is also the cohort effect of historical events or cultural developments, such as the Great Depression or the feminist movement (Stewart, 1994; Strough et al., 2007). Finally, there is a question of how relevant the crossover hypothesis is in industrial societies today. As significantly more women have entered the workforce, particularly in classically male professions, some recent studies have found little or no crossover, or crossover only in traditional families (James et al., 1995).

Believing that autobiographical writings would provide us an uncommon perspective from which to study gender, we wanted to know whether they could help us achieve a greater understanding of how men and women interpret their lives at different ages. Therefore, as we read through each individual's narratives we asked the following questions: 1) Do traditional gender role ideologies explain differences in how men and women interpret their lives? 2) Is there a gender identity crossover at midlife?

METHOD

Participants

The original written narratives of 15 women and 13 men, enrolled in James Birren's Guided Autobiography class between 1981 and 1987, were selected from Birren's archives. At the time the documents were written, each participant was assigned a number to ensure anonymity. All of the original narratives were transcribed onto a disc. A file folder was created for each person, identified by his or her assigned number. The transcribed essays of each person were then placed into separate folders. Thereafter, participants' assigned numbers, their demographic information, and the number of themes they each wrote on were recorded on a Microsoft Excel spreadsheet.

Ages were available for 23 of the participants and ranged from 22 to 72, with a mean age of 50.2 and a median of 57.5. In all instances where birth years were unknown, it was possible to estimate the age of the participant. Consequently, as shown in Table 10.1, age is classified and coded by category.

Table 10.1 Description of sample (n = 28)

Age range	Code	Men		Women	
		n	%	n	%
20–40	3	2	7	6	22
41–65	4	9	32	9	32
>65	5	2	7	0	0

This was a highly educated sample. Only two of the participants (7%) were not college educated. The remaining 93% held college degrees or were enrolled in college at the time of the class. Thirty-two percent had PhD's, 18% had Master's degrees. Two of the participants were ministers and two were nuns. As information on race/ethnicity could not be determined for the majority of participants, it was not taken into consideration. Twenty-five participants were American or Canadian, two were European, and one was Asian.

Procedure

The narratives of all 28 participants were read and outlined in detail by the first author in order to gain an initial understanding of each person and how language was used to describe his or her life. The outlines were set aside for future reference. Several variations on narrative analysis were studied and a new model was developed. An Excel file was created for each participant, with two categories: traditionally masculine and traditionally feminine gender role expectations. To ensure consistency, a separate spreadsheet was devised listing all of the characteristics to be measured in each category. These characteristics were taken directly from the literature review.

A line-by-line appraisal of each participant's narratives was undertaken by the first author with relevant portions of text quoted verbatim and inserted into separate boxes on the spreadsheet under the appropriate category. The manner in which this was done is shown in Table 10.2. All expressions deemed relevant to a particular category were included, without exception. No discretion was exercised. The number of boxes a participant generated corresponds to the number of relevant statements that he or she made.

The spreadsheet of each participant was then independently evaluated by the authors to see whether men and women conformed to gender stereotypes.

Table 10.2 Sample spreadsheet for one participant by categories analyzed

Stereotypical masculine traits	Stereotypical feminine traits
Creating and maintaining a meaningful career is also another way I achieve fulfillment. Working gives my life real meaning.	Since childhood I have followed a path of service to the less fortunate in some way.

In each category, every text box was rated for the strength of the attribute relevant to that category: 1 = weak and 2 = strong. The scores were totaled by category and divided by the number of boxes within that category in order to find the mean. Averaging was necessary as the number of responses varied by both participant and category. If there were no statements under a given category, then it was assigned a zero, but was included in calculating the mean. The mean scores of the authors were then compared for each participant, with discrepancies reconciled.

Following the assessment for strength of attributes, frequency of attributes was measured by counting the number of statements that participants made under each category. Since each statement had previously been assigned a text box (see Table 10.2), the boxes in each category were totaled and then multiplied by .10 to achieve a score. For example, 14 statements in a category would result in a score of 1.4. We measured frequency because we viewed the number of times someone said something as indicative of its importance to that individual.

Once the scores for strength and frequency of attributes were recorded, they were combined for a total score. Because the number of text boxes varied by category and participant, each category's combined maximum score was different. However, since zero was constant for both strength and frequency of attributes, it remained the lowest possible score. In conducting our evaluation, we categorized the scores by high (above 3.0), mid-range (2.0–2.99), and low (zero to 1.99). No statistical evaluation of the level of significance was conducted, since the study is descriptive.

RESULTS

Gender Role Ideologies

Traditional gender norms tell us that men will be high on the masculinity scale and low on the femininity scale, and women will be the opposite. Evidenced by their higher combined mean, as seen in Table 10.3, men,

Table 10.3 Scores for attributes by category (n = 28)

	Strength of attribute		Frequency of attribute		Strength and frequency	
	Masculine	Feminine	Masculine	Feminine	Masculine	Feminine
Men (N = 13)						
Mean	1.6	1.4	1.06	0.5	2.7	1.9
Median	1.6	1.5	0.8	0.5	2.4	1.8
Mode	1.7, 1.6, 1.5	1.7	0.8, 0.3	0.3	2.7, 2.4, 2.0	2
Range	1.3–1.9	1.3–1.9	.03–3.4	0.1–1.0	1.6–5.05	1.1–2.7
Women (N = 15)						
Mean	1.5	1.6	0.9	0.9	2.4	2.5
Median	1.45	1.7	0.8	0.8	2.45	2.35
Mode	1.75, 1.7	1.7	1.1, 0.5, 0.4	1.8, 0.9, 0.8, 0.7, 0.6	2.7, 1.8	3.5, 3.1, 2.0, 2.1
Range	1.0–1.8	1.3–1.9	0.1–1.9	0.3–1.8	1.1–3.35	1.6–3.5

as a group, demonstrated stronger masculine attributes than women. Yet, only .3 points separated the sexes and both groups were in the mid-range of scores.

In other respects, both sexes failed to confirm gender role stereotypes. Individually, only two men could be called strongly masculine. The first had a combined score of 5.05 for masculine traits, greatly exceeding all other participants' scores in the category. However, his score for feminine traits, which should have been low, was 2.1, higher than 62% of the men. The other man, with a masculine score of 3.5, was the only classic example of traditional masculine stereotyping in the sample, with a low score for feminine traits of 1.3. He was the only European man in the study, born just before World War II in a country deeply immersed in cultural norms. Describing his childhood, he stated, "The realization that I was a boy came to me rather early. As I was growing up, I realized my family and relatives treated me differently and it wasn't difficult to realize this treatment was due to sex. It is true in my culture then, and to a certain extent now, that boys were preferred to girls." Here we find traditional gender roles taught and self-integrated, virtually from birth. Out of 28 participants, only four scores (14%) for masculine traits were above 3.0, and two of these were women (3.35, 3.1). Sixty-four percent of participants' scores were in the mid-range. The distribution of masculine traits is shown in Figure 10.1.

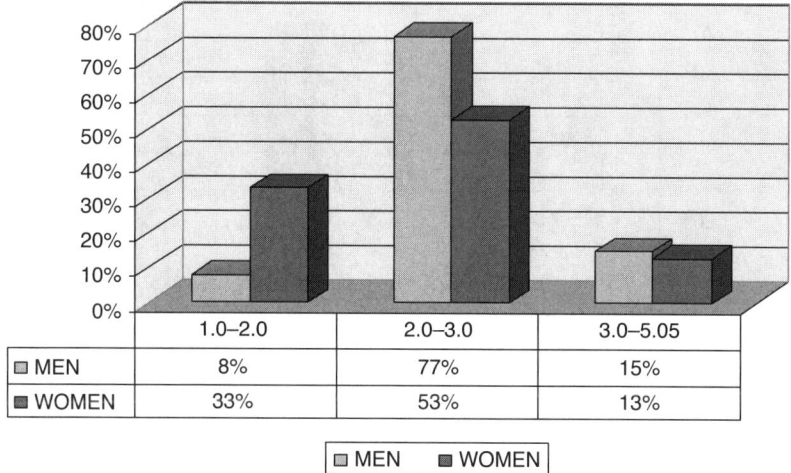

	1.0–2.0	2.0–3.0	3.0–5.05
☐ MEN	8%	77%	15%
◼ WOMEN	33%	53%	13%

☐ MEN   ◼ WOMEN

Figure 10.1 Distribution of masculine traits.

Results for feminine traits were similar. Collectively, women displayed stronger feminine attributes than men, and the distance between men's and women's mean scores (.6) was substantially greater than the spread for masculine traits. The women's mean score was solidly mid-range (2.5), which was lower than expected, while the men's mean, as predicted, was in the low range (1.9).

Consistent with gender stereotypes, women achieved four scores for feminine attributes over 3.0, while men had none. However, only one of the high-scoring women had a low score (1.9) for masculine traits, and the identity of this woman was surprising. She was a 48-year-old PhD, widowed with a child before she was 30, never remarried, and had a distinguished academic career. One would have expected her scores to be the opposite of what they were. Again, though, we see the influence of family. She remarked that her "family of orientation has been a powerful influence on my life. It remains a source of comfort and security." She also attributed her academic success to the belief that she could only gain her mother's "love and approval by being a good student."

The remaining three women had mid-range scores (2.45–2.7). The two highest scores for feminine traits (3.5) were, in both cases, those of nuns. As with masculine traits, 64% of the 28 participants were in the mid-range for feminine traits. The distribution of feminine traits is set forth in Figure 10.2.

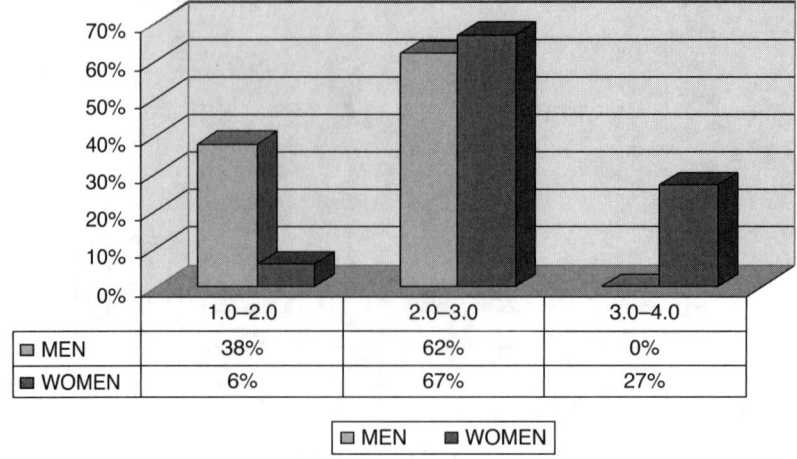

Figure 10.2 Distribution of feminine traits.

	1.0–2.0	2.0–3.0	3.0–4.0
MEN	38%	62%	0%
WOMEN	6%	67%	27%

GENDER IDENTITY CROSSOVER

If the gender identity crossover hypothesis is correct, then the youngest participants should score high in gender-stereotypical traits; middle-aged participants should show signs of androgyny; and the oldest participants should be the most androgynous or should take on the traits of the opposite sex. This did not happen. As seen in Table 10.4, collectively, the youngest men and women and middle-aged women are androgynous. Middle-aged and older men are not. The oldest men are the most masculine. Note, though, that when strength of attribute is segregated out, the whole sample is androgynous.

No evidence of crossover is found in any age-group for either men or women. However, the same is not true individually. Two middle-aged men had higher scores for feminine than for masculine attributes. The point spread for the first man, a minister in his mid-60s, was meaningful ($F = 2.7$, $M = 1.6$), and he was additionally low for masculine traits. The other man, a 58-year-old PhD and college professor, was mid-range for both traits ($F = 2.7$, $M = 2.0$). Two young and four middle-aged women scored higher for masculine than for feminine traits. The youngest, age 22, was essentially androgynous ($F = 2.2$, $M = 2.1$). Two of the middle-aged women had masculine scores over 3.0, and the others scored 2.95 and 2.7, respectively. Their feminine scores ranged from 2.0 to 2.65. Recent research suggests that older women (>70), unlike older men, may not experience gender crossover

Table 10.4 Scores for attributes by age (n = 28)

	Strength of attribute		Frequency of attribute		Strength and frequency	
Code	Masculine	Feminine	Masculine	Feminine	Masculine	Feminine
Men						
3	1.7	1.4	0.8	0.35	1	0.75
4	1.6	1.6	0.9	0.5	3	2.3
5	1.7	1.7	2.1	0.6	3.7	2.3
Women						
3	1.6	1.6	0.6	0.7	2.2	2.3
4	1.4	1.7	0.9	1	2.5	2.7
5	N/A	N/A	N/A	N/A	N/A	N/A

(James, et al., 1995; Strough, et al., 2007). It is interesting to note, however, that one half of our "more masculine" women were over 60.

The woman with the highest masculine score and the greatest spread (M = 3.35, F = 2.3) was an African American in her 60s. She grew up in a poor family with three siblings and was 15 during the Depression. The family lost their home the year she graduated from high school and her parents later divorced. Signs of independence and toughness emerged early on, evidenced by two incidents that she relates. The first occurred in the late 1930s, when she had to decide whether to go to work or to attend the funeral of a teenage boy who had been lynched a half-mile from her home. As she remembers, "Being a female Negro, I went [to work]." She also talks about the only time she "really feared for [her] life." She was the "sole Negro at the polls the first time [she] voted." In her 50s, she got a divorce, enrolled in college, and earned a degree.

DISCUSSION

This was a heuristic and descriptive study. We were seeking, in the first instance, to gain a better understanding of how men and women interpret their lives. In so doing, we also examined whether gender bias could be detected in autobiographical narratives. In the process, we tried to root out the problems inherent in such an endeavor as well as to determine where this exploration ought to go next.

Compatible with the literature, collectively, the men in our study were more masculine than the women and the women were more feminine than the men. On an individual basis, however, gender role ideologies did not explain gender differences. One potential explanation for this is education, which could be gender neutralizing. That is, those with more education might be less likely to adhere to traditional views and gender stereotypes (Adams, Coltrane, & Parke, 2007). In our study, 82% of the participants were college graduates and 11% were undergraduates. The one man without a college education had an extraordinarily high score for masculine traits. This made sense. He was a young man during the Depression, a time when physical strength was valued over intellectual prowess. Now in his 70s, he had worked hard his entire life and had been successful in his civil servant's job. He was proud of being the family breadwinner.

Geography could also be a factor. At least one study has found that residents of urban areas are less traditional in their gender role attitudes than others (Carter & Borch, 2005). All of the individuals writing narratives in this study were urban dwellers, and the great majority of them resided in Los Angeles.

In terms of androgyny or crossover, women in this sample acquired more masculine traits while still retaining feminine traits. Still, mean scores for both were solidly mid-range (M = 2.4, F = 2.5), suggesting that women may have forfeited some stereotypical gender traits in exchange for acquiring others. To understand this, feminism should be considered. From the mid-1960s, the industrialized world underwent dramatic societal change. Birth control, hormone therapy, and books giving women permission to be more than their stereotypical roles liberated women of all ages, sending many back to work and to school (Kipnis, 2006). As the beneficiaries of greater opportunity, the universe of a great many women expanded beyond family. Self-esteem, more egalitarian beliefs, and a new power base followed in due course (Adams et al., 2007; Kipnis, 2006).

We were especially interested to see if this was true of the middle-aged women in our sample, and it was. Of the 10 women aged 40–65 at the time they wrote their narratives, five returned to school in midlife, after marrying and having children. One resumed her career after 22 years, entered feminist therapy, and began Master's degree studies after learning of her husband's infidelity. Another divorced and became a feminist. Many women spoke of gaining control, becoming survivors instead of victims, and becoming more assertive, self-directed, and confident.

That women experienced this kind of personal growth is not surprising, but what about the men? A correspondingly strong rise in feminine traits among the men in our study is not observed until things are broken down by age. Only middle-aged and older men in our sample have mid-range mean scores for feminine traits (2.3). But there is still clear evidence of change. One of the ministers, confronted with controversy over the role of women in his church, stated that he had "become very sympathetic to the concerns of the [feminist] movement." Another man had undergone a life review and concluded that life is too short to pursue goals that did not satisfy him. Two men spoke of becoming more loving. Four others said they had become more relational.

These results seem to support the crossover hypothesis, perhaps not to the extent that Neugarten (1996b), Guttman (as cited in Harker & Solomon, 1996), and Jung (as cited in Harker & Solomon, 1996, and in Neugarten, 1979/1996b) envisioned, but certainly as James et al. (1995) describe it. On the other hand, we cannot characterize these men as androgynous.

Their embrace of more communal beliefs is not accompanied by the abandonment of masculine traits, as evidenced by mean masculine scores exceeding 3.0. It is possible that forfeiting control over outcomes and achievement-oriented behavior is threatening to men's privileged status, or as one study suggests, that masculine identity is a survival mechanism, adapting to circumstances (Heron, 2006).

As for the influence of age, 64% of our sample was middle-aged and we saw more evidence of generativity than of interiority. Risk-taking, empowerment, and restructuring were also present.

There are many limitations to this study. There was never any intention to generalize our results to the population at large, nor to suggest that our findings are definitive. The sample size is small, based on the availability of the original data, and this was a factor in attempting to study the cohort effects for age. Some age categories had only two participants, and there were no women over 65. Additionally, in our original sample, women outnumbered men by three to one. In our experience, fewer men than women sign up for the Guided Autobiography class, which suggests bias. It may also be that writing an autobiography is a typically more feminine activity than it is a masculine one.

Further, as discussed above, most of our subjects were college educated. A more diverse group could have produced an entirely different result. In addition, all of the women were working or had worked at one time, which in some studies has been equated with more egalitarian attitudes (Adams et al., 2007). This in turn raises the issue of the influence of social class on self-view. Each of these areas is worthy of additional research.

There were also issues with respect to measurement. All statements were measured by the same standard (strong/weak), but some statements were more important than others to one's self-identity, even though both may have been relevant to a particular category or trait. Finally, there is the subjective nature of the data itself. Though extreme care was taken to properly categorize and weigh participants' statements, any analysis of this nature remains open to interpretation.

The possibilities for future research are abundant. One question that emerges from the literature review is whether gender identity crossover is unique to middle age or continues into later life. The literature seems to be conflicted, as is our sample. Of the two "old" men, one was androgynous and the other stereotypical.

We also suggest that the development of gender traits does not happen in a vacuum but is strongly correlated with influences occurring early in one's life. An ongoing debate already exists on whether biological or socializing influences are more responsible for differences between men and women and how they interpret their lives. We scrutinized both, and both merit more investigation. As part of this investigation, cultural differences should also be considered.

Finally, locus of control is a useful paradigm for understanding causality in one's life, and it is believed to correspond to gender role stereotypes. Does it? And, if gender stereotypes are changing, will locus of control change as well, or are they unrelated?

CONCLUSION

In this sample, gender role ideologies did not explain differences in how men and women interpret their lives, because substantial and consistent differences between the two genders could not be found. Men were still masculine, women were still feminine, but both were self-attributing of the other's traits. It is our intention, then, to continue this work, using guided autobiography as a unique way to study lifestories, and to explore further the nexus between biological and socializing factors, and gender roles.

REFERENCES

Adams, M., Coltrane, S., & Parke, R. (2007). Cross-ethnic applicability of the Gender-based Attitudes Toward Marriage and Child Rearing Scales. *Sex Roles, 56*, 325–339.

Anthis, K., Dunkel, C., & Anderson, B. (2003). Gender and identity status differences in late adolescents' possible selves. *Journal of Adolescence, 27*(2), 147–152.

Archer, J. (1996). Sex differences in social behavior. *American Psychologist, 51*(9), 909–917.

Barry, D., & Beitel, M. (2006). Sex role ideology among East Asian immigrants in the United States. *American Journal of Orthopsychiatry, 76*(4), 512–517.

Birren, J. (2006). *Benefits of memory priming: Effects of guided autobiography and reminiscence.* Lecture at Joint Conference of the American Society on Aging and the National Council on Aging. (pp. 1–14). San Francisco: American Society on Aging. Retrieved from http://www.asaging.org/asav2/mindalert/pdfs/ booklet_2006.pdf

Birren, J., & Cochran, K. (2001). *Telling the stories of life through guided autobiography.* Baltimore: Johns Hopkins University Press.

Birren, J., & Deutchman, D. (1991). *Guiding autobiography groups for older adults: Exploring the fabric of life.* Baltimore: Johns Hopkins University Press.

Blazina, C., Pisecco, S., Cordova, M., & Settle, A. (2007). Gender Role Conflict Scale for Adolescents: Correlates with masculinity ideology. *Thymos, 1*(2), 191–205.

Brahnam, S., Margavio, T., Hignite, M., Barrier, T., & Chin, J. (2005). A gender-based categorization for conflict resolution. *Journal of Management Development, 24*(3), 197–209.

Carter, J., & Borch, C. (2005). Assessing the effects of urbanism and regionalism on gender-role attitudes, 1974–1998. *Sociological Inquiry, 75*(4), 548–563.

Harker, L., & Solomon, M. (1996). Change in goals and values of men and women from early to mature adulthood. *Journal of Adult Development, 3*(3), 133–143.

Heron, C. (2006). Boys will be boys: Working-class masculinities in the age of mass production. *International Labor and Working-Class History, 69*, 6–34.

Huyck, M. (1999). Gender roles and gender identity in midlife. In S. Willis & J. Reid (Eds.), *Life in the middle: Psychological and social development in middle age* (pp. 209–232). San Diego: Academic Press.

James, J., Lewkowicz, C., Libhaber, J., & Lachman, M. (1995). Rethinking the gender identity crossover hypothesis: A test of a new model. *Sex Roles, 32*(3/4), 185–207.

Lachman, M. (2004). Development in midlife. *Annual Review of Psychology, 55*, 305–322.

Kenyon, G. (2003). Telling and listening to stories: Creating a wisdom environment for older people. *Generations, 27*(3), 30–35.

Kipnis, L. (2006). Something's missing. *Women's Studies Quarterly, 34*(3/4), 22–43.

Moore, D. (2007). Self perceptions and social misconceptions: The implications of gender traits for locus of control and life satisfaction. *Sex Roles, 56*, 767–780.

Mueller, S. L., & Dato-On, M. C. (2008). Gender-role orientation as a determinant of entrepreneurial self-efficacy. *Journal of Developmental Entrepreneurship, 13*(1), 3–21.

Neugarten, B. (1968). *Middle age and aging.* Chicago: University of Chicago Press.

Neugarten, B. (1996a). Personality changes in the aged. In D. Neugarten (Ed.), *The meanings of age: Selected papers of Bernice L. Neugarten* (pp. 256–264). Chicago: University of Chicago Press. (Original work published 1965)

Neugarten, B. (1996b). Time, age, and the life cycle. In D. Neugarten (Ed.), *The meanings of age: Selected papers of Bernice L. Neugarten* (pp. 114–127). Chicago: University of Chicago Press. (Original work published 1979)

Neugarten, B. (1996c). Personality and the aging process. In D. Neugarten (Ed.), *The meanings of age: Selected papers of Bernice L. Neugarten* (pp. 270–279). Chicago: University of Chicago Press. (Original work published 1972)

Neugarten, B. (1996d). The changing meanings of age. In D. Neugarten (Ed.), *The meanings of age: Selected papers of Bernice L. Neugarten* (pp. 72–95). Chicago: University of Chicago Press. (Original work published 1987)

Ochberg, R. (1994). Life stories and storied lives. In A. Lieblich & R. Josselson (Eds.), *Exploring identity and gender: The narrative study of lives* (Vol. 2, pp. 113–144). Thousand Oaks, CA: Sage.

Ray, R. (1999/2000). Social influences on the older woman's life story. *Generations, 23*(4), 56–63.

Ray, R. (2000). *Beyond nostalgia: Aging and life-story writing.* Charlottesville, VA: University Press of Virginia.

Snyder, D. (1997). Parental influence on gender and marital role attitudes: Implications for intervention. *Journal of Marital and Family Therapy, 23*(2), 191–202.

Stewart, A. (1994). The women's movement and women's lives. In A. Lieblich & R. Josselson (Eds.), *Exploring identity and gender. The narrative study of lives* (Vol. 2, pp. 230–250). Thousand Oaks, CA: Sage.

Strough, J., Leszczynski, J., Neely, T., Flinn, J., & Margrett, J. (2007). From adolescence to later adulthood: Femininity, masculinity, and androgyny in sex age groups. *Sex Roles, 57*, 385–396.

Eleven

TELLING STORIES: HOW DO EXPRESSIONS OF SELF DIFFER IN A WRITING GROUP VERSUS A REMINISCENCE GROUP?

Kate de Medeiros

Narratives are often described as expressions of self. The stories we tell, composed of events and experiences we select and order, are integral pieces of our identities (Kenyon & Randall, 2001; McAdams, 1997, 2001; McLean, Pasupathi, & Pals, 2007; Neisser, 1994; Pasupathi, 2007; Randall, 1995). Understanding how expressions of self differ in terms of process (i.e., under what circumstances the narratives are produced) and structure (i.e., the narrative form) continues to be a rich area of inquiry (Gubrium & Holstein, 2000). Regardless of whether one subscribes to the concept of a universal self (Kaufman, 1986), multiple selves (Ewing, 1990), or some other construct (de Medeiros, 2005; Gubrium & Holstein, 2000), context also plays an important role in shaping and interpreting how the self is made known.

To explore further how process, structure, and context shape self-expressions, I begin this chapter by briefly discussing views of self and how they differ, underscoring the importance of narrative form in the production of meaning. I then present findings from a small study involving two groups of older adults: a structured autobiographical writing group and an oral reminiscence group. Overall, the writing group members expressed more "self-refining" moments in their narratives, or moments related to individual turning points in their lives (McAdams, 2001), whereas the reminiscence group expressed more "group-defining" moments, or general historical moments shared by the group in which the individual was also a part. Overall, this work points to the need for further, critical exploration into how methods in narrative gerontology can be applied to better understand the limits and opportunities of narrative and, ultimately, the self in old age.

WHAT IS THE SELF?

There are numerous theoretical constructs of the self that differ (sometimes subtly) on how much, if any, of the physical, psychological, emotional, expressed, and/or imaged individual is included (McLean et al., 2007; Ray, 2000). With regard to self-presentations in narratives, much work has focused on the self as a social and linguistic construct, where self-representation relies on the available cultural symbols, such as language. Kaufman (1986) described a "universal self" to characterize the coherence that one can achieve through the process of articulating meaning in his or her life. In this conceptualization, the self is always looking for continuity, reinterpreting a past self so that it "makes sense" in the present. By creating themes, which Kaufman describes as "cognitive areas of meaning with symbolic force" (p. 25), people are able to establish a sense of unity from their experiences. Using a slightly different view of how the self is made known and understood, Ewing (1990) proposed that what is often considered to be a "unified" self is actually a series of fragmented experiences and expressions that are constantly being reordered and/or reassembled at various moments in time in reaction to some stimulus (e.g., a question). The self is experienced as "whole" although it is actually a "shifting" self, composed of constantly changing parts. Continuity is, therefore, an illusion.

Gubrium and Holstein (2000) have described the self as being "crafted in light of the social conditions and biographical particulars of one's life" (p. 9) and proposed that self is "constructed and projected using culturally recognizable images and culturally endorsed formats" (p. 9). These formats include not only the tools available in narrative practice but also the individual's cultural standpoints and the corresponding rules within these various standpoints, which in turn affect the construction and expression of self. Like Kaufman (1986) and Ewing (1990), Gubrium and Holstein's work supports a view that the presented self is crafted through the store of culturally available tools, communicated in ways that are recognizable in some way to others.

I have argued elsewhere (de Medeiros, 2005) that, although presentations of the self are limited by available cultural symbols, the self does not exist solely as a cultural or linguistic construct. Instead, I have described what

I call the "externally presented" self and the "complementary self," which coexist. The externally presented self describes the part of self that is presented through situationally placed cultural constructs. The complementary self suggests a level of awareness by an individual that he or she may have thoughts or feelings that conflict with or challenge cultural norms and therefore are not expressed. This is not to say that the complementary self is a deviant self but rather a part of the self that is aware of the constraints acting to shape a culturally ideal self (to include both dominant and subcultural values) and modifies its presentation on the basis of context. Awareness influences external presentation. The complementary self acts as an agent to navigate and respond, through the externally presented self, in a way that the individual perceives to be culturally acceptable (de Medeiros, 2005).

Given that many of the discussions of self focus not on the self itself but rather on the way in which the self is expressed, I will briefly address how the self is shaped, made known, and ultimately interpreted in written and spoken narrative through a dialogic process (Bakhtin, 1986; Lucius-Hoene & Deppermann, 2000; Ray, 2000). I will then consider what can be said about the expressed self by looking at the narratives created in two groups of older adults.

Regardless of form used, such as an oral interview, conversation, or written memoir, an exchange begins when the actor/speaker/writer introduces an utterance or form of communication through language to an "other," which could be a listener, reader, or even one's self (Cohler & Cole, 1996; Ray, 2000). The narrative form provides the basic framework that structures how an exchange should unfold (de Medeiros, 2005, 2007). For example, in an interview, the interviewer asks a question to which the respondent provides an answer (Mishler, 1986); conversations involve turn-taking among speakers (Schiffrin, 1994); and memoirs are written first-person autobiographical accounts addressing some aspect of personal development and/or accomplishment (Abrams, 1988). Depending on one's familiarity or past experience with a given narrative form, layers of rules may be present that further shape what is included or omitted. After the speaker/writer's utterance, the listener/reader responds. In spoken exchanges, the listener's response is immediate and in turn affects the speaker's next response. Through this interchange, the intent of the speaker's original utterance is altered and the exchange becomes something jointly constructed between speaker and listener (Bakhtin, 1986; Cohler & Cole, 1996). In writing, the writer must anticipate the reader's response beforehand, addressing any potential questions or points of clarification before the reader actually responds. Whether speaking or writing, however, the decision as to what information is included or omitted and the way in which that information is conveyed (e.g., as a funny story versus a serious story) will depend on how the speaker/writer interprets the context or what is appropriate for a given situation (Lucius-Hoene & Depperman, 2000).

SELF-PRESENTATIONS IN GROUP WORK WITH OLDER ADULTS

Although reminiscence and writing groups for older adults have been described in the research literature for many years, the focus has generally been on measurable outcomes such as changes in overall well-being rather than on the content of the narratives produced (Cully, LaVoie, & Gfeller, 2001; Elford et al., 2005; Sherman, 1991; Stones, Rattenbury, & Kozma, 1995). Considering how the self might be presented in narratives within oral reminiscence and writing groups, it is worthwhile to again consider process, structure, and context. Reminiscing has been described as a social construction whereby participants share a concern for the past and an interest in using the patterns and interpretations of the past to better understand the present (Haight & Webster, 1995; Meacham, 1995; Sherman, 1991). Depending on the purpose of the group (e.g., therapeutic or social), participants may be given topics on which to reminisce (e.g., the Great Depression), developmental states (e.g., childhood), or other guidelines (Burnside, 1995; Burnside & Schmidt, 1994; Sherman, 1991; Stones et al., 1995). Group members can build on one another's stories, individualizing a particular story within the overarching group story or defining a group moment. With regard to types and functions of group reminiscence, Koffman (2000) has suggested that the act of storytelling helps people maintain their self-concept in older age by giving them the opportunity to recall and re-evaluate the past in light of the present. In Koffman's description of a reminiscence group, group members were individually focused on a life review or the resolution of past conflicts (Butler, 1963; Haight, Coleman, & Lord, 1995). The group provided a setting for members to conduct and share their own life reviews with each other but not necessarily to collaboratively build on a group memory of the past.

In written narratives, genre provides structure and, like the visible listener in an oral reminiscence group, influences which aspects of the self are withheld and revealed and how (de Medeiros, 2005; Goffman, 1974; Nelson, 2003). The writer must first determine what is appropriate to tell in a given literary genre and then must consider who the potential reader(s) might be and what information should be included or excluded. In an earlier study (de Medeiros, 2007), I examined the themes by genre in a study of older adults who participated in a writing workshop. The purpose of the workshop was to teach participants, most of whom had little previous writing experience, how to use different literary genres (memoirs, letters, poems, and third-person stories) as mediums for writing about their lives. I found that themes differed by genre, with first-person memoirs more likely to be stories about "joys," letters about "social connectedness," and third-person stories about "self-appraisals."

Sherman (1995) has conducted one of the few published studies comparing spoken versus written lifestories. In it, he compared oral narratives of one reminiscence group of older adults with both oral narratives and written journals of a comparison group of older adults also participating in a reminiscence group. In the first group, participants were asked to tell oral autobiographical stories about a given topic area. The second group also participated in the oral storytelling but recorded other memories in a journal. Participants in both groups then completed questionnaires for assessment of well-being and ego integrity. Sherman found no notable differences in the affect-balance or ego integrity scales between the two groups, suggesting no measurable difference in the psychological effect of the type of reminiscence on participants. However, the narratives themselves (i.e., the oral stories and written journals) were not assessed, studied, or compared, so it is not clear whether the content differed by group.

Rather than focus on measurable outcomes alone, it is important to include analysis of content relative to form to know how narrative operates to structure personal experiences and events. Although narrative approaches have the potential to let outsiders understand how the sense of being an "I" is experienced by the individual (Eakin, 1999), expanded uses of narrative interventions and more in-depth analysis of narrative data are needed.

METHOD

The goal of this small, cross-sectional study was to better understand how structure, process, and content shape self-expression in two types of groups of older adults: those participating in a written lifestory workshop and those in an oral reminiscence group. Twenty-one people aged 65 and over were recruited from the Cedar Creek[1] continuing care in retirement community as part of a larger study on memory in old age. Participants were randomly assigned to either a structured writing workshop (n = 11) or an oral reminiscence group (n = 10). Both workshops were led by the same facilitator, who was trained in each approach. The two workshop groups met once a week for 90 minutes each session over the course of 8 weeks. All workshops were audiotaped. Study inclusion criteria were as follows: minimum education of a high school diploma or equivalent, absence of diagnosed dementia, score of 25 or higher on the Mini Mental State Exam (MMSE; Folstein, Folstein, McHugh, 1975), normal vision and hearing (with or without correction), competence in the English language, an interest in writing, and physical ability to write. The study was approved by the Johns Hopkins University School of Medicine's Institutional Review Board. Written informed consent was obtained from all participants. A description of each workshop follows.

WRITING WORKSHOP

The purpose of the writing workshop was to introduce participants to different literary genres as mediums for creating narratives about their past (de Medeiros, 2007; de Medeiros, Kennedy, Cole, Lindley, & O'Hara, 2007). The literary genres in order of presentation were 1) first-person memoirs or any story about a past event told from the subject's perspective using the first-person pronoun *I* (weeks 1 and 2); 2) letters or a story by the subject written to a specific person who is named in the salutation (week 3); 3) poems, loosely defined as a collection of brief thoughts on a given topic, written in stanza form but with optional rhythm, meter, or rhyme (week 4); and 4) third-person stories or autobiographical stories by and about the subject, but narrated from an outsider's point of view, a *he* or *she* instead of an *I* (weeks 5 and 6). For week 7, participants were encouraged to rewrite a piece using a different genre. Participants could write in a genre of their choice for week 8 or could expand on an earlier piece.

During the first meeting, participants received an overview of the writing workshop schedule and process, read and discussed sample works from previous writing workshop participants, and discussed the assignment for the following week. Each week, participants were asked to write about something from their past for the next workshop meeting, using a given genre. The focus of the workshop was on learning how to work with different literary genres, rather than on addressing specific historical or developmental stages in their lives, as in a life review, for example. Participants could, therefore, write about anything related to their past as long as it was in the assigned genre and involved something they personally experienced, instead of retelling stories they had heard, or writing family histories. The majority of workshop time consisted of participants reading their work aloud and receiving comments from the group. All participants turned in copies of their work to the facilitator at the end of each workshop for additional feedback.

REMINISCENCE WORKSHOP

The purpose of the reminiscence group was to provide participants an opportunity to talk about past events and turning points in their lives. The 8 weeks loosely covered five developmental periods: birth to 12 years (weeks 1 and 2); ages 13 to 19 (weeks 3 and 4); 20 to 40 (weeks 5 and 6); 41 to 60 (week 7); and 60 to present (week 8) (Sherman 1991, 1995). Developmental periods were introduced as a way to organize talk within the group and as a structure commonly described in the literature on reminiscence groups (Burnside & Schmidt, 1994; Sherman, 1995). Participants were reminded often that they could bring up any thoughts, memories, or stories from any point in their past regardless of the developmental period being discussed, as long as it related to the group topic and involved something they had personally experienced. At the start of each meeting, the facilitator asked the group for suggestions of possible topics to get started. Once the group decided on a topic (e.g., a first job), a volunteer would begin by relaying an experience or observation. Other group members could then build on that person's comments or add a personal story.

RESULTS

Table 11.1 includes descriptive data for each participant group. The groups had similar ratios of women to men, and there were no significant

Table 11.1 Mean (±SD) age, years of education, and MMSE scores and range for each study group

Group	Sex	Mean age (±SD) Range	Mean years of education (±SD) Range	Mean MMSE* (±SD) Range
Self stories (n = 10)	4 men 6 women	79.9 (6.2) 67–88 years	16.2 (2.4) 11–18 years	28.3 (1.8) 25–30 points
Reminiscence (n = 8)	3 men 5 women	83.4 (6.0) 77–96 years	16.6 (1.4) 16–20 years	28.5 (1.4.) 26–30 points

*MMSE scores can range from 0 to 30, with 30 indicating the highest level of function.

differences between the groups in age, years of education, or MMSE scores. One writing workshop participant (a woman) withdrew because of a time conflict; two reminiscence participants (one man and one woman) withdrew from the study because of illness. There were 10 writing workshop and 8 reminiscence group participants. All participants described their race/ethnicity as "European American." In addition, five of the writing workshop members were married and five were widowed, and three of the reminiscence group members were married and eight were widowed.

Although the writing workshop and reminiscence groups had similar participant characteristics, there were differences between the groups in presentations of self, especially in which aspects of self were emphasized through the recalled event. Not surprisingly, the writing group participants wrote stories in which the main point of the narrative revolved around a personal realization or discovery that was less dependent on the historical context than on how the event affected him or her at that particular point in life, or "self-defining" moments (see Singer & Messier, this volume). The narratives in the reminiscence group tended to focus on events or situations that other group members may have shared, or group-defining moments. The narrative emphasis on the reminiscence group was placed on the larger historical context to which the individual contributed a memory, rather than on the individual. In the following sections, I present examples of self-defining and group-defining moments. I then present instances where two similar topics—changing elementary schools and World War II—were addressed by both groups, to show how "I" within the narratives differed.

Self-Refining and Group-Defining Moments

I make the distinction between self-defining moments in the writing workshop and group-defining moments in the reminiscence group by looking at where the participant places him- or herself within the event retold, the narrative "I." Self-defining moments from the writing workshop include a story by Matthew about miraculously avoiding a truck accident; a poem by Georgie about her stroke; and a third-person story by Virginia about hosting her last piano recital before moving. All three pieces were read aloud to the group by their authors. Matthew, age 76, begins his piece "Saved For?" as follows:

> In the summer of 1946, a family friend gave me a job as a stock boy in the 5 and 10 cent store.... One day, as I was walking to work a large delivery

van turned into the alley. I saw it coming and scrambled up the bank to escape its path. About half way up the bank, gravity took over and I began to slide down towards the rapidly turning back wheels of the truck! There was nothing to hold on to and I knew that soon both of my legs would be crushed at least. Then I stopped sliding for no obvious reason. The truck continued on its way, I rolled down, brushed myself off, and the thought came to me that I had been saved for some reason.

Matthew finishes his story by saying that the mere thought of being saved for some special purpose has been enough to guide and comfort him throughout his life.

Georgie, age 88, wrote a poem about having a stroke 12 years earlier:

> *Congratulations to my brain.*
> *For eighty-eight years it has worked amain*
> *Through thick and through thin.*
> *Doing the job that God ordained.*
> *I never gave it too much heed*
> *Until 12 years ago. Then WHAM!*
> *A stroke laid me low. So now*
> *It receives lots of my attention.*

In the next two stanzas, she describes some of the abilities she has lost, such as singing and applauding after a concert. She concludes her poem as follows:

> *So hats off to my stroke-struck brain.*
> *Now it hasn't an ache or a pain.*
> *It struggles bravely on even when asked a toughie*
> *Like an obscure British poet's middle name.*

Although the poem does not include any details outside of Georgie's experience, such as reactions by others or a sense place or setting when the event occurred, brevity and conciseness are to be expected given the conventions of poetry. I would note, however, that the topic is particularly interesting. As mentioned earlier, participants were simply instructed to write a poem about a moment from their past. Georgie chose a moment that has affected her life since that time.

The last example is from Virginia, age 76, who wrote a third-person story about hosting a final piano recital for her students before moving out of state. She writes:

> It was a hot May week in the home of a piano teacher in Alabama. There were so many arrangements to complete for the piano recital of her 25 students... . This will be the last recital given by Mrs. Hollis' pupils before

she and her family move to Ohio so her husband can begin attending classes and start a new life there.

The recital marked an end to one important phase in Virginia's life, and the beginning of another as she moved to follow her husband's career. Although she provides a very detailed description of the preparations for the event, she ends by mentioning the tears that came after the event.

Group-Defining Moments

In contrast to the self-defining moments from the writing group, stories in the reminiscence group tended to be about group-defining moments. For example, when the subject of childhood games came up, several people shared memories, such as the following exchange:

> *Charles* (age 81): We played a lot of things with old tin cans.
>
> *Marta* (age 83): That's city stuff, you know. I didn't know any of this until we lived in New York for 1 year when I was about nine. I discovered a whole batch of new stuff. Roller skates. We didn't have roller skates. We had ice skates.
>
> *Anna* (age 78): We didn't have too many places, except the local parks where they had a place where they used to put the water and in the winter they filled it with ice water so it couldn't have been much more than an inch or two.
>
> *Marta:* Well, I discovered roller skates and they were real roller skates with wheels and keys. The 1 year I lived in Brooklyn and the streets were paved with a very soft macadam. It was like velvet when your wheels rolled along. I never encountered it since that time, but that was my introduction to roller skating.

Marta continues by describing the difference between trying to roller skate in New York City and in the country. Although the participants offer personal memories, the memories are directed at supporting the general discussion of childhood games that were popular at a given time, rather than on introspective, key moments in the individual's life.

Group-defining moments were not limited to childhood memories but were prominent throughout all of the reminiscence group meetings. In week 8, the suggested developmental stage to address was age 60 to the present. After one woman, Susan, brought up her hobby of identifying rare plants, a hobby that stemmed from her professional career as a botanist, the discussion turned to the subject of women in the workplace:

> *Mary* (age 79): I think all of the women here remember maybe being elected or put on boards or boards of directors. You go to your first meeting and

they're all men. You're the only woman and they immediately pass you a paper and say, "Will you take notes?" I have always said, "No. I don't take minutes."… Did you find that?

Charles (age 84): Well, I was in the class of '51 and the year I graduated was the first girl that was admitted to the engineering school. And the story that went around campus was that she was looking for a boyfriend.

Marta: We all got that.

Roland (age 81): And then when I finally went to work for the firm where I spent the rest of my life, the senior partner, he was really a great guy, but he would not hire a woman. He said when you have led an organization which is essentially all men and you have one or two women in there, that causes trouble.

In addition to the general topic, an interesting aspect of this exchange is how the speakers appeal to the general members of the group to confirm their experiences. Mary uses the pronoun *you* to stress the similarities among the group members. She asks, "Did you find that?," referring to her being asked to take notes. The men in the group distance themselves from sex discrimination in the workplace by acknowledging that it did occur and by citing examples. This enables the men to contribute to the group moment without implicating themselves in the behavior.

Group Differences, Similar Topics

To further explore self-defining moments and group-defining moments, I present here excerpts from narratives that were similar in topic in the two groups, "changing schools often" and "World War II." In the writing workshop, Robert, an 86-year-old participant, first wrote a poem about changing elementary schools. Later, he rewrote his poem as a first-person narrative with slightly different details. Table 11.2 presents Robert's poem in one column and his story about the same experience in the other to better illustrate the similarities and differences.

Robert's two pieces provide an interesting comparison of how form may affect the telling of the same story. Points of emphasis in the poem differ from those in the first-person memoir, including the mention of Old Man Flynn's death in third grade in the memoir and the absence of any memories for that same grade in the poem.

In the reminiscence group, the topic of changing schools was brought up in the first meeting as an offshoot of a discussion about outhouses.

Table 11.2 Two versions of the same story presented side by side

Poem: "Five Years, Five Schools"	First-person story: "Five Years, Five Schools"
Started out in Chicago School just a block away Able to walk home for lunch Just about every day.	The first year of grade school was at Bonfield Elementary, just a block from home. On the days that mother packed a lunch, usually because of bad weather, it consisted of a sandwich wrapped in paper (no Saran back then), a piece of fruit, and a slice of cake or a couple of cookies all neatly packaged in a sheet of newspaper and tied together with a piece of string, just like all the other kids' lunches.
Began second in Springfield Where we moved in'29 New kid in school Adjusted just fine	It was into the second year that we children were told that Daddy would be leaving to take a new job and, as there was not enough money for the whole family to go with him, we would be moving in with our half-sister and husband until the money could be saved to make the move.
Next stop was Mt. Pleasant, A town that borders D.C. Don't remember much of third grade Blame a poor memory	One occasion I'll always remember is when Old Man Flynn died. He was our landlord and lived directly across the street... My first experience looking at a corpse.
Moved back to Springfield Same town—different school Teacher started a harmonica band I thought that just cool	It was then back to Springfield.... Our fourth grade teacher, Mrs Forshee, organized the harmonic band. The only requirement to participate in the band was to bring a dollar to pay for the Hohner instrument.
Then on to Hillsdale Where I stayed through the seventh year Served on the School Boy Patrol Many memories so dear.	During the summer we moved into our fifth house in 5 years. Mom became a room mother and I remember her showing up at lunchtime with a big tray of taffy apples on a stick she had made that morning.
I recall the words of my father Words I'm certain he meant. Words I'll never forget "Tis cheaper to move than to pay rent."	Should anyone mention the several moves our family had made in those first 5 years, Dad would jokingly replay, "Well, I always believe it was cheaper to move than to pay rent."

The conversation began with Mary, an 84-year-old participant's, mention of schools. James, age 79, then provided details:

> *Mary*: My one-room school had two outhouses, one for the boys and one for the girls, and they were within easy walking distance of the school house proper.
>
> *James*: I went to 14 grade schools in nine different states.
>
> *Gene*: They kicked him out. [laughs]
>
> *James*: My father was in the construction business; my mother was trained to be a language teacher. They met at the University of Illinois. I was the first child and for 9 years their only child, but he was in the business of building factories to manufacture automobile batteries at the time when the crank had just been replaced by automatic starting batteries. It took about 6 months to build one and get it started and off we'd go to San Antonio, or Lancaster, New York, or somewhere. And there was a routine that one went through when entering the school… schools and every state—and I went through it so many times. Mom and James would go, and it was never the principal. It was always the assistant principal. And they would speak to me and my mother about "What grade were you in Illinois?" and I would say, "3B," or whatever. "Well, our schools are much better than theirs so you're not in the third grade here, you're in the second grade."

James then commented that he would eventually be switched to the higher grade level, only to be pulled out of school for another move and have the entire situation repeated at the next school. Overall, James's narrative did not include details about how he felt about the experience of changing schools or how those experiences defined him personally. Rather, his story focused on the events—his father's need to move, how the schools reacted to him when he arrived, the particulars of learning how to read, and other particulars on which the group could comment and build.

Since all of the participants had lived through World War II, and many had served in it in some capacity, it was another topic that emerged. In the writing workshop, Roland, an 83-year-old man, wrote a letter to his parents, which he dated March 13, 1945, about his experiences in flight school. He begins by writing: "We are still doing very interesting things here. Every day our time on the flight line depends on what the weather is doing… . My training has progressed to the point where they think I am ready to fly solo, so this was the day." Roland describes his plane, the procedures for checking its safety, and then how his flight was aborted due to a fuel cap that had been improperly secured. He adds in his letter, "This could have been a whole lot worse when you think of all that can go wrong with these little training planes. If nothing worse than this happens, I'll be very lucky." Of course, in writing the letter some 64 years after the event, Roland knows that everything did turn out okay. It's curious that he chose to write about such a seemingly small event, which suggests it was an experience that held personal significance, perhaps because of the fear he had about flying and the war, or perhaps because of other reasons he did not express.

Several people in the reminiscence group told brief stories about their memories of World War II. Mary, an 84-year-old woman, talked about her experience in the Signal Corps. She described how she and the officers would play ping-pong at lunch: "There were no females in this population. They were all 6 feet 10 or something, but I was able to run around the table faster than anybody." Others in the group talked about discrimination of soldiers prior to the war, racial discrimination within the military, and the use of V-mail. Robert talked about serving in the Army Corps of Engineers. "The Corps of Engineers had a motto," he said: "The difficult we do immediately, the impossible takes a little longer … . When I went to college, I did enroll in the ROTC and the basic was for 2 years and then if you stayed for 2 more years you came out a commissioned officer and so at the end of the second year, I went to sign up to be commissioned in the Corps of Engineers." Robert continued to detail how he surveyed various bases throughout the world. After he had finished, Rosalie, an 81-year-old woman, described her experiences in the Civil Air Patrol in Arizona. She mentioned jokingly, "We were never attacked in Arizona by the Japanese because we were vigilant." Although the participants all told personal anecdotes, they did not seem to be personally revealing but instead were informative or funny, narratives that seemed to directly relate to and support experiences recalled by other members in the group.

DISCUSSION

If the stories we tell are important pieces of who we are, then what can different narrative approaches and contexts reveal about ourselves? Both narrative approaches require the selection of experiences and the ordering of talk. In the writing workshop, participants had 1 week to give thought and structure to their narratives. Although participants in the reminiscence group also had a week to think about the types of experiences they might want to bring up at the next workshop meeting, the way that talk and events were ordered depended greatly on the previous speaker. In these two groups, the difference between what types of narratives are constructed is perhaps exaggerated, since the individual versus group emphasis can certainly be linked to the individual efforts of the writer versus the group efforts of socially constructed talk. However, what the examples from the two groups do illustrate is that there is a difference in what is presented, what is emphasized, and how speakers/writers may modify their presentations on the basis of context, all of which point to different presentations of self.

For example, Robert's initial poem about changing schools is not particularly introspective but it does rhyme, thus rhyming scheme may have been the organizing structure of this particular piece. He includes relevant biographical details in the poem—names of cities and years—but no evaluation of the experience. In his rewrite of the experience as a first-person narrative, however, his writing appears to be more focused on the details and explanation, not just the events themselves, leading to more insight and personal revelation, such as seeing a corpse for the first time.

Roland's letter about a small mishap during pilot training is another curious example. The story itself is not that interesting. There is little action. Roland isn't hurt. He doesn't mention being disciplined because of the forgotten fuel cap. Yet, of all the details or events he could have written about, he chose this one for some particular reason. In the writing group, the focus appeared in response to the question, "What from my past has made me who I am today?" In contrast, the stories in the reminiscence group were presentations tied to elements presumably common to the other group members. For the reminiscence group, the question seemed to be, "In what ways am I the same and different from you?"

The point that self-presentation is heavily influenced by process, structure, and context is not new, but it is one that is not often critically explored in applied research with older adults. For example, there are few published studies that explore the production of narratives by older adults by looking at how form affects content; instead, the focus is on the wider realm of narrative themes or measurable outcomes. Recently, there has been increased interest in how narrative interventions may be used to improve health and well-being, which is certainly an important area of inquiry. However, also important is an understanding of how different types of narratives, and narratives produced under different circumstances (e.g., writing, one-on-one conversation, group participation), may have different outcomes. While the work reported in this chapter has many limitations, it is intended to provide a rough framework for future inquiries on narrative approaches to understanding the aging self.

NOTE

Work reported in this paper was supported by the Brookdale Foundation, Grant #3101-F08.

[1] Personal identifiers, including the names of the retirement community and study participants, have been changed.

REFERENCES

Abrams, M. (1988). *A glossary of literary terms* (5th ed.). New York: Holt, Rinehart & Winston.

Bakhtin, M. (1986). The problem of speech genres (V. McGee, Trans.). In C. Emerson & M. Holquist (Eds.), *Speech genres and other late essays* (pp. 60–102). Austin, TX: University of Texas Press.

Burnside, I. (1995). Themes and props: Adjuncts for reminiscence therapy groups. In B. Haight & J. Webster (Eds.). *The art and science of reminiscing: Theory, research, methods, and applications* (pp. 151–164). Washington, DC: Taylor & Francis.

Burnside, I., & Schmidt, M. (1994). *Working with older adults: Group process and techniques.* Sudbury, MA: Jones & Bartlett.

Butler, R. (1963). The life review: An interpretation of reminiscence in the aged. *Psychiatry, 26,* 65–76.

Cohler, B., & Cole, T. (1996). Studying older lives: Reciprocal acts of telling and listening. In J. Birren, G. Kenyon, J. Ruth, J. Schroots, & T. Svensson (Eds.). *Aging and biography: Explorations in adult development* (pp. 61–76). New York: Springer.

Cully, J., LaVoie, D., & Gfeller, J. (2001). Reminiscence, personality, and psychological functioning in older adults. *The Gerontologist 1*(1), 89–95.

de Medeiros, K. (2005). The complementary self: Multiple perspectives on the aging person. *Journal of Aging Studies, 19,* 1–13.

de Medeiros, K. (2007). Beyond the memoir: Telling life stories using multiple literary forms. *Journal of Aging, Humanities, and the Arts, 1,* 159–167.

de Medeiros, K., Kennedy, Q., Cole, T., Lindley R., O'Hara, R. (2007). Autobiographical writing and memory performance in a group of highly functioning older adults: A preliminary investigation. *American Journal of Geriatric Psychiatry, 15*(3), 257–261.

Eakin, P. (1999). *How our lives become stories: Making selves.* Ithaca, NY: Cornell University Press.

Elford, H., Wilson, F., McKee, K., Chung, M., Bolton, G., & Goudie, F. (2005). Psychosocial benefits of solitary reminiscence writing: An exploratory study. *Aging and Mental Health, 9*(4), 305–314.

Ewing, K. (1990). The illusion of wholeness: Culture, self, and the experience of inconsistency. *Ethos, 18,* 251–278.

Folstein, M., Folstein, S., & McHugh, P. (1975). Mini-mental state: A practical method for grading the cognitive status of patients for the clinician. *Journal of Psychiatric Research, 12,* 189–198.

Goffman, E. (1974). *Frame analysis: An essay on the organization of experience.* York, PA: Maple Press.

Gubrium, J., & Holstein, J. (Eds.). (2000). *Institutional selves: Troubled identities in a postmodern world.* New York: Oxford University Press.

Haight, B., Coleman, P., & Lord, K. (1995). The linchpins of a successful life review: Structure, evaluation, and individuality. In B. Haight & J. Webster (Eds.), *The art and science of reminiscing: Theory, research, methods, and applications* (pp. 179–189). Washington, DC: Taylor & Francis.

Haight, B., & Webster, J. (Eds.). (1995). *The art and science of reminiscing: Theory, research, methods, and applications.* Washington, DC: Taylor & Francis.

Kaufman, S. (1986). *The ageless self: Sources of meaning in late life.* Madison, WI: University of Wisconsin Press.

Kenyon, G., & Randall, W. (2001). Narrative gerontology: An overview. In G. Kenyon, P. Clark, & B. de Vries (Eds.). *Narrative gerontology: Theory, research and practice* (pp. 3–18). New York: Springer.

Koffman, S. (2000). *Reminiscence and gestalt life review: Group treatments of older adults for later life adjustment.* New York: Garland.

Lucius-Hoene, G., & Deppermann, A. (2000). Narrative identity empiricized: A dialogical and positioning approach to autobiographical research interviews. *Narrative Inquiry, 10*(1), 199–222.

McAdams, D. (1997). *The self we live by: Personal meaning and the making of myths.* New York: Guilford Press.

McAdams, D. (2001). Psychology of life stories. *Review of General Psychology, 5*(2), 100–122.

McLean, K., Pasupathi, M., & Pals, J. (2007). Selves creating stories creating selves: A process model of self-development. *Personality and Social Psychology Review, 11*(3), 262–278.

Meacham, J.A. (1995). Reminiscing as a process of social construction. In B. Haight & J. Webster (Eds.), *The art and science of reminiscing: Theory, research, methods, and applications* (pp. 37–48). Washington, DC: Taylor & Francis.

Mishler, E. (1986). *Research interviewing: Context and narrative.* Cambridge, MA: Harvard University Press.

Neisser, U. (1994). Self narratives: True and false. In U. Neisser & R. Fivush (Eds.), *The remembering self: Construction and accuracy in self-narrative* (pp. 1–18). New York: Cambridge University Press.

Nelson, K. (2003). Self and social functions: Individual autobiographical memory and collective narrative. *Memory, 11*(2), 125–136.

Pasupathi, M. (2007). Telling and the remembered self: Linguistic differences in memories for previously disclosed and previously undisclosed events. *Memory, 15*(3), 258–270.

Randall, W. (1995). *The stories we are: An essay on self-creation.* Toronto: University of Toronto Press.

Ray, R. (2000). *Beyond nostalgia: Aging and life-story writing.* Charlottesville, VA: University of Virginia Press.

Schiffrin, D. (1994). *Approaches to discourse.* New York: Blackwell.

Sherman, E. (1991). *Reminiscence and the self in old age.* New York: Springer.

Sherman, E. (1995). Differential effects of oral and written reminiscence. In B. Haight & J. Webster (Eds.), *The art and science of reminiscing: Theory, research, methods, and applications* (pp. 255–264). Washington, DC: Taylor & Francis.

Stones, M., Rattenbury, C., & Kozma, A. (1995). Group reminiscence: Evaluating short- and long-term effects. In B. Haight & J. Webster (Eds.), *The art and science of reminiscing: Theory, research, methods, and applications* (pp. 139–150). Washington, DC: Taylor & Francis.

Twelve

MNËMË AND *ANAMNËSIS*: THE CONTRIBUTION OF INVOLUNTARY REMINISCENCES TO THE CONSTRUCTION OF A NARRATIVE SELF IN OLDER AGE

Philippe Cappeliez and Jeffrey Dean Webster

> In these postmodern times, when so many threats and obstacles to constructing and maintaining a coherent, consistent self abound, the acts of remembering, recalling, reminiscing… may facilitate the kind of coherence, consistency, and sense of identity that each of us so desperately needs.
> —Janelle Wilson (2005, p. 8)

Coherent lifestories enable self-understanding, facilitate growth, and support the pursuit of meaning across the life course (Reker, Birren, & Svensson, in press). Our autobiographies, the parts we tell to ourselves and others, provide a means to make sense of our lives within the broader stories of which we are a part. Sharing ourselves through narrative connects us to our broader cultural group and lets us celebrate both our communal similarities and fundamental uniqueness. Storytelling is a natural human practice.

But where do such well-crafted narratives originate? What are the building blocks that provide the structure and foundation upon which they are built? For our purposes, the most important elements are our memories, those rich and virtually limitless images we have accrued over a lifetime. These autobiographical memories and reminiscences have aroused the interest of researchers, but they have addressed primarily those memories retrieved intentionally and requiring directed cognitive resources. A potentially important omission concerns those memories which arise unbidden, Proustean-like (1913–1927/1999), in a spontaneous fashion (e.g., Webster, Bohlmeijer, & Westerhof, 2010). This chapter concerns the qualities and some consequences of such involuntary recall.

Involuntary memories stand in contrast to voluntary memories. Voluntary memories are prompted, intended, searched for, whereas involuntary memories come to mind spontaneously, automatically, without control or effort. Because researchers in cognitive psychology are mainly interested in goal-oriented activities, they have concentrated their investigations primarily on voluntary memory, with scant attention paid to involuntary memory.

This relative neglect is also apparent in the fields of autobiographical memory and reminiscence research. In the field of autobiographical memory, involuntary memories have, until recently, been studied primarily from the perspective of psychopathology, as a symptom of psychological disorders (e.g., in post-traumatic stress disorder). By contrast, the functionalist perspective that dominates contemporary research on reminiscence in later life has naturally oriented the investigation toward voluntary reminiscence. Indeed, the premise of that approach is that, to understand the phenomenon of reminiscence, it must be recognized first and foremost that it serves a variety of functions or purposes in the life of the older person. These functions in turn depend on such factors as personality dispositions and life circumstances. The taxonomy of reminiscence that Webster (1993, 1997) developed is a prime example of a theoretical and methodological advance based on the notion that personal memories are called up to serve particular life purposes. This research led to the creation of the Reminiscence Functions Scale, a self-report instrument that asks respondents to reflect on their reminiscences and produce a global judgment on how frequently they reminisce for various specific purposes (Webster, 1993, 1997). While this approach has undoubtedly led to significant progress in our understanding of the roles played by reminiscence for adaptation in later life (e.g., Coleman, 2005; Cappeliez & O'Rourke, 2006), it leans toward reminiscences involving awareness and intended uses, i.e., voluntary reminiscences. This contemporary emphasis on voluntary recall stands in contrast to an early position suggested by Aristotle.

Aristotle distinguished between voluntary and involuntary memory in his short treatise best known under its Latin title, "De Memoria et Reminiscentia,"[1] one of the nine essays included in *Parva Naturalia* (Aristotle, 1955). As the French philosopher Paul Ricoeur (2000) points out, Aristotle used two different words of ancient Greek, *mnëmë* and *anamnësis,* to theorize about the fundamental question, "What is a memory?" *Mnëmë* designates a memory that appears almost passively, to the point that Aristotle characterizes its coming to mind as an affective state, a *pathos*. Interestingly, modern French has kept this notion of an affectively charged memory at the core of the everyday use of the word *reminiscence*. In contrast to *mnēmē*, *anamnēsis* refers to memory as the object of a quest. This is what we name "recall" or "recollection" in ordinary language. Essentially, the opposition between *mnēmē* and *anamnēsis* is between simple evocation (memory as an experience) and search (memory as the outcome of an effortful process). Ricoeur (2000) emphasizes that it is precisely by opposition to search that evocation connotes an affective or emotional state. Keeping in mind this line of thought, we note that, etymologically, *ana* in *anamnēsis* implies a process of "returning on." In itself, it opens the possibility of reappraising what has been seen, felt, or learned before. Actually, Aristotle stated that recollection essentially involves a kind of reasoning process. This reflexive notion has been kept in modern languages. Indeed, in French we speak of *"se souvenir"*; in English we say *"re-member."* We will revisit these early insights at several points later in the chapter.

We can now turn to the objectives and the structure of this chapter. First, we will review the current state of knowledge on involuntary reminiscences in older age. As we will see, this account rests on the analysis of naturally occurring reminiscences, as recorded by the research participant. We will complement this literature by the findings of two of our recent studies. The first study investigates the contents of reminiscences as spontaneously reported by a sample of older adults. The second study takes the original approach of exploring how older adults themselves view reminiscing—i.e., their implicit theories of reminiscence. In reporting the findings of these studies, we will note the correspondences with the early insights of Aristotle and delineate some of the ways involuntary autobiographical memories contribute to the construction of the narrative self.

THE CHARACTERISTICS OF INVOLUNTARY REMINISCENCES IN OLDER AGE

The typical method used in research on autobiographical memory has consisted of asking participants to respond with an autobiographical memory either to a word or a phrase (i.e., the cue-word technique), to a particular instruction (e.g., from a specific period of life), or to a characteristic of the memory (e.g., the most positive or most vivid). In all of these cases, the retrieval of autobiographical memories is requested. In other words, remembering is voluntary, deliberate, and purposeful. In contrast, involuntary autobiographical memories, those that come to mind spontaneously and without any conscious or deliberate retrieval effort, have typically been investigated using a diary method. Participants are asked to keep a diary for a set period of time (e.g., 1 week), in which they describe their involuntary autobiographical memories as they occur, providing additional information on the content of the memory and conditions of occurrence, such as location and activity involvement, presence/absence of a trigger, accompanying mood, and emotional valence.

Research carried out with older adults by means of this methodology has led to several interesting insights about involuntary reminiscences in older age (Berntsen, 1996; Schlagman, Kvavilashvili, & Schulz, 2007). First, it appears that the majority of these memories occur when the person is involved in activities characterized as automatic, that is, activities not requiring much concentrated attention, such as washing the dishes or walking. Second, the vast majority of these memories seem to be linked to an identifiable trigger. Most often this trigger is an abstract cue, such as a spoken word or a thought, or a sensory/perceptual cue, such as a sound, or the sight of an object. It is interesting to note that very few of these triggers are state-based cues, such as mood or physiological state. This finding stands in contrast to the central status often attributed to sensory cues and moods, in the footsteps of Proust's (1913–1927/1999) literary description of reminiscence in his novel, *A la recherche du temps perdu* (In Search of Lost Time). Most of these cues seem intrinsically related to the memory content. This may explain why the triggers are relatively easy to identify.

Regarding content, research provides information limited to broad categories. These involuntary memories pertain predominantly to specific episodes rather than to general events or classes of events. It is interesting to note the contrast with voluntary memories, which, in later adulthood, are typically general. Finally, we have some information about the temporal distribution of these involuntary memories. The phenomenon of the reminiscence bump, a tendency to recall memories from the time when participants were approximately 10 to 30 years of age, seems to apply to involuntary memories. Indeed, older adults seem to manifest a marked bias toward the spontaneous retrieval of personal memories about events dating from that period of their life.

A STUDY ON THE CONTENTS OF SPONTANEOUS REMINISCENCES

Except for general descriptions, research says little about the contents of these spontaneous reminiscences: What are they about? We recently tried to shed light on this issue in a study conducted with a sample of 36 older adults, a large majority of whom were women (74%). These persons were, on average, 74 years of age, lived autonomously in the community, and functioned well both physically and cognitively (Cappeliez, 2008). Participants were interviewed on a recent episode of naturally occurring reminiscence. Questions were limited to a description of its features (i.e., the situational context, the contents of the memory, and the emotions before and after the reminiscence). Interviewers were explicitly instructed to refrain from further probing and from inciting participants to re-evaluate the memory. Contents of the interviews were transcribed verbatim and then analyzed in terms of both theme and type of reminiscence. Changes in emotions were also examined, but they are not discussed here (see Cappeliez, Guindon, & Robitaille, 2008, for a study on the interaction between reminiscences and emotions).

Two raters, who were different from the interviewers and who were not informed of the goal of the study, independently identified the type of reminiscence. For this purpose, they used a template with eight functions of reminiscence, which is modeled after Webster's taxonomy (Webster, 1993, 1997) and has gained consensus in the field (Webster & Haight, 1995). Briefly stated, an account of reminiscence was identified as *integrative* if it reflected an evaluation of the past leading to a sense of coherence, meaning, or self-worth, or the acceptance of the past as lived and the integration of the past with the present. An example would be a person recalling the time of her life when she made ginger cookies for her children and stating, "At my age I cannot have big goals in life because I know that the end is near. I am content with all the good moments of daily life when my children and grandchildren come to visit." A report of reminiscence was regarded as *instrumental* if it referred to past episodes of coping with life challenges, solving problems, or reaching goals. As an example, a person recalls the surgery that her daughter underwent, how sad she was, and how she coped with that experience, "which made me stronger, capable of overcoming difficulties." An account of reminiscence was labeled *transmissive* when it entailed sharing a memory containing an instructive story or a life lesson built on personal experience. An example would be a person who recalls his wife's illness and the last moments of her life, commenting on the lesson he derived from that experience: the importance of taking care of one's health and of maintaining an active social life. A reminiscence episode with a purely descriptive content and no manifest evaluative intent, in the form of telling a personal memory like a simple story, was identified as *narrative*. An example would be a person remembering an old TV program that she watched with her siblings and how much they enjoyed it. A reminiscence about difficult moments, unresolved issues, and ongoing inner struggles was classified as *obsessive*. As an example, a person remembers when a priest took money away from her, and expresses her bitterness and generalized disappointment about people in positions of authority. A reminiscence account involving a magnified or glorified past, a contrast between the "good old days" and the present, with the desire to return eventually to the past, was considered a manifestation of *escapist* reminiscence. An example of such reminiscence would be a person remembering past Christmases with envy and longing, expressing the desire to return to that "lost paradise." Reminiscence for *intimacy maintenance* referred to an episode of reminiscence characterized by the wish to keep alive memories of intimate partners with whom the person was no longer in contact: for example, a person recalling her life with her husband, now deceased, and commenting, "To talk about him keeps me alive. His presence helps me." Reminiscences for *death preparation* were memories that reflected taking a perspective on death or dealing with the issue of life's ending. An example would be a person remembering the death of her mother, how she approached it with serenity, and extending this line of thinking to her own situation. Inter-rater reliability, as assessed by Cohen's kappa, ranged from .72 to .83 for the coded measures of emotions and reminiscences. Raters resolved disagreements about categorization through discussion.

The first main finding was that, although the procedure purposely did not ask participants to reappraise or search for insights, virtually all reminiscences appeared in some way to be the product of an appraisal or evaluation. Actually, in the large majority, the reminiscences were memories that participants spontaneously identified as having led to self-acceptance and a sense of coherence and purpose in one's life. These features connote what is known as *integrative reminiscence*. Furthermore, in the manner they were presented, such memories emerged as extracts from a well-developed lifestory. In other words, when specifically asked to report a discrete episode of recent reminiscence, with no prior warning or opportunity of rehearsal, it is as if these older persons proceeded to open a chapter of their lifestory. A similar finding has been reported about memories of life turning-points (Cappeliez, Beaupré, & Robitaille, 2008; Webster & Gould, 2007). When expressly asked to describe a specific memory that represented a turning point in their life, participants of both studies were inclined to provide a response in which they described a series or a category of events—that is, a response more akin to life review or integrative reminiscence.

With strikingly few exceptions, the difficult life circumstances of the past were viewed in retrospect as growth experiences, with the emphasis placed on the ultimate benefits and opportunities they had generated. The participants of our sample thus appeared to engage in reminiscing for the very purpose of reaching the conclusion that their life had been well lived, the successful experiences gaining importance as a basis for the reconstruction of personal identity and sense of coherence. In that sense, our sample appears mostly representative of the 42% or so of older adults who show evidence of interest in life review, a figure based on previous research (Wink & Schiff, 2002). The fact that our sample was largely constituted of women is another factor to consider, as it is known that women are typically more prone to life review than men (Wink & Schiff, 2002).

In the second-most important category of reminiscences, we found memories of lost spouses or family members (i.e., intimacy maintenance). Importantly and unsurprisingly, these memories naturally led to some redefinition of life priorities and purposes. They also prompted thinking about one's death (a form of death preparation). These considerations were, in a number of cases, presented as lessons of life (transmissive reminiscence). Interestingly, integrative reminiscences themselves often evolved subtly into a lesson of life and a path leading to humanistic pursuits, which raters identified as instances of transmissive reminiscence. This eagerness to teach and inform others about lessons of life reflects the pursuit of objectives that go beyond the confines of one's life, such as care for future generations.

INTERPRETATIONS OF FINDINGS WITH THE NARRATIVE APPROACH

The narrative approach to the study of self can help us interpret these findings. Such an approach considers the development of the self as consisting of the integration of autobiographical experiences into a coherent lifestory (e.g., Bluck & Habermas, 2000; Habermas & Bluck, 2000; McAdams, 2006, 2008a; McLean, 2005; Pasupathi & Mansour, 2006). The lifestory enables a sense of coherence across time. This process appears particularly crucial in old age (Pasupathi, Weeks, & Rice, 2006) and it has been linked with physical and psychological well-being (Cappeliez & O'Rourke, 2006).

These findings fit well with three aspects of narrative gerontology that are broadly interconnected. Specifically, emerging findings in the areas of wisdom (e.g., Webster, 2007), emotions management (e.g., Carstensen, Fung, & Charles, 2003), and personality (Hooker & McAdams, 2003;

McAdams, 2008a) all provide important insights. Space limitations preclude an equal discussion of all three, and so we only briefly discuss wisdom and emotions management and then focus on McAdam's lifestory approach to personality development as the most directly relevant of the three.

For several theories and models of wisdom (e.g., Ardelt, 2003; Kenyon, this volume; Randall & Kenyon, 2001; Webster, 2007), critical life experiences are the forge within which wisdom is cast. Life events including loss, fear, anger, and related negative emotions require evaluation, analysis, and eventual assimilation if they are to serve as lessons learned, rather than as triggers of chronic, destructive rumination. Wise persons not only grow through and beyond such negative vicissitudes but also share their hard-won insights with others. For instance, Webster (2003, 2007) has shown that wise individuals score significantly higher on measures of generativity than less wise persons. Generativity (see below) is the Eriksonian impetus to guide, nurture, and mentor upcoming generations. Distilling life lessons from autobiographical memories (and then sharing such revelations with younger adults) is one means, therefore, by which older individuals can engage in this later-life task. As such, when older adults reflect on earlier painful life events, their resolution and integration of these reminiscences is most likely contributing to the development and maintenance of wisdom. Certainly in our sample, the types of integrative reminiscences displayed, the reinterpretation of past sorrows, faults, and limitations as growth experiences, and the propensity for teach/inform functions constitute compelling evidence that wisdom development entails an ongoing synthesis of autobiographical content.

Work conducted within the framework of socioemotional selectivity theory (e.g., Carstensen et al., 2003) has shown that older adults are adept at managing their emotions through a variety of techniques. Older-adult samples, for example, often exhibit a "positivity" effect, wherein emotional balance is achieved via selective recruitment of autobiographical memories (e.g., episodes in which the emotions of pride, happiness, and exhilaration are prominent). Negative memories in later life have been reworked and contextualized, allowing a broad sense of perspective. The painful sting of past hurts, humiliations, and injustices dissipates as these scenes are woven into evolving lifestories (e.g., Charles, Mather, & Carstensen, 2003). For some elderly individuals, this ability to confront negative chapters in their lives leads to a richer, more coherent narrative. Again, our findings are highly consistent with such emotional acumen. With the exception perhaps of bitterness-revival types of recall, our participants were able to employ memories in ways that contributed to increased serenity, closure, and even happiness. Even memories with strong negative valence (e.g., of loss, depression, embarrassment) were often ultimately reinterpreted as strengths, evidence of a type of problem-solving reminiscence that may have contributed to increased self-esteem. This type of narrative emotional management has much in common with important facets of McAdams' work on personal narratives, to which we now turn.

McAdams and colleagues (e.g., Bauer & McAdams, 2004; Hooker & McAdams, 2003; McAdams, 2008a, 2008b) define a lifestory as an "internalized and evolving narrative of the self that provides a life with some degree of coherence and purpose" (McAdams, 2008b, p. 20). It synthesizes a reconstructed past, a perceived present, and an anticipated future into a readily understood story template. Lifestories consist of a number of literature-inspired elements. These include genre (e.g., comedy, tragedy), tone, characters or images, and themes. The latter refers to recurrent goal sequences in narratives that elucidate wants, desires, drives, and other motivational states and processes that move the story forward.

One of the most researched themes to date is redemption, in which "very negative scenes and events give way, sometimes suddenly, to positive life outcomes" (McAdams, 2006, p. 66). In this version of the lifestory, narrators tell of an early beginning in which they possessed some form of gift—be it musical, athletic, intellectual, or social abilities—and a precocious sense of suffering among others less fortunate than themselves. These two traits then became invariably entwined, such that the narrators came to believe that they must use their "gifts" to help others. Hence, the vast majority of redemptive stories have a powerful generative theme.

Using McAdams' (2006) terminology, we can say that our participants told "redemptive stories": a bad, affectively negative scene turns good; the character is saved or redeemed by a later positive outcome of some sort. As Tedeschi and Calhoun (2004) have pinpointed, struggle with traumatic events typically leads to such a revised lifestory. McAdams has shown that the capacity to read and tell one's life in this manner is associated with increased life satisfaction, sense of life coherence, and self-esteem, and with decreased depression (e.g., Adler, Skalina, & McAdams, 2008; McAdams, 2006, 2008a), a finding consistent with the positive contribution of integrative reminiscence to physical and mental health (Cappeliez & O'Rourke, 2006).

As in text recall research, where older adults tend to remember the gist of a passage of text better than specific details (e.g., Bluck, Levine, & Laulhere, 1999), older adults go beyond mere autobiographical recall; rather, they seem compelled to take a broader stance on their memories, to search for fundamental patterns, and to extract some sense of purpose or meaning from life events.

The importance of believing in a life that followed a trajectory of improvement has also been stressed by Ross and Wilson (Ross & Wilson, 2003; Wilson & Ross, 2001, 2003). These authors have investigated how autobiographical memory contributes to the construction of personal identity, largely by maintaining a favorable view of self. And they have underlined the widespread tendency of believing in a forward personal progress, typically at the expense of deprecating our former selves. This sense of an improving trajectory even in the face of actual decline may be particularly active in old age.

The clear conclusion is that, when requested to report a recent reminiscence as it had occurred spontaneously in daily life, older adults automatically embedded it in a structure, that of their lifestory. In that sense, we are dealing here with a process of reappraisal and integration akin to *anamnësis*. But what about the elusive *mnëmë*?

To explore that issue, we resorted to questioning older adults directly on their thoughts and views about reminiscence. Indeed, as Ross (1989) has pointed out, implicit theories about mental phenomena influence recall of these experiences themselves.

IMPLICIT THEORIES OF OLDER ADULTS ABOUT REMINISCENCE

We were specifically interested in discovering how older adults define the phenomenon of *reminiscence*—the context in which it occurs, the triggers, and the role they ascribe to this mental activity in their daily life. For this purpose, we interviewed eight older adults, five women and three men, on average 77 years old, presenting with good physical and cognitive functioning. Three were married and five were widowed, with an average of 12 years of schooling. The individual interviews followed a semistructured format with a series of questions prompting for experiences identified as "reminiscence," the situational context and triggers, the frequency, the relative importance of reminiscing and its impact on life present and future, the role of others in reminiscence, and the type of emotions felt during reminiscing. The contents of the interviews were transcribed verbatim and then submitted to qualitative analysis, using the method of grounded theory (Auerbach & Silvenstein, 2003). This method proceeds in seven distinct stages: 1) identification of the research questions and specification of the research objectives; 2) transcription and revision of the verbatim from the interviews; 3) identification of relevant text; 4) identification of repeated ideas; 5) identification of themes; 6) identification of theoretical constructs; and 7) creation of the theoretical narratives.

Nineteen themes were identified at stage 5 (see Table 12.1). They were regrouped under five theoretical constructs (stage 6):

1. Emotions are intrinsically linked with reminiscence (themes 2, 3, 7–9).
2. Identity is the function of reminiscing that predominates, closely followed by transmission (themes 6, 10–16).
3. Interpersonal relations are central to reminiscence (themes 3, 5, 17, 19).
4. Some reminiscences are spontaneous, whereas others are intentional, each with its particular context and triggers (themes 1–6).
5. The mere capacity to reminisce is a positive index of cognitive aging (theme 18).

Table 12.1 List of themes

1. Sensory stimuli act as triggers of reminiscence.
2. Emotional states induce reminiscence.
3. The death of close family members and family reunions facilitate reminiscences.
4. Moments of solitude are opportune for reminiscence.
5. Situations of transmission of life lessons naturally trigger reminiscence.
6. Retirement and advancing age in general are linked with increased frequency of reminiscence.
7. The emotional nature of certain events of the past makes them salient and thus matter for reminiscence.
8. The emotion felt at the time of recall differs in function of the emotional valence initially associated with the memory.
9. An effort is made to consciously control negative reminiscences or those that could turn out to be problematic.
10. Reminiscences are intrinsically linked with self-concept, since they constitute the story of one's life.
11. Putting the past to rest, making peace with it, is important to living in the present.
12. Good memories are important: they allow reliving in order to live better.
13. Reminiscences are used to predict the future; they provide continuity, stability.
14. Memories are revisited to provide ways of coping better with current life problems.
15. Reminiscences are used as points of reference for identity.
16. Reminiscences about the way society was in the past help in contextualizing identity.
17. Reminiscences reaffirm links with other people.
18. Reminiscences constitute a marker of memory functioning: having reminiscences is reassuring regarding the fear of Alzheimer's disease; reminiscences are a way to exercise memory.
19. The main contents of reminiscences are about family and the period of youth.

The final step in the qualitative analysis consists in pulling everything together in the form of a theoretical narrative that synthesizes the theoretical constructs. Following the procedure, the theoretical narrative about these theoretical constructs is presented here in relation to the initial research questions (stage 7).

Definition of Reminiscence

Reminiscence was defined as a personal memory that has an emotional impact. But participants went further: they expressly identified the emotional loading of certain events as what made them "matter for memory." The emotional component of the reminiscence is so important that it is viewed as the *raison d'être* of the reminiscence. This description of reminiscence corresponds to the Aristotelian notion of *mnëmë* in terms of a memory at the interface of the emotional and cognitive realms.

Reminiscences were considered intimately linked with the self-concept in the sense that reminiscences are labeled as "elements of the story of life." Remembering the past is regarded as an important activity, because forgetting the past is considered equivalent to the loss of self.

All instances of reminiscence provided as examples by the participants appeared very detailed and vivid, as if they were presenting a well-elaborated account of a slice of their life. These occurrences characteristically related to the family as topic and to youth as period of life. This finding is congruent with the phenomenon of the reminiscence bump described earlier (Rubin, Rahhal, & Poon, 1998). Higher accessibility of autobiographical memories from the bump period is typically explained by the intimate connection of these memories with life goals and identity. It thus seems that events occurring in that period of life act as identity markers for the rest of life whenever autobiographical memories are retrieved (Conway & Holmes, 2004; Holmes & Conway, 1999). They are the building blocks of a lifestory that acts as an organizational structure for recalling other important life events, i.e., a lifestory schema (Bluck & Habermas, 2000; Glück & Bluck, 2007).

Impact of Reminiscences

As indicated earlier, emotions are intrinsically linked with reminiscences. Reminiscences and emotions have reciprocal relationships, meaning that emotions trigger reminiscences and, in turn, reminiscences generate emotions. Interestingly, a form of voluntary control is exercised on some reminiscences after they come to mind. For memories of negative events, it takes the form of either intentional forgetting or a purposeful attempt to use these memories to improve life. For positive memories, it takes the form of using these reminiscences to reach an acceptance of the past. This reflects the predominance of the identity function of reminiscence (i.e., integrative reminiscence). The self-concept that emerges is characterized by both stability and growth. On the one hand, the past is revisited as an anchor point to project into personal future (stability). On the other hand, the past is reviewed as a guide for self-improvement (growth).

Another influence of reminiscence is on the maintenance of interpersonal relationships. Reminiscing reinforces social links, either privately through the recall of that other person's life and shared history or socially via the communication of a lesson of life (i.e., transmissive reminiscence).

Triggers

Intriguingly, a clear distinction is made between reminiscences that occur spontaneously and others that are intentionally solicited. Moments of solitude are identified as particular contexts for deliberate reminiscences. Reminiscences are also sought in situations where the person wishes to transmit a lesson of life. The death of a close family member or a friend and a family gathering are typical circumstances for such reminiscing.

Spontaneous reminiscences are associated with a state of diffuse attention. In those cases, an image or some words from somebody else are sufficient to trigger a personal memory. These findings closely parallel those of the research on involuntary reminiscences reviewed earlier.

An emotional state is also mentioned as a possible trigger of spontaneous reminiscences. The analogy with dreams is naturally evoked for spontaneous reminiscences. Again, these are features of *mnëmë*.

Metamemory and Reminiscence

Metamemory refers to attitudes and beliefs about one's memory processes and performance. For example, the conscious intention to use memories as an explicit strategy to combat cognitive decline is an instance of metamemory. In that respect, our participants noted that connecting with one's personal past through reminiscences is a mental activity that increases with advancing age. This echoes a finding from empirical research. Middle-aged and older adults are indeed more likely than younger adults to demonstrate autobiographical reasoning—that is, to make connections that link experiences to the person's sense of self (Pasupathi & Mansour, 2006). The mere occurrence of these reminiscences provides a reassurance that memory is functioning well. The capacity to reminisce is viewed as a positive sign. Voluntary reminiscences constitute a way of exercising memory to counteract certain negative consequences of aging and possibly to ward off dementia. Also, and more important, because reminiscing sustains a sense of identity, it affords a degree of protection against a disease that is expressly viewed as a loss of self.

SYNTHESIS AND CONCLUSION

This chapter was prompted by a curiosity about the role of involuntary reminiscences in the life of older adults. We first consulted the embryonic research literature on the characteristics of involuntary reminiscences. That line of research informed us about how these reminiscences may occur in everyday life but told us very little about their purposes. Consequently, we launched our own investigation, first by interviewing older adults on a recent occurrence of reminiscence. This method led directly to the report of personal memories that presented all the characteristics of a chapter of one's life review. As we have seen, the links with the narrative construction of the self were patently evident. What was communicated to the listener was the product of this synthesis. Furthermore, the context of the interview promoted the subtle transfer from the integrative mode to the transmissive mode, a phenomenon that Randall and colleagues (Randall, Prior, & Skarborn, 2006) have discussed. Deriving a lesson of life from one's memories and sharing it with younger generations was the fitting conclusion of almost all accounts. Typically, this process of giving back involved transcending the negative in the pursuit of individual and collective betterment.

The original reminiscences might well have occurred spontaneously but, in the interval, had been interpreted and integrated into the lifestory. This is an interesting finding in its own right, but, clearly, our first attempt had missed involuntary reminiscences in their immediacy. Asking older adults themselves what they thought of the role of reminiscences, either voluntary or involuntary, opened up an interesting avenue. They helped us understand that as soon as involuntary reminiscences come to mind they are in many instances subjected to some form of control. Indeed, the line separating involuntary and voluntary reminiscences is a fine one. That exploration of involuntary memories reaffirmed the importance of reminiscences in later adulthood along familiar lines. In brief, our older participants told us that reminiscences help them to manage emotions and consolidate their identity. Reminiscences contribute to a narrative of stability coupled with growth, two complementary facets of "successful aging." Reminiscences are regarded as components of the story of life, the building blocks of identity, their occurrence being in itself a reassurance against the threat of the loss of self, magnified by dementia. The relevance of the social context was once again reaffirmed. Reminiscences reinforce social links through the sharing of one's most personal heritage, the story of one's life.

Before concluding, a word of caution regarding the interpretation and generalization of the findings is in order. Indeed, some characteristics of the participants and the choice of procedure for collecting memories could have potentially introduced biases in responding. Even though we are confident that our recruitment reached participants from somewhat heterogeneous educational and social backgrounds, it could still have included self-selected individuals with personal characteristics of higher openness to experience, introspection, and interest in narrating experiences and life review. Also, the majority of the sample in both studies was women, who, as mentioned earlier, are generally more inclined to life review than men. In the study on the contents of spontaneous reminiscences, participants were explicitly asked on the spot about a recently experienced episode of *naturally occurring* reminiscence. Nevertheless, the possibility remains that this procedure of "remembering about remembering" may have opened the door to some control and oriented participants toward somewhat more voluntary memories. As reviewed above, an alternative method of collecting spontaneous memories that other researchers have used is the daily diary, but this procedure is itself not immune to the same potential bias. Future research needs to examine these issues carefully.

In conclusion, we have seen that, echoing the interest of Aristotle, a few contemporary researchers are beginning to address the question concerning the distinction between voluntary and involuntary memories. Limited evidence suggests that there may indeed be differences, for instance, in terms of quality, frequency, and emotional valence. As a psychosocial process drawing from a common memory pool, there are, of course, similarities as well. The research we have reported here also suggests an intriguing possibility, namely the fluidity, or interactional nature, of *mnēmē* and *anamnēsis*. Specifically, each type has the potential to trigger the other. Consciously recalling earlier times to retrieve a particular memory can often instigate the spontaneous remembering of related events, times, and episodes. Moreover, as indicated by the findings in our second study, involuntary memories are often incorporated into a broader narrative. Further analysis of the shifts between *mnēmē* and *anamnēsis* will help us understand the ways in which our unique memories are woven into our organic and evolving lifestory.

NOTES

The study on implicit theories of reminiscence was supported by a grant from the Social Sciences and Humanities Research Council of Canada (SSHRC #410-2006-0124) to Philippe Cappeliez, who acknowledges the contributions of Héloïse Drouin and Marilyn Guindon in data collection and analysis for that study.

[1] The Greek words *mnëmë* and *anamnësis* have usually been translated in the philosophical literature, respectively, in Latin as *memoria* and *reminiscentia*, in English as *memory* and *recollection*, and in French as *mémoire* and *réminiscence*. In line with Ricoeur's interpretation, we believe that the essential distinction made by Aristotle between *mnëmë* and *anamnësis* is between a memory coming almost passively to the mind (i.e., an involuntary autobiographical memory or involuntary reminiscence) and one that is the product of an effortful recollection (i.e., a voluntary autobiographical memory or voluntary reminiscence).

To make the matter even more complicated, there are important nuances between the English term *reminiscence* and the French term *reminiscence*. In English, *reminiscence* is defined simply as the act of recalling past experiences. This meaning is close to autobiographical memory. In French, *réminiscence* is defined as the return to mind of an image not recognized as a memory. This corresponds to involuntary memory. In everyday language, it refers to a vague, imprecise memory, in which the affective tonality dominates. In both senses, *réminiscence* is thus closest to *mnëmë*.

REFERENCES

Adler, J., Skalina, L., & McAdams, D. (2008). The narrative reconstruction of psychotherapy and psychological health. *Psychotherapy Research, 18*, 719–734.

Ardelt, M. (2003). Empirical assessment of a three-dimensional wisdom scale. *Research on Aging, 25*, 275–324.

Aristotle. (1955). De memoria et reminiscentia (On memory and reminiscence). In W. Ross (Ed.), *Parva naturalia (Short treatises on nature)*, (pp. 234–252). London: Oxford University Press.

Auerbach, C., & Silvenstein, L. (2003). *Qualitative data: An introduction to coding and analysis.* New York: New York University Press.

Bauer, J., & McAdams, D. (2004). Personal growth in adults' stories of life transitions. *Journal of Personality, 72*, 573–602.

Berntsen, D. (1996). Involuntary autobiographical memories. *Applied Cognitive Psychology, 10*, 455–460.

Bluck, S., & Habermas, T. (2000). The lifestory schema. *Motivation & Emotion, 24*, 121–147.

Bluck, S., Levine, L., & Laulhere, T. (1999). Autobiographical memory and hypermnesia: A comparison of younger and older adults. *Psychology and Aging, 14*, 671–682.

Cappeliez, P. (2008). *Nostalgia and beyond: Themes, affects, and meanings of spontaneous reminiscences.* Paper presented at the annual meeting of the Canadian Association on Gerontology, London, Ontario, Canada.

Cappeliez, P., Beaupré, M., & Robitaille, A. (2008). Characteristics and impact of life turning points for older adults. *Ageing International, 32*, 54–64.

Cappeliez, P., Guindon, M., & Robitaille, A. (2008). Functions of reminiscence and emotional regulation among older adults. *Journal of Aging Studies, 22*, 266–272.

Cappeliez, P., & O'Rourke, N. (2006). Empirical validation of a comprehensive model of reminiscence and health in later life. *Journal of Gerontology: Psychological Sciences, 61B*, P237–P244.

Carstensen, L., Fung, H., & Charles, S. (2003). Socioemotional selectivity theory and the regulation of emotion in the second half of life. *Motivation and Emotion 27*(2), 103–123.

Charles, S., Mather, M., & Carstensen, L. (2003). Aging and emotional memory: The forgettable nature of negative images for older adults. *Journal of Experimental Psychology: General, 132*, 310–324.

Coleman, P. (2005). Uses of reminiscence: Functions and benefits. *Aging & Mental Health, 9*, 291–294.

Conway, M., & Holmes, A. (2004). Psychosocial stages and the accessibility of autobiographical memories across the life cycle. *Journal of Personality, 72*, 461–480.

Glück, J., & Bluck, S. (2007). Looking back across the life span: A lifestory account of the reminiscence bump. *Memory & Cognition, 35*, 1928–1939.

Habermas, T., & Bluck, S. (2000). Getting a life: The development of the lifestory in adolescence. *Psychological Bulletin, 126*, 748–769.

Holmes, A., & Conway, M. (1999). Generation identity and the reminiscence bump: Memories for public and private events. *Journal of Adult Development, 6*, 21–34.

Hooker, K., & McAdams, D. (2003). New directions in aging research: Personality reconsidered. *Journal of Gerontology: Psychological Sciences, 58B*, 296–304.

McAdams, D. (2006). *The redemptive self: Stories Americans live by*. New York: Oxford University Press.

McAdams, D. (2008a). Personal narratives and the lifestory. In O. John, R. Robins, & L. Pervin (Eds.), *Handbook of personality: Theory and research* (3rd ed., pp. 242–262). New York: Guilford Press.

McAdams, D. (2008b). American identity: The redemptive self. *The General Psychologist, 43*, 20–27.

McLean, K. (2005). Late adolescent identity development: Narrative meaning-making and memory telling. *Developmental Psychology, 41*, 683–691.

Pasupathi, M., & Mansour, E. (2006). Adult age differences in autobiographical reasoning in narratives. *Developmental Psychology, 42*, 798–808.

Pasupathi, M., Weeks, T., & Rice, C. (2006). Reflecting on life: Remembering as a major process in adult development. *Journal of Language and Social Psychology, 25*(3), 244–263.

Proust, M. (1999). *A la recherche du temps perdu* [In search of lost time]. Paris: Gallimard. (Original work published 1913–1927)

Randall, W., & Kenyon, G. (2001). *Ordinary wisdom: Biographical aging and the journey of life*. Westport, CT: Praeger.

Randall, W., Prior, S., & Skarborn, M. (2006). How listeners shape what tellers tell: Patterns of interaction in lifestory interviews and their impact on reminiscence by elderly interviewees. *Journal of Aging Studies, 20*(4), 381–396.

Reker, G., Birren, J., & Svensson, C. (in press). Restoring, maintaining, and enhancing personal meaning in life through autobiographical methods. In P. Wong & P. Fry (Eds.), *The human quest for meaning* (2nd ed.). Mahwah, NJ: Erlbaum.

Ricoeur, P. (2000). *La mémoire, l'histoire, l'oubli* [Memory, history, forgetting]. Paris: Éditions du Seuil.

Ross, M. (1989). Relation of implicit theories to the construction of personal histories. *Psychological Review, 96,* 341–357.

Ross, M., & Wilson, A. (2003). Autobiographical memory and conceptions of self: Getting better all the time. *Current Directions in Psychological Science, 12,* 66–69.

Rubin, D., Rahhal, T., & Poon, L. (1998). Things learned in early adulthood are remembered best. *Memory and Cognition, 26,* 3–19.

Schlagman, S., Kvavilashvili, L., & Schilz, J. (2007). Effects of age on involuntary autobiographical memories. In J. Mace (Ed.), *Involuntary memory* (pp. 87–112. Malden, MA: Blackwell Publishing.

Tedeschi, R., & Calhoun, L. (2004). Posttraumatic growth: Conceptual foundations and empirical evidence. *Psychological Inquiry, 15,* 1–18.

Webster, J. (1993). Construction and validation of the Reminiscence Functions Scale. *Journals of Gerontology: Psychological Sciences, 48,* 256–262.

Webster, J. (1997). The Reminiscence Functions Scale: A replication. *International Journal of Aging and Human Development, 44,* 137–148.

Webster, J. (2003). An exploratory analysis of a self-assessed wisdom scale. *Journal of Adult Development, 10,* 13–22.

Webster, J. (2007). Measuring the character strength of wisdom. *International Journal of Aging and Human Development, 65,* 163–183.

Webster, J., Bohlmeijer, E., & Westerhof, G. (2010). Mapping the future of reminiscence: A conceptual guide for research and practice. Manuscript submitted for publication.

Webster, J., & Gould, O. (2007). Reminiscence and vivid personal memories. *International Journal of Aging and Human Development, 64,* 149–169.

Webster, J., & Haight, B. (1995). Memory lane milestones: Progress in reminiscence definition and classification. In B. Haight & J. Webster (Eds.), *The art and science of reminiscing: Theory, research, methods, and applications* (pp. 273–286). Washington, DC: Taylor & Francis.

Wilson, A., & Ross, M. (2001). From chump to champ: People's appraisals of their earlier and present selves. *Journal of Personality and Social Psychology, 80,* 572–584.

Wilson, A., & Ross, M. (2003). The identity function of autobiographical memory: Time is on our side. *Memory, 11,* 137–149.

Wilson, J. (2005). *Nostalgia: Sanctuary of meaning.* Lewisburg, PA: Bucknell University Press.

Wink, P., & Schiff, B. (2002). To review or not to review? The role of personality and life events in life review and adaptation to older age. In J. Webster, & B. Haight (Eds.), *Critical advances in reminiscence work: From theory to application.* (pp. 44–60). New York: Springer.

Thirteen

ACHIEVING NARRATIVE COHERENCE

FOLLOWING TRAUMATIC WAR EXPERIENCE:

THE ROLE OF SOCIAL SUPPORT

Karen Burnell, Peter Coleman, and Nigel Hunt

The concept of narrative underpins how we interpret ourselves and the world around us as we move through the transitions of life. We talk to each other in story form, and this activity shapes our identity, our narrative identity (Bruner, 1990). As McAdams (2001) argues, we are continually creating and editing our personal *lifestory*, a structure that provides meaning and continuity despite the natural, age-related changes that come with growing old. Our natural propensity to interpret events in terms of stories and to situate our self within these stories allows us to make meaning of our experiences and to have a sense of identity and purpose.

This same propensity is true, not only for everyday events but also for threatening and traumatic ones. Undergoing a traumatic experience, such as war, challenges our ability to make meaning through the creation of a coherent narrative, for such experiences shatter long-held assumptions about self and world (Janoff-Bullman, 1992; Joseph & Linley, 2005). It is important that we create a coherent personal narrative, something that is often achieved through social support, through the presence of a supportive audience. Yet with traumatic experience, we lose the concept of the audience. There is no one to listen to the story of the trauma; no one worthy of hearing it; no one who should be exposed to it—all of which makes it that much more difficult for the traumatized individual. However, the presence of a supportive audience aids the meaning-making process, which then may lead to the reconciliation of the event within the greater lifestory and the ability to grow from the event (Pennebaker & Seagal, 1999).

Narrative theory and methodology provide a suitable and valuable approach to understanding how traumatic memories are managed, integrated, and ultimately reconciled into the lifestory by providing insight into the meaning-making process (Chase, 2008; Crossley, 2000; Polkinghorne, 1988). Our aim in this chapter is to discuss the ways in which war research can benefit from such an approach by providing insight into the role of social support in the reconciliation of traumatic memories and the interpretation of social changes that challenge identity. To achieve this, we present a two-level model of analysis concerning social support and narrative coherence, along with excerpts of interviews conducted with British veterans (aged 23 to 86) of World War II (WWII) through to the Iraq War. We also present an analysis of interviews with Soviet WWII veterans (ages 73 to 91) that addresses social change and challenges to narrative identity. Such research has implications, we believe, not only for reconciliation in later life but also for the potential reconciliation that can occur earlier in life.

TRAUMA THROUGHOUT THE LIFE COURSE

Traumatic events can affect veterans in the immediate aftermath of conflict and/or later in life. Unreconciled trauma may have been prevalent throughout life (Hamilton & Workman, 1998; Schreuder, Kleijn, & Rooijmans, 2000). Alternatively, post-trauma symptoms may present for the first time only in later life (Lindman Port, Engdahl, & Frazier, 2001). The (re)emergence of trauma in later life is due to a number of possible factors, such as retirement (Busuttil, 2004) or a decline in physical health (Ong & Carter, 2001). Of interest to our discussion here is the likely loss in later life of social-support resources that previously may have aided the avoidance of memories (Hunt & Robbins, 2001).

The presence of traumatic war memories can affect the process of reminiscence and life review in later life (Coleman, 1999) because of a natural unwillingness to reflect on past events (Bender, 1997). Since reminiscence and life review are linked to meaning-making, the avoidance of looking back can have an impact on the ability to find meaning in events (Krause, 2005). As one ages, it becomes harder to avoid remembering the past because of age-related changes in cognition. In the absence of social support, this problem is only exacerbated. As argued by Baltes and Lang (1997), the degree to which individuals cope with change over the life course is due in part to available resources.

Research has generally focused on difficulties associated with traumatic memories in later life, perhaps because it is then that such memories can be triggered, and the process of life review provides a natural opportunity for reflection and reconciliation. Staudinger (2001) suggests, however, that life reflection occurs throughout the adult life course, once concepts of coherence (Habermas & Bluck, 2000) and story *factors* (McAdams, 2001) have been learned: in other words, once a person is able to see his or her life as a story. Indeed, McAdams (1993) suggests that Butler's (1963) concept of life review as the *pinnacle event of life* actually involves reflecting on the personal narrative that has been created throughout the life course rather than creating an entirely new story in later life. For this reason, there has been a drive towards understanding the potential for early life reconciliation through the creation of a coherent personal narrative (Burnell, Coleman, & Hunt, 2006, 2010).

TRAUMA AND NARRATIVE COHERENCE

The concept of the lifestory, along with that of narrative intelligence (Randall, 1999), is based on the principle that we are naturally predisposed to structure our lives into a story. From birth, we develop within a culture of storytelling, with main characters, plotlines, twists, and motivations. During adolescence, we are driven to construct our own personal narrative, perhaps because for the first time we have an understanding of our past, an awareness of our present, and a sense of our future (McAdams, 1993). Or, it is the first time that our coherent childhood narrative is disrupted, which necessitates actively constructing an adult one. Either way, through this process, we create a sense of coherence, continuity, and purpose.

It is the extraordinary nature of war experience that makes meaningful integration problematic within our personal narrative and with other autobiographical memories (Bluck & Habermas, 2001). Janoff-Bullman's influential theory of shattered assumptions suggests that a traumatic event is difficult to integrate because of disparity between the traumatic event and other autobiographical memories (Janoff-Bullman, 1985, 1992). It is only over time that the event emerges as an explicit and integrated personal narrative (van der Kolk & Fisler, 1995). As Michelle Crossley (2000) asserts, while traumatic experiences produce a fragmented narrative, the ability to rebuild and reconstruct through narrative, or through the lifestory schema

(Bluck & Habermas, 2000), can aid reconciliation. Only when the memory can be recalled explicitly as an important and emotional memory relating to other experiences does it lose its threatening and unconscious nature.

While some individuals may make meaning using only internal personal resources, others rely on external social resources, such as social support, to aid the management of traumatic memories. Cohen and Wills (1985) proposed two social-support hypotheses: main effect and buffering. According to the main-effect hypothesis, social support is sought by individuals to allow them to talk about and process experiences. In terms of narrative, this would help them in the meaning-making process to move toward a more coherent and reconciled narrative and maintenance of narrative identity. According to the buffering hypothesis, the type of social support sought by an individual allows the avoidance of experiences, providing a safe haven away from traumatic memories. Arguably, this may result in the perpetuation of traumatic memories and symptoms, since the narrative would remain fragmented and incoherent, and identity would not be renegotiated or maintained (Burnell et al., 2006; Hunt & Robbins, 2001).

TRAUMA AND NARRATIVE INQUIRY

Narrative inquiry has been used to understand the ways in which individuals make meaning of traumatic and challenging events and the resources they employ to do this. The following section presents a two-level model of grounded narrative analysis that we have developed to provide insight into the types of social support that either aid or hinder the meaning-making process and lead to a coherent personal narrative (Burnell, Hunt, & Coleman, 2009). Analysis occurred at two levels. First, narrative form was analyzed and defined in terms of narrative coherence; second, narrative content was analyzed with attention given to social-support resources.

Despite the quantity of research dedicated to narrative coherence, there is no agreed-upon definition of the concept (Mishler, 1995). Baerger and McAdams (1999) define *coherence* as the presence of a story structure, affect, and integration. Others define it more loosely as a structural property of a good story and a social obligation to be fulfilled as a competent member of society (Linde, 1993). In addition, it is argued that a narrative should be structured in a way that captures an audience (Mandler, 1984), because an audience is needed to help the individual derive feelings of identity and meaning (McAdams, 2006).

While important, structure is not the only component required for a complete definition of coherence. There must also be emotional evaluation in order to convey understanding of the personal significance of an event (Androutsopoulou, Thanopoulou, Economou, & Bafiti, 2004; Coleman, 1999; Singer & Rexhaj, 2006). Integration is also a vital aspect of narrative coherence because it highlights the complexities of a narrative (see also Tromp, this volume). If stories are perceived as being too simple, they cannot realistically reflect lived experience (Rosenwald, 1992). Coleman (1999) argues further that, in order for a person to work through traumatic memories and to reach reconciliation, a story must integrate events through a common, uniting theme.

To analyze narrative coherence, we synthesized these definitions into a model of coherence with criteria relating to structure, emotional evaluation, and integration. We based our model on the work of Baerger and McAdams (1999), but adapted it to reflect the theoretical and clinical literature regarding trauma narratives. Table 13.1 contains the coding criteria of the model.

The orientation and structure criteria (O1/O2, S3a) were applied to local coherence (i.e., individual sentences) in order to identify basic storytelling principles. Criterion S3b was an original addition to the model and was inspired by a WWII veteran's explicit awareness of temporal coherence when using phrases such as "it broke part of the hinge of the ramp... ah... but I've jumped a gun."

Affect reflects the emotional evaluation of an event and its impact on an individual and the ability to express congruent emotions arising from traumatic events. This is especially indicative of reconciliation. Specifically, A4 captured emotional evaluation of an event through explicit statements of emotion, whereas A5 concerned the consistency of emotion, displayed either verbally or nonverbally. Taken together, these two affect criteria enabled a holistic evaluation of the emotional content of the narrative.

Integration was split into three criteria: the presence of a uniting theme (I6), the explanation or absence of contradictions (I7), and the presence of fragmentation (I8) within the narrative. Criterion I6 related to the presence of a theme within the narrative that provides meaning and advances lived experience through a meaningful message to future generations (McAdams, 2006). From the perspective of trauma, a theme is necessary to give meaning to events that challenge the plotlines and coherence of the lifestory, as well as narrative identity.

Furthermore, it was necessary for the uniting theme to be positive, rather than negative and maladaptive. Research on the narratives of veterans with Gulf War Syndrome (GWS, a term widely used to describe unexplained illness experienced by Gulf War veterans) reveals that poor health may be associated with narratives that revolve around the perpetual nature of GWS

Table 13.1 Narrative coherence criteria

Elements of narrative form	Coding criteria and definitions
Orientation (O)	O1 Introduction of main characters (scene setting) O2 Temporal, social, historical, and personal context
Structure (S)	S3a Structural elements of an episodic system presented with causal and temporal coherence (does not include contradictions). Structural elements include an initiating event, an internal response, an attempt, and a consequence. S3b Explicit recognition of temporal coherence, i.e., "I've jumped the gun/where was I?" Explicit recognition of storytelling
Affect (A)	A4 Past or present emotional evaluation of what described events mean to the narrator communicated through explicit statements of emotion A5 Consistency of verbal and nonverbal content within a meaning unit
Integration (I)	I6 Meaning of events and experiences is expressed within the context of the larger story. This includes a coherent theme linking all the events (theme may be explicit and/or implicit). I7 Contradictions between events or the narrator's personality traits or values, emotional evaluation, or changes in attitudes are acknowledged and explained in a causally coherent manner. I8 Fragmentation defined as broken speech and unfinished sentences, and incongruent information contained within the context of the larger narrative (unless otherwise stated, the narrative is fluid). If fragmentation is found within a narrative, the narrative is coded as incoherent.

(Kilshaw, 2004). Thus we argue here that reconciliation is not achieved by making a negative narrative central to the lifestory but, rather, by integrating the experience into the lifestory as a coherent chapter that one may grow from. In this way, the memory loses its threatening and unconscious nature, can be recalled explicitly as an important and perhaps emotional memory, and yet also relates to other experiences that have occurred in one's life.

Analysis of logical and functional contradictions within the narrative (I7), at both the global and local levels, was included to assess the consistency of integration within the narrative. The presence of unexplained contradiction within the narrative indicated that traumatic war memories had not been fully integrated into the narrative and remained unreconciled.

Finally, the inclusion of fragmentation (I8) reflected findings from clinical research indicating that the presence of fragmentation and disorganization within the narrative is indicative of unreconciled trauma. Fragmentation was defined as the presence of broken speech and/or unfinished sentences, or the presence of incongruent material.

Narratives were considered to be coherent if all criteria were present and there was no evidence of fragmentation (I8 absent from narrative coding). No criterion was perceived as being more important than another. Without orientation and structure, capturing a supportive audience to aid reconciliation would be more difficult and, without this audience, consistent emotional evaluation and integration would be harder to achieve. Once the criteria were applied to each narrative, groups were formed on the basis of coherent, reconciled, and incoherent narratives (see Table 13.2 for definitions and analysis protocol). The narrative content was then thematically analyzed to highlight common social support themes within and across the groups.

Themes were defined as specific patterns of interest (Joffe & Yardley, 2004) and were exclusively applied to units of meaning at the manifest (directly observable material) and latent (material requiring interpretation) levels. Deductive themes were applied to the narratives using a coding manual from previous research (Burnell et al., 2006), but inductive themes were also identified. Thematic analysis focused on social support from comrades, family and friends, and society as a whole, and the communication that took place with members of these groups. The co-authors were independently consulted to assess the credibility of the analysis. The combination of these two levels of analysis allowed insight into potential relationships between the specific types of social support that may be associated with narrative coherence.

The model was applied to the narratives of 30 British male veterans ranging in age from 23 to 86 years of age and representing a range of specialties, ranks, and years of service within the British Army, Royal Air Force, Royal Navy, and Royal Marines. Between them, these men had served in WWII, the Suez Crisis, Korea, Aden, Radfan, Cyprus, Malaya, Northern Ireland, Borneo, Falklands/Malvinas, the Gulf War, and Iraq.

SOCIAL SUPPORT AND NARRATIVE COHERENCE

Table 13.3 describes the number of veterans with coherent, reconciled, and incoherent narratives, along with an indication of their age and the wars in which they served. As Table 13.3 shows, no cohort differences were found

Table 13.2 Analysis protocol

Stage	Description
1. Transcription	• Natural pauses in speech represented as an ellipsis (…) • Emotions represented using brackets, e.g., (laughs). Nonverbal actions also enclosed in brackets, e.g., (claps). Added information or anonymous information enclosed in brackets and in italics, e.g., *(name of town)*

2. Narrative coherence analysis	• Transcripts analyzed for narrative coherence by means of narrative coherence model for the elements' orientation and structure, affect, and integration
	• Coded into coherent, reconciled coherent, or incoherent:
	  • *Coherent:* All elements of narrative coherence present (except I8) and no presence of traumatic memories as determined through narrative content
	  • *Reconciled coherent:* All elements of narrative coherence present (except I8), but presence of past traumatic memories that are no longer traumatic (ascertained from content)
	  • *Incoherent:* Absence of at least one element of narrative coherence and/or presence of I8 or traumatic memories (ascertained from content)

3. Narrative content: Thematic analysis	• Themes defined as specific patterns of interest and applied to units of meaning, e.g., either whole sentences and/or paragraphs • Analysis at the manifest (directly observable material) and latent (material requiring interpretation) levels • Initial themes coded within the interviews • Interview revisited and coded into exclusive "in vivo" categories; only one code applied to one unit of meaning, using the wording of the veteran as a label • Application of in vivo categories applied to the remaining interviews • Within original, in vivo categories were split (splicing) or were linked together (linking) • Finalized themes then applied to each interview transcript, using color coding and labels
4. Exportation of quotes	• Exportation of narrative content quotes into an Excel spreadsheet with participants in columns (with biographical information) and narrative content themes and coherence elements in rows, thus enabling exploration of the data within and between participants.

Table 13.3 Description of British veterans across groups

	Coherent	Reconciled	Incoherent
Number of veterans	9 male veterans	7 male veterans	14 male veterans
Age range (mean)	42–84 years (68.2)	40–86 years (60)	23–86 years (64.1)
Wars/conflicts	WWII (Western Europe, Burma), Korea, Suez, Aden, Radfan, Northern Ireland, Falklands/Malvinas	WWII (Burma), Suez, Cyprus, Northern Ireland, Falklands/Malvinas, Gulf War, Bosnia, Kosovo, Iraq	WWII (South East Asia, Western Europe, Burma), Suez, Cyprus, Malaya, Borneo, Northern Ireland, Falklands/Malvinas, Gulf War, Iraq

across groups, which further emphasizes the importance of social support in the reconciliation of traumatic war memories.

Comradeship

All veterans spoke positively of the importance of comradeship, but different patterns of communication with comrades emerged from each of the groups. Communication had taken place for some of the veterans with coherent narratives, but this was certainly not the norm. A number of veterans with coherent narratives indicated that they had avoided communication during service, but this had changed in later life:

> Very often people would talk to me about [my war experience].... Obviously a lot of my friends... knew... what I'd done... and many of them had shared the same sort of experience... and we'd talk about them. (Served from 1965 to 1975; Aden and Northern Ireland veteran)

It is important to note that veterans with coherent narratives did not report a need to communicate in quite the same way as veterans with reconciled or incoherent narratives, who emphasized the need to communicate but lacked the opportunity to do so. This was particularly the case during service, when military norms dictated the avoidance of communication:

> He's [a comrade] probably thinking the same thing... and he daren't mention it to you and you daren't mention it to him because of... what he may think. (Served from 1943 to 1947; WWII veteran, Burma)

Or there was a lack of opportunity in later life due to a loss of social support:

> I had to wind [the veterans' association] up.... No one was prepared to step in and help... and I wasn't prepared to do it all by myself... so... it wound up, which didn't help me at all. (Served from 1943 to 1947; WWII veteran, Burma)

Family and Friends

Interactions with family and friends seemed to differ across the groups. Veterans with coherent narratives reported positive interactions with family and friends in earlier and in later life and most had felt able to talk to friends and family about their experiences. Once again, it is important to note that these veterans emphasized that they had not been affected by their experiences:

> Oh no, I was very happy to talk about them [experiences]... yes... I'm sure that's a help. (Served from 1940 to 1946; WWII veteran, Middle East and Burma)

Veterans with reconciled narratives reported some positive, but also some negative interactions. However, relationships with family and friends had improved with time, and these veterans had started to share their experiences with others after an initial period of avoidance. This may explain the fact that, while rarely processing memories with comrades, the veterans with reconciled narratives had, at some stage, communicated with family and friends:

> I don't actually remember discussing personal experiences until 2002 when we had the 20th anniversary [of the Falklands/Malvinas war].... That was the first time I really ever discussed personal experiences with anybody. (Served from 1979 and currently serving at the time of the interview; Northern Ireland, Falklands/Malvinas, Kosovo, Gulf War veteran)

Veterans in the incoherent group reported negative interactions both in earlier and later life, along with the need to talk about their experiences. However, they also emphasized the absence of a supportive family environment in which to communicate:

> My children don't know.... I should think it's more a question of when you start talking about that [war experiences]... you see them falling asleep... so it isn't a matter that comes up. (Served from 1939 to 1957; WWII veteran)

Societal Support

Once again, thematic differences were found in perceptions of societal support across levels of coherence. Veterans with coherent narratives highlighted positive interactions and communications with members of the public and reported feeling appreciated and understood, even when they had served in controversial wars:

> I think people felt that… Korea had to be done…. I did once go to a… reception in London a long time after Korea and the Ambassador said to me… "You were in Korea, were you?"…. And he was incredibly… forthcoming and grateful, and then I thought to myself, "Well perhaps it was [necessary]." (Served from 1947 to 1978; Korea, Suez, Aden, and Radfan veteran)

For veterans with reconciled narratives, perceptions of support and interactions were mixed. For most, societal support provided a way of justifying actions, which aided reconciliation:

> I've never had anybody say anything negative about it [Falklands/Malvinas war], and that's good… and that's… very comforting if you're gonna [sic] do that kind of thing. (Served from 1979 and currently serving at the time of the interview; Northern Ireland, Falklands/Malvinas, and Gulf War veteran)

For others, perceptions of societal support remained negative, which had perhaps hindered reconciliation by challenging the veteran's perception of the justification of and motives for war:

> So I'm stood on the station feeling ever so proud and this woman came to me…. "Excuse me," she said…. "Were you in Suez?"… And I said, "Yes I was."… And do you know what she said?… "You're no better than Nazis."… I was totally flummoxed. It took me literally 10 years to really understand [why she said that]. (Served from 1954 to 1956; Cyprus and Suez veteran.)

These negative interactions seemed to strengthen the view that civilians are unable to understand conflict, which may lead to feelings of being misunderstood and unappreciated:

> I don't think a lot of civilians grasp that, oh, you're trained to do it…. Doesn't mean you're always going to pull the trigger… because most of us have consciences…. If you shoot a man… it [goes] round through your head…. It's not something you forget about… ever. (Served from 2001 to 2005; Iraq veteran)

SOCIAL SUPPORT AND NARRATIVE IDENTITY

Social support also has implications for the continuation of narrative identity. As we have seen from the previous discussion, when one's role in an event is challenged by criticism or change, this can have an impact on narrative identity, which is also created through the meaning-making process. A particular aspect of narrative identity is the generative identity, which is formed through our ability to understand the choices we make and the consequences of these actions beyond our individual life course (McAdams, 1990).

The creation of generative identity results in an imagined future that links key events through personal beliefs and values. If the imagined future changes and loses credibility, which may result from traumatic events or social change, then future identity is also threatened, rendering the narrative incoherent. Consequently, the individual must make meaning from this disruption to create a coherent narrative to maintain identity. As discussed earlier, generativity is an aspect of the integration criterion I6 within the model of narrative coherence previously described.

An example of disruption of narrative identity is provided by Coleman and Podolskij (2007), who examined the ways in which 50 Russian and Ukrainian Soviet World War II veterans (aged 73–91 years) had renegotiated personal identity following the fall of Communism. During the qualitative interviews conducted with them, veterans identified events affecting the (dis)continuity of identity and subsequent renegotiation.

Thematic qualitative analysis of the veterans' narratives revealed that most of the veterans had successfully created or maintained a coherent narrative identity despite feeling negatively about the change in national identity. The importance of family throughout the life course appeared to aid identity maintenance with grandchildren in particular, providing a source of hope and purpose:

> What has changed is that I have lived under Soviet power, and now it is democracy, a change for the worse. What has not changed is my attitude to my family. I love them as before and take care of them.

Those who had been unable to renegotiate identity also appeared to have experienced loss or bereavement and, therefore, loss of family to provide support and purpose in the face of change:

> The basic condition of my life is loneliness…. My children call on me often, but they have their life. I have lived at their house, but I couldn't help and have come back here…. Life has passed quickly as if I haven't lived at all.

Once again, the research of Coleman and Podolskij (2007) highlights the importance of social-support resources such as family support, even when perceptions of societal support change drastically, as for these Soviet war veterans.

LIMITATIONS AND FUTURE RESEARCH

Despite the ability of the two-level narrative and thematic analyses to reveal interesting patterns of social support across levels of coherence and continuation of identity, it is difficult to infer causality from the retrospective qualitative data obtained. It may be that social support directly influences the ability to make meaning of events, resulting in a coherent narrative and identity. Alternatively, the ability to find meaning may result in positive perceptions of social support. For this reason, conclusions here are tentatively drawn.

To understand how meaning is made post-trauma, it is also important that we understand an individual's narrative processes pre-trauma. Currently, it unknown to what extent the experience of trauma changes the natural processes, if at all. It may be that people affected by trauma are those who find it difficult to find meaning even in daily events or who find meaning through a passive audience, rather than an active audience. For instance, it is not uncommon for veterans to keep diaries or write autobiographies about their experiences. Some may prefer to find meaning through these individual processes, which makes it important that we gain an understanding of why a veteran might prefer this approach and of the differences in narratives that each such approach produces.

Future research should focus on exploring the meaning-making process by investigating pre-trauma narrative processes, the role of active and passive audiences, and changes in narrative coherence and identity after taking part in an informal intervention, which promotes communication with comrades and family members.

IMPLICATIONS

Despite these limitations, the findings of the research presented here highlight the importance of social support in achieving reconciliation and maintaining identity. Since the ability to reconcile traumatic events and maintain identity has implications for well-being (Coleman, 1999), these findings have implications for developing therapeutic interventions for individuals who experience trauma and significant social change.

A number of interventions have used the concepts of narrative and reminiscence effectively (Fielden, 1990; Haight, 1991; Maercker, 2002). Westwood has found success in using the principles of restorying and guided autobiography in conjunction with social support to promote reconciliation in a group of young Canadian peace-keeping returnees (Westwood, Black, & McLean, 2002) and Canadian veterans of WWII (Shaw & Westwood, 2002).

In addition, narrative exposure therapy (NET) has been found to be an effective intervention for child victims of war and refugee populations and may be a suitable intervention for war veterans as well (Neuner, Schauer, Klaschik, Karunakara, & Elbert, 2004).

Despite the presence of social support in these therapies, they remain formal interventions facilitated by professionals. The research presented in this chapter suggests the opportunity for a more informal intervention promoting social-support resources to reconcile challenging and threatening experiences. Such an intervention would focus on narrative development, or restorying, through communication with supportive others, particularly those who have had similar experiences. Such interventions are known as peer support interventions, and there is evidence to indicate that they may improve the psychological health and well-being of individuals with mental or physical illness (Hogan, Linden, & Najarian, 2002). Peer support interventions differ from naturally occurring social support interactions with peers in that they involve an individual newly affected by an experience or diagnosis being matched with a peer who is experientially similar to the person they are supporting but with more experience. In other words, peers have completed the journey on which the newly affected individual is only just embarking. In addition, a peer would normally be trained by a health professional to ensure the quality and usefulness of the interaction.

This concept of structured peer support is becoming increasingly prevalent within the armed forces. For instance, Royal Marines coming to the end of their service careers may train as welfare officers to provide support to recently deployed personnel and their families, with a particular focus on encouraging communication within natural support systems. Combat Stress (the Ex-Services Mental Welfare Society) also trains formerly serving personnel as welfare officers to provide practical support to veterans in the community and help veterans identify and use naturally occurring social support.

It would appear that peer support is positively perceived by veterans and presents a very natural therapeutic opportunity. Academic and clinical research into peer support interventions for veterans is limited, however. The two key studies taking place are a peer mentoring service for newly discharged personnel conducted by King's Centre for Military Health Research, and a peer support program for formerly serving personnel conducted through the National Health Service. Clearly, peer support models have sound theoretical underpinnings, and there is potential for them to be adapted for use with currently and formally serving veterans. However, in both cases, the intervention focuses on individuals who present with clinical symptoms or are identified as being at risk. Specific attention should be given to developing more informal peer support interventions that help all veterans restory war experiences into a chapter of the coherent personal narrative. The research findings suggest that some veterans have achieved coherence through peer and family support without the need for a formal intervention. It is apparent, however, that others are not as fortunate. Future research should focus on systematically investigating the feasibility, appropriateness, and effectiveness of narrative peer support interventions for veterans.

CONCLUSIONS

The impact of war on veterans' narrative coherence and identity is an important area of research. Research has shown the potential narrative mechanisms of meaning-making and reconciliation throughout the life course, as well as the importance and possibility of reconciliation in earlier rather than later life. It is important that future research at both the theoretical and applied levels of narrative gerontology focuses on the specific factors that support the creation of a coherent narrative throughout the life course. Such research has implications for the development and provision of targeted narrative therapies for veterans of war and conflict.

REFERENCES

Androutsopoulou, A., Thanopoulou, K., Economou, E., & Bafti, T. (2004). Forming criteria for assessing the coherence of clients' life stories: A narrative study. *Journal of Family Therapy, 26*(4), 384–406.

Baerger, D., & McAdams, D. (1999). Life story coherence and its relation to psychological well-being. *Narrative Inquiry, 9*(1), 69–96.

Baltes, M. & Lang, F. (1997). Everyday functioning and successful aging: The impact of resources. *Psychology and Aging, 12*(3), 433–443.

Bender, M. (1997). Bitter harvest: The implications of continuing war-related stress on reminiscence theory and practice. *Aging and Society, 17*(3), 337–348.

Bluck, S., & Habermas, T. (2000). The life story schema. *Motivation and Emotion, 24*(2), 121–147.

Bluck, S., & Habermas, T. (2001). Extending the study of autobiographical memory: Thinking back about life across the life span. *Review of General Psychology, 5*(2), 135–147.

Bruner, J. (1990). *Acts of meaning*. Cambridge, MA: Harvard University Press.

Burnell, K., Coleman, P., & Hunt, N. (2006). Falklands War veterans' perceptions of social support and the reconciliation of traumatic memories. *Aging and Mental Health, 10*(3), 282–289.

Burnell, K., Coleman, P., & Hunt, N. (2010). Coping with traumatic memories: Second World War veterans' experiences of social support in relation to the narrative coherence of war memories. *Ageing and Society, 30*, 57–78.

Burnell, K., Hunt, N., & Coleman, P. (2009). Developing a model of narrative analysis to investigate the role of social support in coping with traumatic war memories. *Narrative Inquiry, 19*(1), 91–105.

Busuttil, W. (2004). Presentation and management of post traumatic stress disorder and the elderly: A need for investigation. *International Journal of Geriatric Psychiatry, 19*(5), 429–439.

Butler, R. (1963). The life review: An interpretation of reminiscence in the aged. *Psychiatry, 26,* 65–76.

Chase, S. (2008). Narrative inquiry: Multiple lenses, approaches, voices. In N. Denzin & Y. Lincoln (Eds.), *Collecting and interpreting qualitative materials* (3rd ed., pp. 57–94). Thousand Oakes, CA: Sage.

Cohen, S., & Wills, T. (1985). Stress, social support, and the buffering hypothesis. *Psychological Bulletin, 98*(2), 310–357.

Coleman, P. (1999). Creating a life story: The task of reconciliation. *The Gerontologist, 39*(2), 133–139.

Coleman, P., & Podolskij, A. (2007). Identity loss and recovery in the life stories of Soviet World War II veterans. *The Gerontologist, 47*(1), 52–60.

Crossley, M. (2000). Narrative psychology, trauma and the study of self/identity. *Theory and Psychology, 10*(4), 527–546.

Fielden, M. (1990). Reminiscence as therapeutic intervention with sheltered housing residents: A comparative study. *British Journal of Social Work, 20,* 21–44.

Habermas, T., & Bluck, S. (2000). Getting a life: The emergence of the life story in adolescence. *Psychological Bulletin, 126*(5), 748–769.

Haight, B. (1991). Reminiscing: The state of the art as a basis for practice. *Journal of Aging and Human Development, 33,* 1–32.

Hamilton, J., & Workman, R. (1998). Persistence of combat-related posttraumatic stress symptoms for 75 years. *Journal of Traumatic Stress, 11*(4), 763–768.

Hogan, B., Linden, W., & Najarian, B. (2002). Social support interventions: Do they work? *Clinical Psychology Review, 22*(3), 381–440.

Hunt, N., & Robbins, I. (2001). World War II veterans, social support, and veterans' associations. *Aging and Mental Health, 5*(2), 175–182.

Janoff-Bullman, R. (1985). The aftermath of victimization: Rebuilding shattered assumptions. In C. Figley (Ed.), *Trauma and its wake: The study and treatment of post-traumatic stress disorder* (pp. 15–35). New York: Brunner/Mazel.

Janoff-Bullman, R. (1992). *Shattered assumptions: Towards a new psychology of trauma.* New York: The Free Press.

Joffe, H., & Yardley, L. (2004). Content and thematic analysis. In D. Marks & L. Yardley, (Eds.), *Research methods for clinical and health psychology* (pp. 56–68). London: Sage.

Joseph, S., & Linley, P. (2005). Positive adjustment to threatening events: An organismic valuing theory of growth through adversity. *Review of General Psychology, 9*(3), 262–280.

Kilshaw, S. (2004). Friendly fire: The construction of Gulf War syndrome narratives. *Anthropology and Medicine, 11*(2), 149–160.

Krause, N. (2005). Traumatic memories and meaning of life: Exploring in three age cohorts. *Ageing and Society, 25*(4), 501–524.

Linde, C. (1993). *Life stories: The creation of coherence*. New York: Oxford University Press.

Lindman Port, C., Engdahl, B., & Frazier, P. (2001). A longitudinal and retrospective study of PTSD among older prisoners of war. *American Journal of Psychiatry, 158*(9), 1474–1479.

Maercker, A. (2002). Life-review technique in the treatment of PTSD in elderly patients: Rationale and three single case studies. *Journal of Clinical Geropsychology, 8*(3), 239–249.

Mandler, J. (1984). *Stories, scripts, and scenes: Aspects of schema theory*. Hillsdale, NJ: LEA.

McAdams, D. (1990). Unity and purpose in human lives: The emergence of identity as a life story. In A. Rabin, R. Zucker, R. Emmons, & S. Frank (Eds.), *Studying persons and lives* (pp. 148–200). New York: Springer-Verlag.

McAdams, D. (1993). *The stories we live by: Personal myths and the making of the self*. New York: Oxford University Press.

McAdams, D. (2001). The psychology of life stories. *Review of General Psychology, 66*(5), 1125–1146.

McAdams, D. (2006). The problem of narrative coherence. *Journal of Constructivist Psychology, 19*(2), 109–125.

Mishler, E. (1995). Models of narrative analysis: A typology. *Journal of Narrative and Life History, 5*(2), 87–123.

Neuner, F., Schauer, M., Klaschik, C., Karunakara, U., & Elbert, T. (2004). A comparison of narrative exposure therapy, supportive counselling, and psychoeducation for treating posttraumatic stress disorder in an African refugee settlement. *Journal of Consulting and Clinical Psychology, 72*(4), 579–587.

Ong, Y., & Carter, P. (2001). Grand rounds: I'll knock elsewhere—The impact of past trauma in later life. *Psychiatric Bulletin, 25*(11), 435–436.

Pennebaker, J., & Seagal, J. (1999). Forming a story: The health benefits of narrative. *Journal of Clinical Psychology, 55*(10), 1243–1254.

Polkinghorne, D. (1988). *Narrative knowing and the human sciences*. Albany, NY: SUNY Press.

Randall, W. (1999). Narrative intelligence and the novelty of our lives. *Journal of Aging Studies, 13*(1), 11–28.

Rosenwald, G. (1992). Conclusion: Reflections on narrative self-understanding. In G. Rosenwald & R. Ochberg (Eds.), *Storied lives: The cultural politics of self-understanding* (pp. 265–289). New Haven, CT: Yale University Press.

Schreuder, B., Kleijn, W., & Rooijmans, H. (2000). Nocturnal re-experiencing more than forty years after war trauma. *Journal of Traumatic Stress, 13*(3), 453–463.

Shaw, M., & Westwood, M. (2002). Transformation in life stories: The Canadian war veterans life review project. In J. Webster & B. Haight (Eds.), *Critical advances in reminiscence work: From theory to application* (pp. 257–274). New York: Springer-Verlag.

Singer, J., & Rexhaj, B. (2006). Narrative coherence and psychotherapy: A commentary. *Journal of Constructivist Psychology, 19*(2), 209–217.

Staudinger, U. (2001). Life-reflection: A social-cognitive analysis of life review. *Review of General Psychology, 5*(2), 148–160.

van der Kolk, B., & Fisler, R. (1995). Dissociation and the fragmentary nature of traumatic memories: Overview and exploratory study. *Journal of Traumatic Stress, 8*(4), 505–525.

Westwood, M., Black, T., & McLean, H. (2002). A re-entry program for peacekeeping soldiers: Promoting personal and career transition. *Canadian Journal of Counselling, 36*(3), 221–232.

Fourteen

USING SELF-DEFINING MEMORIES IN COUPLES

THERAPY WITH OLDER ADULTS

Jefferson A. Singer and Beata Labunko Messier

The dynamic increase in the number of older adults that is due to medical advances has profound implications, not only for health care providers, but also for providers of mental health care in particular. Worldwide, the number of people aged 65 and older was estimated at 506 million as of midyear 2008, and it is projected that in 2040 the number will increase to 1.3 billion, representing 14% of the world population (U.S. Bureau of the Census, 2009). Consequently, it is not surprising that therapists are increasingly treating older clients for individual, family, and marital problems. Working with older adults in couples therapy can involve many similar concerns to those of younger clients, but may also raise challenges not common in couples therapy with younger individuals. These challenges include issues surrounding physical decline and illness, cognitive impairment, dependency, and loss, as well as shifting gender and caretaking roles. As noted by Carter and McGoldrick (1980, 1999), these developmental changes challenge older couples to learn how to preserve their marital functioning and interest in each other by exploring new partnership, familial, and social constellations.

Although this developmental perspective takes both the gains and losses of older life into account, many researchers have pointed out that psychotherapy with older adults has been hampered by the prevalence of a loss–deficit model, highlighting cognitive losses, as well as physiological and psychological illness related to the aging process (Knight & McCallum, 1998;

Satre, Knight, & David, 2006). However, recent research, based on the theoretical and methodological advances in gerontology and life span psychology, has started to portray aging in a more positive light (Knight, Nordhus, & Satre, 2003).

Even as the preponderance of memory research on older individuals continues to focus on problems of decline and impairment, contrasting studies have detected surprising resilience and strength. For example, while numerous scientific investigations have confirmed that working memory generally declines with age (Light, 1990; Salthouse, 1991), several studies have revealed that when older adults process emotionally and personally meaningful information, there are no significant differences between younger and older individuals in their memory performance (Craik & Trehub, 1982; Hultsch & Dixon, 1990; Smith, 1996). Moreover, more recent scientific investigations on autobiographical memory in aging have yielded some encouraging findings that can contribute to the development and use of therapeutic interventions with older adults.

Piolino et al. (2006) examined the effect of aging on two different components of autobiographical memory: *episodic memory*, which consists of specific personal events, and *semantic memory*, which refers to general knowledge about one's past and is often linked to critical components of personal identity (Conway, Singer, & Tagini, 2004). The results revealed some decline in the recall of episodic memories and better preservation of personal semantic memories in older adults. This finding is congruent with previous research on autobiographical memories (Levine, Svoboda, Hay, Winocur, & Moscovitch, 2002; Piolino, Desgranges, Benali, & Eustache, 2002) that has demonstrated that older individuals are more likely to recall semantic memories than they are episodic memories. This study also found that older adults expressed a greater subjective sense of remembering for events from the remote past, especially those related to the period of the "reminiscence bump"—that is, adolescence and early adulthood (Berntsen & Rubin, 2002; Cappeliez & Webster, this volume). In addition, as stressed by Piolino et al., the ability of older individuals to "travel back into their past" to relive experiences can contribute to a stronger sense of identity and continuity across the life span.

Martinelli and Piolino (2009) further explored the properties of episodic and semantic memory in an older population and compared both types of memory to a unique subcategory of autobiographical memories, called "self-defining memories." As defined by Singer and Salovey (1993), *self-defining memories* are characterized by vividness, affective intensity, repetition, linkage to similar memories, and connection to a person's most enduring concerns or unresolved conflicts. Over multiple studies, researchers have been able to demonstrate that personally important self-defining memories are linked to an individual's central themes of identity and to enduring goals or conflicts within personality (Blagov & Singer, 2004; Moffit & Singer, 1994; Singer, 1990; Sutin & Robins, 2005). The results of the Martinelli and Piolino study, consistent with previous findings, demonstrated that, compared to younger participants, older participants displayed impaired retrieval of episodic memories. However, no difference was found between younger and older adults in the retrieval of semantic and self-defining memories. The preservation of self-defining memories in normal aging suggests that older individuals can compensate for their difficulties in retrieving episodic memories by recovering self-defining memories that contain specific details from their past and that are particularly relevant to their central identity concerns.

Systematic investigation comparing the self-defining memories of older and younger adults has led to several interesting insights about narrative identity and the nature of self-defining memories in older age. Singer, Rexhaj, and Baddeley (2007) collected self-defining memories from 49 college students and 44 older adults (50 and older) and examined potential differences in their affect, specificity, integrative meaning, and content. On average, the older participants perceived their memories as more positive and less negative in emotional tone than did the students. This finding is consistent with previous research on autobiographical memories that has demonstrated a tendency in older individuals to emphasize positive experiences from their lives and to diminish or reframe negative ones (Bohlmeijer & Westerhof, this volume; Carstensen & Mikels, 2005; Levine & Bluck, 1997; Schlagman, Schultz, & Kvavilashvili, 2006). In addition, self-defining memories of older adults were more summarized and less detailed. Most importantly, congruent with the related research on reminiscence and life review with older adults (Cappeliez & Webster, this volume; Webster & McCall, 1999; Wong & Watt, 1991), the memories of older participants included more meaning-making and lesson-learning statements that reflected their propensity to integrate life experiences into their larger life narratives.

McLean (2008) also examined the narrative identity of 85 young adults and 49 older adults (over 65) in an extensive self-defining memory interview. She found that as they narrate their lifestories, older and younger individuals employ different kinds of narration. Older participants constructed the self more in terms of stability, providing a means for resolution, in contrast to younger participants, who constructed the self more in terms of change, giving them opportunity for greater self-exploration and potential revision. McLean noted that the focus on stability in the narratives of older adults may be an adaptive process that reflects their effort to preserve a coherent sense of self in the face of physical, cognitive, relational, and occupational life changes. These results suggest that certain self-defining memories may have taken on a more "iconic" and enduring status for older individuals, but that shifting the meaning or interpretation of these memories might also be more challenging.

Taken together, studies on self-defining memories in older adults suggest that older adults have a rich capacity to recall personally meaningful memories from their past, providing therapists with a practical tool to assist them in communicating salient themes and concerns from their lives. The articulation of older adults' self-defining memories can support their efforts to construct a coherent lifestory; at the same time, it can also promote intimacy and compassion through their sharing of these memories with significant others. The value of mutual sharing of personal past stories in older adults has been highlighted in the work of Pasupathi and Carstensen (2003). In a first study of 129 adults, they found that age was related to increases in positive emotion during mutual reminiscing. A second study of 132 adults expanded this finding, revealing that age was indeed associated with increases in positive emotions, but only while individuals were retelling positive events. Such results suggest that mutual reminiscing by generating positive emotional experiences can provide older adults with a potential method of emotion regulation. This study raises the question of whether the exchange of negative reminiscences, along with positive memories, if mediated by a therapist, could go beyond emotion regulation and result in greater mutual understanding and more compassionate connection within a dyad.

In a previous clinical case study examining this possibility, Singer (2004) presented the results of exploring an autobiographical memory shared in common by an older couple. The husband, who was terminally ill with cancer, had contacted the therapist in the hopes of narrowing the rift between himself and his wife before his death. There had been a long history of distance and subdued conflict between them, stemming back to his years of alcohol abuse. Although he had been sober for a decade, the battle lines had been drawn long before then, and they had relied on silence and separate activities to keep a fragile truce between them. In describing the history of their relationship, each partner returned to the same memory of a drive home from a substance abuse treatment center. During the drive, the wife reached out to take her husband's hand; he pulled back his hand and then she pulled back as well. They both noted that in the 17 years since, they had shared not a single moment of physical intimacy. This memory was indeed a touchstone event that seemed to haunt them both. In the course of treatment, after employing many different forms of intervention, including cognitive-behavioral exercises, the therapist returned to the memory and engaged the couple in a reverse role play. They each took their partner's part and recreated the now infamous "drive home." By expressing the imagined thoughts and fears of the other, they were each able to forge a greater sense of understanding and forgiveness around this pivotal event. Their ability to give the memory a new and different ending coincided with the multiple efforts that they had begun to make toward a more loving relationship. Many times before the husband's death, approximately 10 months after the start of therapy, the couple returned to their memory work, using it as "an emotional handle" (Greenberg, 2004). They held onto this memory as a concrete expression of the pain and separation that would return if they did not continue to reach out to each other in their final days together.

In this case, the important memory emerged spontaneously and then became a point of emotional entry for addressing complex feelings and attitudes that were creating conflict within the relationship. In the following case study, our goal in working with an older couple was to demonstrate that the systematic recruitment of self-defining memories can be an effective clinical tool in couples therapy with older adults. In contrast to the previous intervention, the clinician asked each member of the couple to generate his or her personal self-defining memories. These individual memories were then supplemented by a shared "relationship-defining" memory.

CASE HISTORY

Background of the Couple

Adam and Deborah Sowell are a couple in their early 60s who entered therapy with the first author (JAS) to work on their repetitive fights and mutual threats to dissolve their relationship. Adam has two adult sons from a previous marriage; his first wife died roughly 15 years earlier from a congenital heart condition. Deborah was married twice before and has two adult children, a daughter and a son. Her first marriage ended when her children were very young, and her second husband succumbed to cancer 14 years ago. Adam and Deborah were introduced to each other by a mutual friend 11 years ago and after a swift courtship were married less than a year later.

Looking back over the past 10 years of their marriage, Adam remarked that perhaps one of the reasons for their ongoing conflicts was that they had leapt into their life together and did not take enough time to get to know each other before making a full commitment to each other. It is true that, temperamentally, Adam and Deborah are very different people, leading to a low threshold for flare-ups between them. Adam is on the taciturn side, not one to air his feelings easily; Deborah is vivacious, sensitive, and highly expressive of her changing moods. On the one hand, their contrasting styles of displaying and communicating emotion have strained their relationship on many occasions. On the other hand, they are capable of exuding a pleasure and excitement about being in each other's company. Both are attractive, physically fit, and social; they enjoy bicycling, travel, and gatherings with friends. With his silver hair and ruggedly handsome features, Adam could fit a Hollywood casting call for the part of a senator or CEO. Deborah, with her stylish cardigan sweaters and quirky jewelry, looks like she could be on her way to a trendy restaurant in Manhattan. Adam is retired from a highly successful law firm, and Deborah has scaled back her real estate practice to focus more on her landscape painting. Their financial comfort has afforded them opportunities to take extended trips to tropical places, tour with their sailboat on cruises up and down the Eastern seaboard, and decorate a home with the finest furniture and art. Part of what is perplexing for them is that with ample time and resources to savor their life together, why do they spend so much time fighting and making each other miserable?

The catalyst for many of their conflicts was often Deborah's perceptions of imbalances or inequities in the relationship, particularly centering on issues of allocation of their time to each other and their children. On numerous occasions Deborah perceived herself as putting herself out to accommodate Adam's sons' visits, at the expense of her own needs and her own children. She would clean, cook, and host his "boys," along with their wives and children, but felt she received little in return for all of her effort. Adam had a great deal of trouble accepting this version of the visits, or her characterization of inequity in the relationship. His anger would slowly build up until he responded in a surly and defensive manner, negating her complaints and bemoaning the fact that she has little trust in his good will. An argument of this kind could escalate into a period of sustained unspoken resentment. They would go around the house making only the most perfunctory comments to one another, and Adam would sleep in the guest bedroom. These festering rifts could last a few weeks and even drag into a month or two before they would put aside their hurt and self-righteousness.

For all couples we treat, our initial assessment includes an evaluation of the degree of "we-consciousness" that the two members of the couple possess. We-consciousness is the couple's awareness that they belong to a larger entity that transcends each of them as individuals, and that good relationships require attention to the needs of this third entity (the relationship), along with respect for each individual that makes up the dyad. We are always interested to know how much attention couples have given to the question, "What is best for us?" In other words, "How will my and my partner's words and deeds contribute to the health of our relationship and the strengthening of the bond we have forged together?" Couples who put this question in the foreground, along with concerns for individual fulfillment, are more likely to build a strong momentum for mutual satisfaction, an empathy for one another's needs, and a recognition of the importance of balancing personal goals with mutual goals that the couple sets together (Clark & Mills, 1979; Mills & Clark, 1982; Mills, Clark, Ford, & Johnson, 2004; Reid, Doell, Dalton, & Ahmad, 2008; Sarnoff & Sarnoff, 1989; Sharpe, 2000; Shem & Surrey, 1998). Fundamental for a strong sense of "we-ness," and often most problematic for couples in treatment, is the degree of trust and vulnerability shared by the members of the couple. To reach a point where each partner is willing to embrace the mantra of "couple first," a deep reservoir of good will and trust must be established. While it is not the focus of this chapter to detail how to assess this level of mutuality within couples (Labunko Messier et al., 2008), the critical point is that a distrust or refusal to become vulnerable in the relationship is likely to sabotage most efforts in couples therapy to bring about greater satisfaction, intimacy, and we-oriented thinking.

Clearly, Adam and Deborah entered treatment lacking a foundation of trust in each other. Adam has always carried a little bit of a chip on his shoulder that dates back to a modest upbringing in a factory town in Massachusetts. Over time, his parents had done well enough to rent a small cottage on the seashore in Rhode Island, and they would spend a good portion of the summer there. Adam felt that the wealthier kids looked down on him and that he could never quite fit in. His family's situation worsened at the end of his time in high school when his father suffered a stroke from which he never fully recovered. Adam remembered scrambling for money and his mother's continued anxiety during his years at the state university. His college days were far from idyllic; instead they were filled with shame and efforts to conceal his relative poverty from his classmates. Throughout law school, the building up of his practice, and the creation of his own firm, a persistent theme was his dogged determination to prove that he was just as good as the "Ivy Leaguers" and the well-heeled set from Boston and New York. Adam's first marriage had a rough start, but over time he felt a devotion to his wife Sue and his two sons. When Sue's heart condition worsened and eventually proved to be fatal, he went through an extended period of sadness and depression over this loss. His firm also faced some economic challenges in the years before he met Deborah. His relationship with his sons has generally been very positive, although both boys have had phases of rebellion and testing him. They now both work together in a contracting business in Idaho and visit a couple of times a year with their families.

Deborah grew up under traumatic family circumstances. Her parents divorced when she was a teenager and both suffered from alcohol abuse. She remained with her mother, but her mother experienced a series of hospitalizations for depression and substance abuse, leaving Deborah to spend extended periods with her grandparents. Her father also played an inconsistent role in her life and seemed to markedly favor her brother throughout her growing up. Deborah also recalled an episode of molestation by an older cousin who babysat for her, a memory that has increasingly troubled her since her discussion of it in her individual therapy. Deborah married young, in part to escape her immediate family, and had two children with her first husband. They divorced after 5 years, and Deborah was left to raise the children on her own. Finally, when she was 30, she met her second husband, Cliff, and enjoyed a much happier marriage, although both Cliff and she drank regularly. Cliff died of colon cancer after 10 years of marriage together, and Deborah was devastated by this loss. Approximately a year later, however, a close friend who was also a friend of Adam's encouraged the two of them to get to know each other. Deborah and Adam spoke on the phone for several weeks and then finally agreed to meet. They clicked strongly on this first meeting and, within the year, their relationship blossomed rapidly toward marriage. Despite an intense sense of passion for one another, it did not take long after the wedding for a consistent pattern of conflict and fighting to emerge.

At the time of entering treatment, they were displaying the following pattern of interaction. They were able to get along well for a while, but Adam could not seem to figure out how to make Deborah see that he cares and is committed to her in his daily behavior. As a result, he withdrew and isolated himself from her. She, in turn, took this frustration and withdrawal as a confirmation that he did not truly love her and could not be trusted. Her complaints and criticisms would increase in volume, only leading to more withdrawal on his part. Finally, they were likely to have a full-scale conflagration in which threats about ending the marriage were hurled back and forth. This pattern reached a crisis point when a fight resulted in their decision to put their ocean-view $3 million house on the market, the very house that they had designed together, the most concrete symbol of their decade-long commitment to each other.

After some initial crisis intervention, we began to work on their communication patterns, drawing on Gottman's identification of ways in which both partners can sabotage good dialogue (Gottman, & DeClaire, 2001; Gottman, & Silver, 1999), as well as the steps they could take to build more positive daily interactions and to redirect negative interactions. Although these therapeutic interventions helped to stabilize and improve the relationship, it often seemed that the couple reached an impasse around themes of trust and compassion.

One vital factor contributing to this impasse seemed to be that they had come to their relationship much later in life. Each partner had such an extensive history, connecting to their previous marriages, their offspring (both as children and adults), and their traumatic losses, that their ability to step out of these pasts and find a mutual resting place of compassion for each other was often taxed. In theory, the fact that they had both suffered the loss of a spouse seemed like a valuable starting point for connection, but the overlay of other past hurts and resentments frequently undermined their efforts at understanding and instead drew them back from one another into separate places of sadness and anger. To address their rift in empathy that continued to impair their mutual trust and hope for the marriage, I (JAS) proposed an intervention based on the use of self-defining memories.

The Self-Defining Memory Intervention in Couples Therapy

As the first step, I gave the couple a brief overview of our research into the role that important personal memories can play in individuals' self-understanding and sense of identity. I explained what self-defining memories are and outlined the five criteria of vividness, emotional intensity, repetition, linkage to similar memories, and connection to enduring themes or unresolved conflicts. I indicated that some individuals write about specific events and some choose to write in more general terms. I also told them that individuals vary in making explicit statements about what the memory has taught them or how it reflects a particular theme or value important to them. I emphasized that there was no one right way to go about writing about their memories. I requested only that they take their time and do their best to record 10 self-defining memories that might be helpful in explaining who they are to their partner. Once they had written down their memories, they were not to share them with their partner but to bring them in for me to review first, and then we would take the next step in the exercise. Since they were about to leave for a vacation, they had more than 2 weeks to work on this assignment before I saw them next.

Both partners took this project very seriously and came in to our next session with typed memories, a paragraph or two in length, and each described in some detail. The Appendices at the end of this chapter present excerpted versions of their memories (initially, Adam produced nine memories, but subsequently generated a tenth) with one memory apiece, in bold, presented in entirety. Collecting the memories from them, I promised to read through them thoroughly and to apply coding criteria based on my research that would help me to interpret them (Blagov & Singer, 2004; Singer & Blagov, 2002; Singer & Bonalume, in press).

Interpreting the Self-Defining Memories

Adam's Self-Defining Memories

The most striking features of Adam's memories were that they were all summarized and that he chose to attach a "lesson-learned" statement to every one. I checked with him to see if he had misinterpreted my instructions and thought that it was required to supply these lessons. He indicated that he knew that the lesson-stating was optional, but he felt that it helped to clarify his choices by adding these statements. Prior research (Blagov & Singer, 2004) has demonstrated an association between better adjustment and the tendency to produce memory narratives that include statements of meaning or lesson-learning. On the other hand, this same research also illustrated the connection between over-general memories and higher levels of defensiveness with regard to strong emotion (see also Steunenberg & Bohlmeijer, this volume). The structure of Adam's memories, along with the aphoristic statements at the end of each memory, suggested a rather over-controlled and avoidant coping style, especially in relation to experiences that might evoke sadness and feelings of shame and/or embarrassment.

The content and emotional trajectory of the memories reinforced my sense of a defensive posture, but also an underlying determination to go forward with his life in a positive fashion. Out of the 10 memories, Adam had 4 positive, 5 negative, and 1 mixed in overall tone. Across several memories, he showed a tendency to start with a negative circumstance, such as his parents' life of hard work, his mother's frustration with his complaints of boredom, his father's stroke, and his wife's passing, yet end in a more uplifting place by indicating ways in which he overcame his negative beginning. McAdams and colleagues have explored this narrative pattern of "redemption" in several studies (McAdams, Diamond, de St Aubin, & Mansfield, 1997; McAdams, Reynolds, Lewis, Patten, & Bowman, 2001) and found it to be associated with better physical and mental health and greater personal resilience.

What also emerged from Adam's memories was a somewhat simplistic and idealizing depiction of his family that placed an emphasis on their strong work ethic, shared leisure time, and rituals of family meals. Even with this "Norman Rockwell" gloss, he managed to convey information about his critical mother and his struggles with acceptance and rejection in social interactions. His response to these negative interactions was to withdraw and shut down. This emerged most powerfully and poignantly in his tenth memory (of which I will say more later) and in the lesson statement at the end of his eighth: "While I am willing to do anything for anyone, I am sensitive to feedback. If I get negative or no feedback, I have a tendency to back away."

Deborah's Self-Defining Memories

Deborah ended up producing 19 separate memories, of which 13 were negative in theme and 6 positive. Structurally, she recorded 10 specific memories and 9 summary ones. Only two of her memories contained lesson-learning or meaning-making statements. In contrast to Adam, Deborah's higher number of specific memories suggested a greater availability to her emotional life and a less defensive style. On the other hand, the predominance of negatively toned memories highlighted the depressive cast of her interior life, while the sparse number of meaning-making statements pointed to more problematic adjustment and a tendency to impulsivity and lower levels of self-restraint (Blagov & Singer, 2004; Weinberger, 1998). This memory analysis supported my clinical impressions of Deborah's emotional volatility, susceptibility to substance abuse, and conflict-laden interpersonal life.

The actual content of her memories contrasted some loving and nurturing memories of her grandparents and, occasionally, of her father with several memories of devastating disappointment and neglect inflicted on her primarily by her mother but at times by her father, other relatives, and peers at school. Although Adam had a number of redemptive memories, Deborah generated only one redemptive memory (her one positive memory of her mother), as well as five "contamination memories" in which her narrative began on a positive note and ended in a negative place. Individuals with high numbers of contamination memories share a pessimistic worldview, are more prone to psychological and physical symptoms, and are more likely to suffer from depression (McAdams et al., 1997, 2001).

Despite these dysphoric indicators in Deborah's memories, she wrote, "I find as I write these memories down, it has allowed me the freedom to go back, to open my eyes and to realize that, yes, there were sad memories that made a huge impact in my life, but also to realize and remember that there was joy along the way." In taking the memories as a whole, I would agree with Deborah that there is a theme of strength, resilience, and a tremendous longing for a loving and safe connection with others in her life. This is expressed powerfully in her last memory of her mother, which seeks to salvage some goodness from what had been the most painful and disappointing relationship in her life.

Interestingly, in both sets of memories written independently, there is a similar idealization of a loving home with good cooking, shared time in the evening, and a sense of security and safety. In Adam's memories, there is also explicit mention of Deborah and his desire to build a loving life with her. For better or worse, and in revealing irony, he describes her "beautiful smile," the same physical attribute he identifies in his mother as "her infectious smile." Perhaps he sees in Deborah both the warmth he found in his mother's love and the more problematic tendency to scrutinize and judge him that has challenged his sense of adequacy. Having completed this preliminary analysis of the memories, I was ready to discuss these findings with Adam and Deborah and lead them through an exchange of their memories with each other.

The Couple's Exchange of Self-Defining Memories

To begin this session of memory exchange, I first reviewed with Adam and Deborah what I had learned from reading and coding the memories. I pointed out how Adam's memories had a more summary structure and that he had been very systematic in applying a meaning or lesson to each memory narrative. I suggested that these characteristics expressed a strong tendency toward control of emotion in Adam and the logical tendency of his legal mind. He was able to acknowledge that he had held back to a certain degree from engaging too emotionally with his memories and that he preferred to emphasize the meaning-making rather than the feeling dimension of the exercise. In reviewing Deborah's memories, I pointed to the balance between specific and summary memories, and a greater tendency to jump to the emotional rather than to the intellectual import of her recollections. Her memories were much more evocative in their imagery and elicited an immediate response in readers, given their powerful and often painful content. The couple found it amusing to see the parallels between their memories and their own daily dispositions and shared some smiles over this. I then moved on to highlighting the patterns in the memories that reflected the frequent conflicts and traps that would emerge in their interactions. For Adam, I identified his pattern of presenting interactions in which he felt judged unfairly and his tendency to respond defensively or justify himself. I indicated that his strong tendency to move to a moral lesson protected him from engaging with possible emotion and vulnerability evoked by the memory's details. He seemed to be more able to move to a posture of resentment than linger in places where sadness might emerge.

In talking with Deborah, I emphasized the emotional intensity and immediacy of many of her memories. They conveyed repetitive themes of being disappointed, abandoned, and even betrayed by family members and friends. In the midst of these traumatic recollections were small glimpses of her grandparents' loving support, her father's intermittent efforts at parenting, and the one shining moment of her mother's single act of kindness. This memory tableau expressed her deep distrust of others' intentions and the possibility of consistency in relationships, as well as her significant self-doubt about her own worthiness to be loved in a lasting way.

With these two "memory scripts" laid out, I asked the couple to consider together how easy it was for them to fall into their familiar escalating conflicts. If Deborah felt slighted or ignored, she would try to overcompensate with kindness until she could no longer restrain herself from expressing her pain to Adam. Adam would receive this complaint as "yet another criticism" and move quickly into a defensive mode, leading him to withdraw and stew in anger. His withdrawal threw Deborah into a freefall of rejection feelings, and she doubted that he had ever loved her. Her challenge to the integrity of his affection for her brought his rage to the surface and a full-fledged battle would break out. Mutual withdrawal and despair would follow and linger for weeks. Holding in their hands the tangible evidence of the memories that underlie this destructive dance, the couple seemed to take more ownership of the mutual problem they were facing.

Sharing Deborah's Self-Defining Memories

The solution to this stalemate, I proposed, lay in their willingness to generate compassion for the mutual yet distinctly different wounds they shared. As a step toward increasing their compassion for each other, I asked Deborah to choose a memory of her own for Adam to read out loud. She had him read Memory #12, the "riding cap" memory (see Appendix A). As he read about her efforts to win the riding cap and the dashing of her hopes (when, despite her success, her friend's uncle did not present her with the promised hat), his voice trembled and he reached out to take her hand. He commented quietly to her about how many times she has been let down by her family, and how he understood how hard it must be to experience that from him.

I then asked Deborah to read her last memory to Adam (Appendix A, Memory #19). The memory involved her mother addressing her daughter's fear of the wicked witch in *The Wizard of Oz* by introducing Deborah to the actress who played this character. Deborah explained to Adam that this was the only distinct memory she had from childhood of her mother coming through for her and showing her that she loved her. As Deborah finished the story of her backstage encounter with Margaret Hamilton, the actress who played the Wicked Witch of the West, she began to cry about the "special-ness" she felt that day from her mother's efforts to dispel her fear. We all shared the deep irony that her mother, who often loomed as a wicked pres-ence in Deborah's childhood memories, could express her humanity by revealing the decency in the actress who portrayed the most famous witch in film. Once again, Adam seemed to move closer to Deborah and conveyed an enhanced compassion for her fragility in relationships. At this point, we were out of time and agreed to take up Adam's memories in the next meeting. Their homework was to read together through both sets of memories and continue to discuss them with each other.

Sharing Adam's Self-Defining Moments

When they returned for the next meeting, they explained that they had fol-lowed my instructions and something unexpected had occurred—namely, Adam had recalled a tenth memory. Not only had he recalled one more memory, but it was highly specific and emotionally raw for him. He pro-ceeded to share it with me; I have transcribed this narrative as his final memory listed in Appendix B. Even more than his previous memories, it tells the story of how he could feel caught in a position of being wrongly accused and coming up short. Even though he had not caused his father to fall from the ladder and learned later that the stroke had preceded his tumble to the ground, what remained with him were those first moments when his mother scolded him and identified him as the culprit in his father's accident. Even though his family soon realized that this was not the case, Adam's mother had never apologized or withdrawn her words. They all just went on with their lives. Both in their discussion of the memory outside of the session and in the repetition of the narrative for my benefit, Deborah emphasized her need to recognize Adam's fear of being misrepresented and wrongly judged. She saw more deeply how easily she could provoke this reaction in their seemingly minor squabbles. This insight allowed her to understand why what she perceived as the mentioning of "pet peeves" or "minor annoyances" could quickly catch fire and become arguments between them.

After some further discussion of these dynamics, I asked them to partake in one last memory exercise. Instead of recalling separate self-defining memories, I asked them to provide me with a shared memory that they felt could help define their relationship or express an important theme. They both joked about their first meeting after several long phone conversations. Adam showed up at Deborah's door with a Groucho Marx nose, mustache, and glasses on. Once he took them off, Deborah said she was struck by how Adam looked exactly the way she might have hoped. More seriously, they then recalled and agreed on the following memory (here described by Adam with Deborah filling it in):

> When we were first dating, we would stay together at a condo by the ocean. I remember that we had a lot of romantic nights together, but one night in particular we went for a midnight walk. The sky was clear except for two large black clouds overhead. We both looked up and each of us felt like we could see the shapes of angels in them. We decided that those angel clouds were Sue and Cliff looking down on us, and that they were okay with us being together. We felt like we got their blessing that night in a funny kind of way.

With this powerful shared memory as touchstone, I encouraged the couple to hold this image in their minds and to rely on it in moments of conflict. I assured them that conflict is inevitable, especially for two older people who have laid down strong patterns in their lives and who have had many more separate than shared experiences in their lives. Nevertheless, this final memory revealed the depth of connection and hope that exists at the core of their relationship, and it can be a continual reminder to place priority on their union rather than on their discord.

CONCLUSION

In the months since the self-defining memory intervention for this older couple, they have been able to make repeated reference to the memories and insights gained from the exercise. They seem to grasp the dynamic of Deborah's need for affirmation and Adam's defensive withdrawal in a deeper and more compelling fashion. Increasingly, we are able to joke that the problem is no longer the destructive "dance" but instead the timing of when their awareness of this pattern will kick in. With each passing month, they have moved closer to anticipating and cutting short their tendencies to engage in these painful conflicts. Most of all, they have increasingly mastered the ability to move more quickly to a place of compassion, understanding, and forgiveness when either one or both show a tendency to go back to these old wounds.

Based on the gathering evidence in the laboratory studies of Piolini and others, as well as the examples from our clinical practice, self-defining memories can indeed play a meaningful and constructive role in treatment of older adults. Even as recall for other episodic memories appears to fade, these memories, so central to identity and of such long-standing nature in the life narrative, retain their vividness and emotional resonance. In couples treatment, they can help to remind older partners of the origins of enduring emotional wounds that can trigger fear and conflict in the relationship. Through a carefully guided intervention to identify these memories, and supportive discussion of their implications for each partner's self-under-standing and sense of identity, the clinician can build greater compassion and common understanding in the couple.

Two important clinical questions to consider are as follows: 1) When might it be appropriate to use this self-defining memory exercise with an older couple? 2) Are the memories the couple shares likely to be already familiar to each other, or do new and previously undiscussed experiences emerge? With regard to the application of this intervention, we have found that the memory exercise is helpful in building compassion and intimacy for virtually any couple, but it is of particular potency for couples who are stuck in repetitive conflicts. As long as no member of the couple has an organic memory or language impairment, the couple generally embraces the exercise and brings a sense of curiosity and passion to the exercise of reviewing their respective lives.

The answer to the second question connects to our response to the first. One of the reasons for the utility of the self-defining memory exercise for many couples is that often memories that have not been previously shared are revealed and discussed for the first time. In the case of Adam and Deborah, both his memory of his mother blaming him for his father's fall *and* her memory of the visit with the "wicked witch" had not been previ-ously shared with each other. Considering the powerful messages that each of these memories conveyed to their respective partners and the subsequent enhanced mutual understanding, a strong argument can be made for the value of the self-defining memory exercise.

As Singer et al. (2007) found in their study of older adults compared with college students, the former may recall fewer specific details in their overall self-defining memories, but their capacity to make sense of their memories and extract lessons from them is greater. Too often we associate memory in older individuals with an emphasis on deficits and what is lost. The clinical case study presented in this chapter argues that older individuals may indeed display some memory advantages over younger individuals in their capacity to distill the most meaningful essences from a lifetime of recollections. Both individual and couples therapists would be wise to avail themselves of this valuable resource in their work with older individuals.

APPENDIX A

Deborah's Self-Defining Memories

1. Positive memory of paternal grandparents and holiday celebration.
2. Positive memory of going with father on errand, playing with cousins.
3. Positive memory of father, aunt, and playing with her cousins.
4. Negative memory of being molested by older male cousin who babysat for her.
5. Negative memory of mother being drunk and brought home by police. The next day, Deborah had minor surgery at the local hospital and her mother was not there to support her.
6. Negative memory of being the go-between in parents' fights.
7. Negative memory of winning a game of solitaire and her mother refusing to believe that she had won.
8. Negative memory of her mother having a breakdown just as Deborah had her first period. Her mother was not present to help her through this milestone in her life.
9. Negative memory of mother's second breakdown, seeing her in the locked hospital unit.
10. Negative memory of pouring out vodka bottles in the sink.
11. Negative memory from eighth grade of her friends borrowing her clothes and only returning them when they were ruined.
12. Negative memory of her friend's uncle promising her a riding cap if she rode in a horse show. She rode in the show, but he never followed through with the promised cap.
13. Negative memory of a "peeking Tom" in a bathroom stall, scaring her when she was a college student.

14. Negative memory from her sophomore year of college when she learned that her grandmother had died.
15. Positive memory of sharing meals with this same grandmother.
16. Negative memory of being promised she could go to the same private school that her brother went to, but ultimately not being able to go because of parents' divorce.
17. Negative memory of father repeatedly favoring brother.
18. Positive memory of paternal grandparents and their benign presence in her life.
19. Positive memory of mother taking care of her. Full text of memory is as follows:

> As I write this last memory, for now, it helps me to understand my mother. She loved me in her way, she was a sick woman with a disease, but she loved me. She did her best. I never could watch *The Wizard of Oz*. I was so afraid of the witch. My parents got tickets to go see the play at Starlight Musical, an outside amphitheater in Indianapolis. I was maybe 9 or 10. The real witch from the movie was the witch in the play. My mom somehow got me backstage to meet the witch without her makeup on, I was never afraid to watch the movie from then on. That was one of the very few times she took care of me, she found a way to cure my fears. Something in that day was about me for me, one of the very few times *I felt special* with my mom. I am so thankful to have the memory.

APPENDIX B

Adam's Self-Defining Memories

1. Negative memory about times when he and other children would call each other names, teaching him not to judge or stereotype others.
2. Negative memory of feeling inadequate compared to the wealthy Rhode Island summer people he got to know when his family would rent a beach cottage.
3. Negative memory of his father having a stroke before he could enjoy his retirement, teaching him a lesson about having balance in his life.
4. Positive memory of his parents making a good home for him through their hard work and frugality, reminding him how much intolerance he has for people who whine or complain.

5. Positive memory of how his mother would threaten him with chores when he claimed to be "bored"; he would always go outside and find something to do.

6. Extremely positive memory of growing up with family meals every night. He always insisted on this when he raised his own children.

7. Positive memory of playing board games instead of watching TV with his parents and then with his children.

8. Negative memory of how difficult it was to please his mother, realizing that he is not going to please everyone all the time in his life, but also noting his tendency to back away when he gets negative feedback.

9. Mixed memory: negative emotion about his wife's death and subsequent loneliness, but ending with description of meeting Deborah, his love of her beautiful smile, and his hopes for their life together.

10. Negative memory of his mother initially blaming him for his father's fall and not apologizing to him for her mistake. Full text of memory is as follows:

> My family and I had just arrived for the summer in Rhode Island and we had brought down a ladder on top of the station wagon to work on the house. I took it down with my father, but then ran off to the beach to look for my friends. When I was down at the water, a neighbor came and found me and told me that I better go back to the cottage, my father had fallen. I went back and the ambulance was on the way. My father was lying at the foot of the ladder, unconscious and not responsive. The paramedics showed up and got him off to the hospital. He had had a stroke. We did not know this at first and we thought he had injured himself by falling off the ladder. My mother blamed me for not being there to spot him. I felt horrible. Even though we learned soon after that he had had the stroke first and then stumbled to the ground, nothing more was said. She never apologized for wrongly blaming me for his collapse.

REFERENCES

Berntsen, D., & Rubin, D. (2002). Emotionally charged autobiographical memories across the life span: The recall of happy, sad, traumatic and involuntary memories. *Psychology and Aging, 17*(4), 636–652.

Blagov, P., & Singer, J. (2004). Four dimensions of self-defining memories (content, specificity, meaning, affect) and their relationship to self-restraint, distress, and defensiveness. *Journal of Personality, 72,* 481–511.

Carstensen, L., & Mikels, J. (2005). At the intersection of emotion and cognition: Ageing and the positivity effect. *Current Directions in Psychological Science, 14,* 117–121.

Carter, E., & McGoldrick, M. (1980). *The family life cycle: A framework for family therapy.* New York: Gardner Press.

Carter, E., & McGoldrick, M. (1999). *The expanded family life cycle* (3rd ed.). Boston: Allyn & Bacon.

Clark, M., & Mills, J. (1979). Interpersonal attraction in exchange and communal relationships. *Journal of Personality and Social Psychology, 37,* 12–24.

Conway, M., Singer, J., & Tagini, A. (2004). The self and autobiographical memory: Correspondence and coherence. *Social Cognition, 22,* 491–529.

Craik, F., & Trehub, S. (1982). *Aging and cognitive processes.* New York: Plenum Press.

Gottman, J., & DeClaire, J. (2001). *The relationship cure.* New York: Three Rivers Press.

Gottman, J., & Silver, N. (1999). *The seven principles for making marriage work.* New York: Three Rivers Press.

Greenberg, L. (2004). Emotion-focused therapy. *Clinical Psychology and Psychotherapy, 11,* 3–16.

Hultsch, D., & Dixon, R. (1990). Learning and memory in aging. In J. Birren & K. Schaie (Eds.), *Handbook of the psychology of aging* (3rd ed., pp. 259–274). New York: Academic Press.

Knight, B., & McCallum, T. (1998). Adapting psychotherapeutic practice for older clients: Implications of the contextual, cohort-based, maturity, specific challenge model. *Professional Psychology: Research and Practice, 29,* 15–22.

Knight, B., Nordhus, I., & Satre, D. (2003). Psychotherapy with the older client: An integrative approach. In I. Weiner (Series Ed.) & G. Stricker & T. A. Widiger (Vol. Eds.), *Comprehensive handbook of psychology: Vol. 8. Clinical psychology* (pp. 453–468). New York: Wiley.

Labunko Messier, B., Singer, J., Alea, N., Baddeley, J., Vick, S., & Sanders, R. (2008, July). Measuring relationship mutuality: Development of marital engagement-type of union scale and partners apperception test. Poster presented at the biennial conference of the International Association for Relationship Research, Providence, RI.

Levine, L., & Bluck, S. (1997). Experienced and remembered emotional intensity in older adults. *Psychology and Aging, 12,* 514–523.

Levine, B., Svoboda, E., Hay, J., Winocur, G., & Moscovitch, M. (2002). Ageing and autobiographical memory: Dissociating episodic from semantic retrieval. *Psychology and Ageing, 17,* 677–689.

Light, L. (1990). Interactions between memory and language in old age. In J. Birren & K. Schaie (Eds.), *Handbook of the psychology of aging* (3rd ed., pp. 275–290). San Diego: Academic Press.

Martinelli, P., & Piolino, P. (2009). Les souvenirs définissant le soi: dernier bastion de souvenirs épisodiques dans le vieillissement normal? [Self-defining memories: Last episodic memories bastion in normal aging?]. *Psychologie et Neuropsychiatrie de Vieillissement, 7,* 151–167.

McAdams, D., Diamond, A., de St. Aubin, E., & Mansfield, E. (1997). Stories of commitment: The psychological construction of generative lives. *Journal of Personality and Social Psychology, 72,* 678–694.

McAdams, D., Reynolds, J., Lewis, M., Patten, A., & Bowman, P. (2001). When bad things turn good and good things turn bad: Sequences of redemption and contamination in life narrative, and their relation to psychosocial adaptation in midlife adults and in students. *Personality and Social Psychology Bulletin, 27,* 472–483.

McLean, K. (2008). Stories of the young and the old: Personal continuity and narrative identity. *Developmental Psychology, 44,* 254–264.

Mills, J., & Clark, M. (1982). Exchange and communal relationships. In L. Wheeler (Ed.), *Review of Personality and Social Psychology* (Vol. 3, pp. 121–144). Beverly Hills, CA: Sage.

Mills, J., Clark, M., Ford, T., & Johnson, M. (2004). Measurement of communal strength. *Personal Relationships, 11,* 213–230.

Moffit, K., & Singer, J. (1994). Continuity in the life story: Self-defining memories, affect, and approach/avoidance personal strivings. *Journal of Personality, 62,* 21–43.

Pasupathi, M., & Carstensen, L. (2003). Age and emotional experience during mutual reminiscing. *Psychology and Aging, 18,* 430–442.

Piolino, P., Desgranges, B., Benali, K., & Eustache, F. (2002). Episodic and semantic remote autobiographical memory in aging. *Memory, 10,* 239–257.

Piolino, P., Desgranges, B., Clarys, D., Guillery-Girard, B., Taconnat, L., Isingrini, M., & Eustache, F. (2006). Autobiographical memory, autonoetic consciousness, and self-perspective in aging. *Psychology and Aging, 21,* 510–525.

Reid, D., Doell, F., Dalton, E., & Ahmad, S. (2008). Systemic-constructivist couple therapy (SCCT): Description of approach, theoretical advances, and published longitudinal evidence. *Psychotherapy Theory, Research, Practice, Training, 45,* 477–490.

Sarnoff, I., & Sarnoff, S. (1989). *Love-centered marriage in a self-centered world.* New York: Hemisphere Pub. Corp.

Salthouse, T. (1991). *Theoretical perspectives on cognitive aging.* Hillsdale, NJ: Erlbaum.

Satre, D., Knight, B., & David, S. (2006). Cognitive-behavioral interventions with older adults: Integrating clinical and gerontological research. *Professional Psychology: Research and Practice, 37,* 489–498.

Schlagman, S., Schultz, J., & Kvavilashvili, L. (2006). A content analysis of involuntary autobiographical memories: Examining the positivity effect in old age. *Memory, 14,* 161–175.

Sharpe, S. (2000). *The ways we love: A developmental approach to treating couples.* New York,: Guilford Press.

Shem, S., & Surrey, J. (1998). *We have to talk: Healing dialogues between women and men.* New York: Basic Books.

Singer, J. (1990). Affective responses to autobiographical memories and their relationship to longterm goals. *Journal of Personality, 58,* 535–563.

Singer, J. (2004). A love story: Self-defining memories in couples therapy. In A. Lieblich, D. McAdams, & R. Josselson (Eds.), *Healing plots: The narrative basis of psychotherapy.* (pp. 189–208). Washington, DC: American Psychological Association.

Singer, J., & Blagov, P. (2002). *Classification system and scoring manual for self-defining autobiographical memories. A scoring manual.* Unpublished manuscript, Department of Psychology, Connecticut College, New London, CT.

Singer, J., & Bonalume, L. (in press). Autobiographical memory narratives in psychotherapy: A coding system and case study analysis. *Pragmatic Case Studies in Psychotherapy.*

Singer, J., Rexhaj, B., & Baddeley, J. (2007). Older, wiser, and happier? Comparing older adults' and college students' self-defining memories. *Memory, 15,* 886–898.

Singer, J., & Salovey, P. (1993). *The remembered self: Emotion and memory in personality.* New York: Free Press.

Smith, A. (1996). Memory. In J. Birren & K. Schaie (Eds.), *Handbook of the psychology of aging* (4th ed., pp. 236–250). San Diego: Academic Press.

Sutin, A., & Robins, R. (2005). Continuity and correlates of emotions and motives in self-defining memories. *Journal of Personality, 73,* 793–824.

U.S. Bureau of the Census (2009, June). *An aging world: 2008.* Retrieved on November, 24, 2009, from http://www.census.gov/prod/2009pubs/p95-09-1.pdf.

Webster, J., & McCall, M. (1999). Reminiscence across adulthood: A replication and extension. *Journal of Adult Development, 6,* 73–85.

Weinberger, D. (1998). Defenses, personality structure, and development: Integrating psychodynamic theory into a typological approach to personality. *Journal of Personality, 66,* 1061–1080.

Wong, P., & Watt, L. (1991). What types of reminiscence are associated with successful aging? *Psychology and Aging, 6,* 272–279.

Part 3   Interventions

Fifteen

ON SUFFERING, LOSS, AND THE JOURNEY

TO LIFE: TAI CHI AS NARRATIVE CARE

Gary Kenyon

> On the new earth, old age will be universally recognized and highly
> valued as a time for the flowering of consciousness.
> —Eckhart Tolle (2005, p. 288)

> You know that the element with which you can create love is
> our own suffering, and the suffering we experience every day
> around us.
> —Thich Nhat Hanh (1999, p. 165)

> Soul respects another's failure to find perfection, resistance to
> enlightenment, sheer ignorance of absolute truth, misguided
> attachments, and unrelenting meandering.
> —Thomas Moore (1994, p. 30)

In what follows, I want to reflect further on three interrelated themes that
I have explored in previous writings (Kenyon, 1991; Kenyon & Randall, 1997;
Randall & Kenyon, 2001). The first concerns the way in which the
narrative metaphor, or life as story, provides insight into the *inside* of aging,
which in turn highlights a different understanding of the human journey
from that using the dominant metaphor of decline, particularly in terms of
our experience of time. Second, I want to present examples of how narrative
gerontology allows us to observe the inside story of suffering and loss,

a story that often results in instances of acceptance, meaning, and wisdom, and even in moments of peace.

Third, I want to explore how we can consciously read our inside story and, in a sense, *restory* our journey by means of the art of Tai Chi—a discipline in which I am trained and, in fact, teach a course on at my home institution, St. Thomas University. Through Tai Chi, I believe, we can co-create a wisdom environment that both enhances our personal journey to life and helps others become better travelers in their journeys, too. A *wisdom environment* can be defined as a biographical encounter that facilitates acceptance, nonjudgment, and the expression of our personal stories (Randall & Kenyon, 2001, pp. 169–173), and in the process promotes narrative openness (Freeman, this volume). As such, it is a form of "narrative care." For its part, the term *journey to life* (as opposed to the more familiar term *journey of life*) refers to a combination of such phenomena as acceptance, meaning, wisdom, spiritual insight, connectedness, and peace. I have become convinced that this change of preposition merits further attention as suggesting a possible *telos* of the human experience.

THE INSIDE AND OUTSIDE OF AGING

The process of aging as viewed from the outside—that is, *outer* aging—is in many ways not an inviting story. In much of the world it is dominated by an ethic of control, achievement, and accumulation, and by expectations of continued material and physical growth. In addition, we tend to believe that if only we had this person, or that thing, or that job, we would be happy. What is more, the journey of life is fraught with many forms of change. The longer we live, the more chance for change there is. Many of these changes, of course, are perceived as loss and involve pain, suffering, separation, and grief. From a physical point of view, aging does indeed involve decline to some degree or other. As biologists remind us, every day we are alive decreases the probability of our continued survival. There is less and less clock time available to us. For many of us, then, the outside story of aging leads to resistance and fear, as evidenced in the "anti-aging" movement. By means of cosmetics, medications, or brain exercises (though, in moderation, such interventions have a place), we attempt to turn back the clock, or at least to slow it down. Indeed, we attempt to deny death itself. An emphasis on such interventions and attitudes makes some sense, of course, since, from an outer perspective, the human journey can be characterized as short in duration, as meaningless and absurd, as an invitation to despair.

But is this story of the human journey accurate or complete? From the perspective of narrative gerontology, a perspective that is sensitive to inner aging and to which we gain access (as Plato suggested long ago) by asking those who are living the aging journey themselves—and by looking at our own lives as stories too—we see something different. We see lives that are "restoried" (Kenyon & Randall, 1997) toward acceptance and meaning, toward spiritual insight and wisdom, toward narrative openness (Freeman, this volume), and toward the awareness of a story that is larger than that of their individual selves. We see a journey to *more* life, not less.

The inside of aging provides, among other things, the following fundamental insight: human beings do not have an age identity. The "old," that is, is usually the "other." Regardless of their chronological age, most older adults will refer to those older than them as the "old ones." To take one example: a nun I know, herself in her 80s, told me that she cared for "the old nuns in the nursing home." Stories like this abound. As Simone de Beauvoir (1973) has noted, there is no switch that turns on to tell us that we are old at a particular age. When asked, many older adults will say that, inside, they feel as though they are still in their 30s or 40s. Another source of support for this insight comes from narrative research that asks older adults to "just tell me your story." Some will say, "I need to start at the beginning," whereas others will start with the birth of a child, or their marriage, or some other major point in their life. Moreover, as has been demonstrated repeatedly since Sharon Kaufman's (1994) *The Ageless Self*, being a certain age does not feature as a major theme in their lifestory (Black, 2006; Caissie, this volume; Kuhl & Westwood, 2001). There is also evidence that some oldest old persons live in a vibrant or eternal present (Nygren, Norberg, & Lundman, 2007; Randall & Kenyon, 2001). And, while older persons have an awareness of finitude, it is generally accepted in gerontology that, as a group, they tend not to fear death nor be preoccupied with the thought of it (Randall & Kenyon, 2001).

The foregoing highlights the insight that, as we age, we live more according to narrative time, or story time, than we do clock time. The experience of time is a function of our lifestory and of personal meaning. From a narrative perspective, time is open; the past and the future are capable of being restoried in the present. While some of us may live more according to clock time and live more in either the past or the future, a narrative perspective expands our understanding of the experience of time as it is lived by older persons (Randall, this volume). This is not to say that we do not have or need a relationship to outer time and the realities that go with it. The larger societal story that we live within, for instance, often includes a powerful ageist element. But my point is that this is not, and need not be, the whole story of aging.

CHANGE, SUFFERING, AND LOSS

A narrative perspective gives us an inside story, not only of aging and time but also of change—in particular, its negative aspects. What are we to make of the myriad forms of change that take place throughout the journey of our lives? Some changes are pleasant and joyful, and we do not usually need to make an issue of them: falling in love, the birth of a child or grandchild, the start of a new career. We value these changes and are thankful for them. It is change we do not expect, or change that alters our story in an unpleasant way, that we spend more time trying to deal with. As noted earlier, the longer we are alive, the greater the chance that we will experience many such changes. Again, from the outside of aging, we resist, avoid, deny, or otherwise prefer to have nothing to do with them, for they are painful and cause us suffering. In the words of philosopher and humanitarian, Jean Vanier (2005), "Our spontaneous reaction to suffering is repulsion. We are frightened of pain; the most common response to the existence of pain is to be scandalized by it and to seek to eliminate it" (p. 86). It is this perspective that makes it difficult for many of us to be comfortable with persons who are disabled, dementing, or in any way perceived to be frail or "old." As illustrated by the various examples I want to outline now, however, a narrative perspective presents us with a rather different story: an inside story of loss along the journey.

Dementia

The stories of dementia survivors demonstrate very powerfully the possibility of discovering meaning in suffering through acceptance or surrender. Here are three examples. The first concerns a gentleman, now deceased, who was a guest lecturer in my Introduction to Gerontology class. After surviving the shock of diagnosis and problems early on with medication, he began volunteering through the local Alzheimer's Society and giving public talks. He told us that until he was diagnosed with the disease, he had never given such a talk in his life. As you can imagine, after listening to him there was hardly a dry eye in the room.

The second example has to do with a colleague, recently retired, who is a professor emeritus in the philosophy department of my university. Several years ago he was diagnosed with Alzheimer's. Like the first gentleman, he has visited my class on two occasions and, in fact, with his partner, has written a book on his illness experience. In his own words, "at first it was incredible, but hard things take time to be *fully* accepted. There is also a natural tendency to save face by keeping silent about some unfortunate things that happen to us. We want to conceal them; yet once we accept the truth, what is there to hide? We are indeed free" (Drew & Ferrari, 2005, p.73). The diagnosis of Alzheimer's, he told me, eventually gave him a new reason and purpose in life: to help others deal with the disease, through writing and speaking and being himself a survivor.

The final example is that of an acquaintance whom I heard speak recently at an Annual Coffee Break organized by our local Alzheimer's Society. I have known this man for many years, as he was on the board of our university's Third Age Centre. In announcing to us that he had been diagnosed with the disease, he explained that one of the worst outcomes was that he had been an accountant all his life, but that now, in his late 70s, he could no longer add or subtract. Still, he felt that he had received much help from the Alzheimer's Society and wanted to share his story for the benefit of others. These three examples illustrate a movement from loss and suffering to surrender and acceptance, to the creation and discovery of new meaning, and to an awareness of a story that is larger than that of our individual concerns.

Holocaust

Several years ago, I was asked to contribute a commentary to a special issue of a journal devoted to research based on analysis of the lifestories of Holocaust survivors (Kenyon, 2005). One finding of such research was that, for many of them, the stereotype of depression, post-traumatic stress, and meaninglessness turned out to be just that, a stereotype. In fact, many had gone on to healthy, meaningful lives, and lives of service to others. This research lends support to the views of Viktor Frankl (1962), himself a survivor, whose life and work demonstrates the ability of the human spirit to create and discover meaning—that is, to restory—amid seemingly hopeless circumstances.

Suffering

As with dementia and the Holocaust, when viewed from a narrative perspective, the phenomenon of suffering in general has both an outside and an inside story. On the outside, it is a topic best avoided and not worthy of attention, for it is about sadness, weakness, vulnerability, and loss, including loss of control. Yet, when older persons are asked about the meaning of suffering, as in a recent study by gerontologist Helen Black (2006), many of them say that it brings people together in meaningful ways. In fact, many report that achievement, success, and power, which tend to strengthen the ego, also tend to separate us from one another. We love each other through our weakness and vulnerability, Vanier (1998) reminds us, not through our strength.

From a narrative perspective, suffering cannot be understood without placing it in the context of our entire lifestory. In other words, the larger story we live within influences the meaning we assign to our suffering. The larger story, in this case, includes our gender, culture, cohort, and family. Then there is the unique inside story of suffering, which is imbued with personal meaning. As narrative gerontologists have discovered with respect to other phenomena, the stories of suffering told by older adults are often complex and paradoxical, illogical and uncertain (Black, 2006).

What this all means is that we cannot understand objectively what counts as an example of suffering for a particular individual. As a psychiatrist colleague once said to me, we all have an Achilles heel, and it is different for each one of us. The experience of a particular trauma or loss will devastate one person, yet hardly phase another. An example of the uniqueness of suffering is offered again by Black (2006). One of her participants had experienced the death of a son and had just been diagnosed with cancer. Yet, suffering for this woman was connected more to the story of an unfaithful partner earlier in her life. Such an example highlights the insight that there is a gap or a space between what happens to us and the meaning that we place on it. There is no necessary connection between the two. It is this space that allows for the possibility of restorying the experience toward less suffering (Kenyon & Randall, 1997; Tolle, 1997).

From this point of view, suffering occurs as a result of attempting to hold on to the story we have been living while that story has inevitably changed. There is a perceived loss and betrayal, whether the loss originates in our physical, mental, or spiritual being. A necessary condition for restorying and suffering less is thus acceptance and surrender. We need to relinquish our control story. We need to be narratively open and not say, "that's my story and I'm sticking with it."

Aging Itself

The aging process itself may offer the opportunity to enhance the journey to life. Author Mary Morrison (1998) was 87 when she wrote the following: "As we age, the old, driving ego becomes increasingly a bore to others, and more importantly, to ourselves. At this point we meet another of old age's paradoxes: lose yourself, find yourself. Pay attention to what you do so you can find out who you are; and try to say goodbye to the old self that wants to make the world meet its demands. For those who will do this work, a new way of being, a new 'me' is accessible and available—one that becomes at home in the world" (p. 41).

Morrison's comments are supported by a study of older persons that was carried out by gerontologists Edmund Sherman and Theodore Webb (1994), who note of the older persons they studied: "Most certainly did display a 'letting-go' quality and an acceptance of their inevitable losses, but they definitely cannot be described as 'resigned.' They appeared to be in a state of being that was quite alive, but that was also more contemplative than they described themselves as being in earlier life stages" (pp. 259–260). The authors go on to point out that the individuals studied felt that the self they used to be was a "hypothesized self" but that now their self-as-being was a larger self.

To quote another writer commenting on the aging process: "A point comes in our lives at which we 'choose' how we go into our last years, how we approach our death. The choice may be painful, requiring (should we choose to continue to 'grow' old, instead of merely sinking into the aging process) that we let go of much that has been central even to our inner lives" (Mowat, cited in Luke, 1987, p. viii). From this point of view, the aging process itself can be considered a gift, or a portal, as author Eckhart Tolle (1997) would say, to our larger story—to our wisdom story.

Similar insights are reported in a recent narrative study of the oldest old. The authors of the study found that their participants possessed an inner strength (meaning, for instance), that they could see something positive coming from the negative in their lives, that they could accept and adjust to a new situation and reach out to others for support, and that they felt themselves part of a greater whole (Nygren et al., 2007).

JOURNEYING TO LIFE

Before continuing with my discussion, I want to address two important issues. First, there will always be stories of despair and of narrative foreclosure (Freeman, this volume). Although always possible in principle, even in one's final moments, not everyone ages well and is able to restory his or her life in the face of the changes and challenges that later life brings. Second, the process of finding new meaning in life through restorying is neither facile nor mechanical. When life presents us with suffering or loss, the initial movement is very often one of denial and closing off, a feeling of separation and alienation. As Black (2006, p. 68) observes, "Suffering can disconnect us from self, body, others, and even God." The title of a journal article from the field of narrative medicine captures this situation in narrative terms: "My Story is Broken: Can You Help Me Fix It?" (Brody, 1994).

The movement from separation and denial to acceptance is not a matter of willpower or of a technique that can be called upon whenever needed. Our lifestories come from somewhere; they contain facticity as well as possibility (Kenyon, Clark, & de Vries, 2001). In other words, we can restory our lives but we cannot make ourselves up at will. Acceptance and letting go have an ineffable quality about them, whether we call it grace, karma, chance, an appropriate narrative environment, or a combination of all of these factors. Yet, it is clear that life brings many of us to the "storying moment" (Randall & Kenyon, 2001), to the awareness of our lives as the story of a journey, even if the path is not one that we would freely have chosen. In fact, perhaps the story is designed that way so that we cannot take credit for any progress we may make, which in the end would result only in slowing us down. That is, by taking credit for this progress, paradoxically, it could simply strengthen our ego by leading us to mistakenly believe that we are solely responsible for the direction of the journey.

That said, restorying, and even radical restorying are nonetheless possible. In fact, after the initial movement just described, it is life itself that often brings us to the point of acceptance and of openness to new meaning, as the previous examples suggest. Without minimizing the "hell" we may experience in the early phase of such changes, this is not necessarily always a bad thing. Loss and suffering can bring us to new meaning, to wisdom, and to the awareness of a larger journey *to* life. Somehow we come to accept life as it is, and not as we want it to be. Alternatively, as my sister recently said to me, having spent the last year with my acutely ill brother-in-law, and using words that echo the spiritual teacher Eckhart Tolle (1997), sometimes we can accept that our situation is totally *un*acceptable, and this, too, can provide a measure of relief.

Florida Scott-Maxwell (1968, p. 65), who wrote her autobiographical book *The Measure of My Days* when she was in her 80s, takes this notion one step further: "I often want to say to people, 'You have neat, tight expectations of what life ought to give you, but you won't get it. That isn't what life does. Life does not accommodate you, it shatters you. It is meant to, and it couldn't do it better. Every seed destroys its container or else there would be no fruition.'" Scott-Maxwell is arguing that the story of the human journey is about change and disillusionment. We are meant to be travelers whose itinerary changes, yet our destination is not necessarily one of desolation and despair, but of meaning and even peace of mind. From a narrative perspective, while we cannot make ourselves up, it is possible for us to become better travelers through reading and restorying our lives.

The way to a more meaningful aging is through our own inner journey, our unique inside story. There is no shortcut and no way to avoid this path. Such a perspective is consistent with many spiritual traditions. Insofar as there is a close connection between the notions of spirituality and meaning, from a narrative point of view, we can indeed speak of aging as a spiritual journey (Bianchi, 1995; Kenyon & Randall 2001; Randall & McKim, 2008). It needs noting, however, that in the present context, spirituality is not connected to particular religious or spiritual traditions per se. Rather, it is connected to the *process* of finding meaning in the journey to life.

TAI CHI AND NARRATIVE CARE

I would now like to explore Tai Chi as a particular approach to both restory-ing and enhancing the journey to life. Tai Chi is an appropriate intervention to consider in this context, for it can be practiced in some form or other by virtually all adults, even by those who are dementia survivors or who are otherwise mentally or physically challenged.

As with the examples I have used so far, within Tai Chi, progress toward wisdom and meaning is not through control, or analysis, or the accumula-tion of intellectual knowledge. It is through softness, loss, vulnerability, and yielding (Huang, 1993; Liao, 2007; Mitchell, 1988). From the perspective of yin and yang, it is the female principle, yin, that, in the end, brings true strength and wisdom. Tai Chi is at once a martial art, a healing art, and a form of moving meditation. Concepts central to it include yielding and adhering, investing in loss, letting go, and becoming soft and empty. Progress in Tai Chi, whether we view it as meditation or as martial art, occurs to the degree that we are able to accept and surrender to what is happening in the present moment.

One way to describe this is to say that when something comes at you, whether it is a training partner or life itself, do not abandon your intention, or disarm before the inevitable. By the same token, do not rigidly or stub-bornly attempt to control the situation. Instead, "follow" what is happening and be flexible. One of my students, herself from China, observes that in Tai Chi "you step back to get a larger view." I call this the Third Way—that is, beyond fight or flight. We attempt to move with changes, and have no expectations from ourselves or from our environment. It is sometimes said that human life itself is yang energy, which means in this case that it is a stressor. Tai Chi is yin energy in that it attempts to balance that stressor by receiving, accepting, and neutralizing. Tai Chi involves a giving-in, but by no means does it involve a giving-up. It is not resignation but acceptance, which means that it involves the attempt to follow the situation until it can be brought to a balanced or healthy conclusion. We are asked to blend with the oncoming force, to meet it, follow it, and eventually direct it. As the author and practitioner Klein (1984, p. 53) advises, in the context of Tai Chi as a martial art, "Never interfere with your partner's momentum (whether physical or emotional); let it flow by you or rechannel it."

In my experience, arriving at the point of yielding takes a great deal of simply showing up to practice, and of losing, time and again, to a partner who has already learned to let go and be empty, and who is able to follow whatever you are giving him or her. It takes time to discover your sources of resistance: physical, emotional, and spiritual. In Tai Chi, to use a saying reminiscent of Jesus, if you try to save yourself, you will lose. However, this is precisely why Tai Chi can be a very effective path to surrender, to wisdom, and to an enhanced journey to life. As with the examples I discussed near the beginning of this chapter, it is a way for us to see that giving in does not mean giving up, to see that there is strength in diminishment and loss. We need to become small in order to allow the larger story we are in to become clear and to guide us. Little by little, I have been able to apply this as a form of restorying my own life, and thus as a narrative intervention in situations of crisis and stress. That said, there can always be situations that take us completely by surprise, in which case the practice goes temporarily out the window. As a result, the journey is always human, all too human, which means that *humility* is an aspect of Tai Chi, as well.

There are other forms of surrender or yielding in Tai Chi. Tai Chi is an art form and, as such, the ego needs to give in to the fact that there is no end point to reach, no ultimate success where I can say "I have *made* it." There is only continuous refinement of the moves and the principles of the art. At some point, the doing of a particular form in Tai Chi is done for its own sake, because it is there. There is always something to learn, both from the form itself and from my fellow practitioners. Even after some 30 years of practice, there are days when I feel that I have only begun to learn what this art is about, and I am in awe of its profundity. Other days, it all seems to come together and I have a feeling of tremendous peace and connectedness with what is around me. Nevertheless, the difference between this kind of practice and many other things in life is that, in Tai Chi, one needs to drop any expectation of progress. In traditional Tai Chi, for instance, there are no belts or other external recognitions of progress. One simply practices for oneself and, little by little, deepens one's art.

This orientation is challenging to many who, as I discussed at the outset, are accustomed to a payoff, to a reward for achievement, and to having an ultimate goal at which to arrive. In my own development as a martial arts practitioner, I was fortunate to have a karate *sensei* (or teacher) who, unlike the more common practice in *karate*, held back our belts, especially the black belt. His hope, he told us, was that by the time we received our black belts we would be training only for our personal growth. This experience helped me to move beyond the tyranny of achievement and competition with which I grew up, where there were always winners and losers, instead of mutual sharing and making your own best effort.

Another way that Tai Chi can lead us through the journey *to* life—that is, from suffering to wisdom and moments of peace—is the group aspect of the practice. In good Tai Chi classes, there is no competition; members are accepted for who they are and where they are in their own practice. The basic human need to be accepted is allowed to express itself. There is no judgment. Rather, there is mutual respect and camaraderie, or what in some traditions is called a *sangha*: a group of kindred spirits. Such a climate is extremely effective in producing moments of peace, especially when the form is performed by the group in total silence, with the sense of acceptance permeating the room. In this way, a sacred healing space is created, a wisdom environment. Each person can feel that he or she need not be someone special, need not measure up. It is the attitude and the effort that matters. In our Western culture, though, it can be difficult for people to do this, to stop comparing, to stop desiring a belt or a medal, to stop feeling inadequate. Once they do, however, a huge load is lifted from their shoulders. They relax and feel free just to be themselves and to refine their own journey—in some cases, for the first time ever in their lives.

Tai Chi is a particularly effective approach for the journey to life because, in addition, it is highly adaptable. I teach and participate in classes where the members range in age from their 20s to their 80s and sometimes 90s. Indeed, my oldest student is 96. From a gerontology perspective, Tai Chi is thus effective in promoting intergenerational connections (Westerhof, this volume). Sometimes, there are participants of this age range within the same class, and sometimes there are special classes. For the past several years, I have extended my teaching to include two special classes in particular. In what follows, I want to describe these two groups and, in the process, demonstrate how Tai Chi can be a form of *narrative care*—that is, a form of restorying in which we help one another on the journey to life.

The first special group meets at a private retirement residence in my home community. The classes last 30 minutes, once a week, and we practice from a seated position. With peaceful music, and with movements adapted to the physical limitations of the residents, a wonderfully relaxed and mostly silent space is created, with very positive feedback coming from participants and staff alike. Periodically, I am asked why I bother to come "to hang out with us old fogies." I respond that it is, in fact, one of the highlights of my week. Without using these exact words, I tell them, "It's how I find my way through my own pain to some moments of peace by sharing with you. So, thank you very much. It wouldn't happen if you weren't here. We are both giving and receiving."

The second and more recent group consists of two classes, held at two different nursing homes. One is at a Veterans' unit and is composed mostly of male residents, many of whom have Alzheimer's. The other includes Alzheimer's survivors, as well as adults who are physically and mentally challenged. Several staff members attend as well, along with a few of the residents' spouses. These, too, are 30-minute classes, once a week. The majority of participants are seated, but those who wish to stand, do so. Some perform all of the movements, some just a few, and some do not move at all.

I have learned from these groups not to make assumptions about what is going on, or *not* going on, inside a given person. While physical and cognitive processes clearly diminish as dementia progresses, emotional and spiritual life may remain very active. One of the most powerful examples of this is a story told by a former student who is now the administrator of another nursing home. One resident in the advanced stages of Alzheimer's was in a fetal position and had not spoken in a long, long time. Except for the provision of basic care, the woman was all but ignored. My colleague decided to bring a puppy to her room as part of the pet therapy program. She placed the animal near the woman's face. To the astonishment of all present, the woman opened her eyes, smiled, and, moving her head slightly, gently caressed it.

The instruction I give is that we can benefit from Tai Chi and feel peace simply from watching the practice, listening to the music, and breathing quietly. Also, we do not have to do anything we cannot do or do not wish to do. This can be a challenge at times, however, when well-intentioned staff members attempt to "get the residents moving." In such instances, I have to call them to one side and gently ask them not to do that in this class, as it is clearly frustrating to some of the participants. An example of this concerns a participant (now deceased) by the name of Monty.

Monty was a regular participant in the Veteran's class. She would some-times just watch me, or even have a nap, and never performed any of the movements. One day, I asked her if she liked the music. She motioned for me to come closer. "Of all things they have us do here in a week," she whispered, "this is my favorite." Another gentleman who did not speak at all, and did not move much during the class itself, responded this way when I asked if there were any questions: "Yeah, how long have you been doing this stuff anyway?" In the case of others who did not move the first day, a finger or a foot was seen to activate over the weeks. A final example is a situation that occurred at the end of one class while I was waiting at the entrance to leave the building. I realized that I needed a special code to open the door. Sitting in a wheelchair nearby was a member of the class who had said nothing during it and not moved at all. When I called out to ask if someone could let me out, the man eased himself over to me and, in a low voice, said "one, five, two, six." I rest my case! In narrative care, it is all about the residents' personal stories and not about what we, as experts, think is "best" for them.

There is something of a "ripple effect" (Noonan, this volume) that occurs as new participants—be they residents, staff, volunteers, or family—hear about the class and decide to try it. When they first arrive, they are usually suspicious, until I explain that you can do just what you like in this class, and even have a nap. Often, they will sit and watch the others and then gradually join in. The soft music, the friendly atmosphere, and the slow speed of Tai Chi itself are also factors, of course, that make the program appealing.

There are at least two ways, then, in which Tai Chi functions as a form of narrative care. First, it brings the participants, and the instructor, to the stillness and peace within their own stories. I believe that such peace is part of our lifestory, but it is without words. I believe, too, that this kind of inter-vention makes participants feel they are experiencing something personal and purposeful and that this, itself, is an important reason why it works. I also believe that Tai Chi can be beneficial for dementing persons, such as perhaps Mark Freeman's mother, as we help them co-author their stories deeper into the disease (Freeman, this volume). It can help to bring them to a more positive experience of the present moment, beyond the thinking mind and its often emotional turmoil, to moments of peace.

Second, Tai Chi is narrative care in that, in my case at least, I always try to be aware of how each participant is doing during each session. That is, I try to connect with each participant's present story. As other chapters in this volume demonstrate, narrative intervention is thus a creative process and is sometimes very simple, provided one is present to the group and considers each member a unique individual (Noonan, this volume; van den Brandt, this volume).

Clifford, for example, can move only one hand. He does not speak except to say "hi." One day I noticed that he was sitting at the back of the room, and he looked very sad. "Clifford," I said, "I think you like to sit in the front, don't you?" He grabbed my hand and held it tight. His eyes brightened. I helped him move to the front. Since then, he has never missed a class and has begun to perform more movements than before. A second example is Woody. A veteran of the Korean War, he and I always bow to one another when he enters the room. Over the past year, however, he has become more frail, and has gone from performing most of the movements to being anxious because he is no longer able to do them. Without saying anything to him, I simply bow to him at the beginning and end of the class and he smiles and brightens up.

CONCLUSION

In the final analysis, we cannot control aging and the fact that our lives will end. However, the life-as-story metaphor offers us the opportunity to grow older and not just get older. We can become better travelers by learning from what life and aging do to us. We can try to stay on the journey and remain narratively open. In this way, the journey can have more meaning and, one hopes, moments of peace. It is peace that we seek, not happiness. The latter presupposes the satisfaction of our expectations or of our preferred story; the former arises from letting that story go. What is more, as narrative gerontologists, we can co-create a wisdom environment in which we can share these insights and experiences, and support one another in the journey to life.

REFERENCES

Bianchi, E. (1995). *Aging as a spiritual journey*. New York: Crossroad.

Black, H. (2006). *Soul pain: The meaning of suffering in later life*. Amityville, NY: Baywood.

Brody, H. (1994). "My story is broken; can you help me fix it?" Medical ethics and the joint construction of narrative. *Literature and Medicine, 13*(1), 79–92.

de Beauvoir, S. (1973). *The coming of age*. New York: Warner.

Drew, L. & Ferrari, L. (2005). *Different minds: Living with Alzheimer disease*. Fredericton, Canada: Goose Lane.

Huang, A. (1993). *Complete Tai-Chi*. Rutland, VT: Charles E. Tuttle.

Frankl, V. (1962). *Man's search for meaning*. New York: Simon & Schuster.

Kaufman, S.T. (1994). *The ageless self: Sources of meaning in late life*. Madison, WI: University of Wisconsin Press.

Kenyon, G. (1991). Homo viator: Metaphors of aging, authenticity, and meaning. In G. Kenyon, J. Birren & J. Schroots (Eds.), *Metaphors of aging in science and the humanities* (pp. 17–35). New York: Springer.

Kenyon, G. (2005). Holocaust stories and narrative gerontology. *International Journal of Aging and Human Development, 60*(3), 249–254.

Kenyon, G., Clark, P., & de Vries, B. (2001). (Eds.). *Narrative gerontology: Theory, research, and practice.* New York: Springer.

Kenyon, G., & Randall, W. (1997). *Restorying our lives: Personal growth through autobiographical reflection.* Westport, CT: Praeger.

Kenyon, G., & Randall, W. (2001). Narrative gerontology: Stories in theory, research, and practice. In G. Kenyon, P. Clark, & B. de Vries (Eds.), *Narrative gerontology: Theory, research, and practice* (pp. 3–18). New York: Springer.

Klein, B. (1984). *Movements of magic: The spirit of t'ai-chi-ch'uan.* North Hollywood, CA: Newcastle.

Kuhl, D., & Westwood, M. (2001). A narrative approach to integration and healing among the terminally ill. In G. Kenyon, P. Clark, & B. de Vries (Eds.), *Narrative gerontology: Theory, research, and practice* (pp. 311–330). New York: Springer.

Liao, W. (2007). *The essence of t'ai chi.* Boston: Shambala.

Luke, H. (1987). *Old age.* New York: Parabola.

Mitchell, S. (Trans.). (1988). *Tao te ching.* New York: HarperPerennial.

Moore, T. (1994). *Meditations on the monk who dwells in daily life.* New York: HarperCollins.

Morrison, M. (1998). *Let evening come: Reflections on aging.* New York: Doubleday.

Nhat Hanh, T. (1999). *Going home: Jesus and Buddha as brothers.* New York: Riverhead.

Nygren, B., Norberg, A., & Lundman, B. (2007). Inner strength as disclosed in narratives of the oldest old. *Qualitative Health Research, 17*(8), 1060–1073.

Randall W. & Kenyon, G. (2001). *Ordinary wisdom: Biographical aging and the journey of life.* Westport, CT: Praeger.

Randall, W., & McKim, E. (2008). *Reading our lives: The poetics of growing old.* New York: Oxford University Press.

Scott-Maxwell, F. (1968). *The measure of my days.* New York: Penguin.

Sherman, E., & Webb, T. (1994). The self as process in late-life reminiscence: Spiritual attributes. *Ageing and Society, 14,* 255–267.

Tolle, E. (1997). *The power of now.* Vancouver, Canada: Namaste.

Tolle, E. (2005). *A new earth: Awakening to your life's purpose.* Toronto: Penguin.

Vanier, J. (1998). *Becoming human.* Toronto: Anansi.

Vanier, J. (2005). *Befriending the stranger.* Toronto: Novalis.

Sixteen

OLDER ADULTS IN SEARCH OF NEW STORIES: MEASURING THE EFFECTS OF LIFE REVIEW ON COHERENCE AND INTEGRATION IN AUTOBIOGRAPHICAL NARRATIVES

Thijs Tromp

"What is the use in looking back? I'm old, my life is over. And here I am, still sitting and waiting for the good Lord to come and take me." This statement, made by one of the participants in a research project that my colleagues and I have been conducting on the effects of life review, touches the very heart of the project: Why look back? Why not simply close the book of the past and look ahead to new opportunities, living in the present without the disturbing memories of the past? The answer to such questions lies in the highly complex connections between historical time, experience, memory, identity, and personal meaning. In this chapter, I will introduce a method for analyzing autobiographical narrative interviews. Following this, I will be presenting some of the results from our project, and then conclude with a discussion of their theoretical implications.

LIFE REVIEW IN THE CONTEXT OF ELDERCARE

Theoretical Background of Life Review

It is Erik Erikson who provided the framework in which the phenomenon of looking back in the later years of life is to be understood (Erikson, 1963, 1982, and especially 1978). Although his theoretical vision on human development has been criticized by many scholars as being predominantly masculine, Western, and Caucasian, not to mention unsupported by empirical evidence (Pieteikainen & Johnson, 2003), his view on the last stage of life is still prominent among both gerontologists and theologians who are dedicated to reminiscence and life review (Kunz & Soltys, 2007; Moody & Caroll, 1997). According to Erikson, the last stage of life is characterized by the outcome of one's ego development. Older adults have to acquire ego-integration, by which he means they should integrate the past into a coherent and meaningful conception of the course of their life overall. To that end, they should be engaged in recalling and evaluating past experiences and trying to integrate those experiences into a meaningful vision of their personal life, and even of the life of all humankind.

A successful outcome of this process of life review would be that one is able to look back on one's life with feelings of happiness, contentment, and fulfillment, as well as a deep sense that one's life has meaning, that one has made a contribution to life, and that there is hope, both for future generations and for humanity as a whole. On the one hand, one should be coming to terms with one's own life history; indeed, from this perspective, doing so is the pinnacle of one's life course and includes the acceptance of death as the completion of life. Simultaneously, however, there is a kind of detachment from the concern for personal identity, by reaching a stage of wisdom in which the importance of one's own life is placed in the context of the destiny of humankind. Some older adults may not reach this stage of integration and hope and as a consequence will despair at their experiences and perceived failures. As they struggle to find a purpose to their lives, they may fear death. Alternatively, they may feel that they have all the answers (not unlike in adolescence) and end with a strong dogmatism that only their view has been correct.

Development of Life Review in Eldercare

In line with this Eriksonian view, in many assisted living homes and nursing homes, reminiscence activities are increasingly being offered to residents (Bohlmeijer & Westerhof, this volume; Noonan, this volume; van den Brandt, this volume). Looking back and talking about the past is no longer regarded as a symptom of senility but as a perfect indication of a healthy process toward ego-integration (Haight & Haight, 2007). Usually, a distinction is made between spontaneous and structured reminiscence. Spontaneous reminiscence occurs, for example, during daydreaming or takes the form of a casual chat during a social encounter. Structured reminiscence is a planned activity with the express purpose of eliciting personal memories, often by means of sensual triggers such as aromas, images, photographs, melodies, or significant objects. A special kind of such reminiscence is *life review*, usually defined as structured reflection on one's entire life course from an evaluative perspective and carried out in an individual setting (Haight & Haight, 2007). One way of doing life review—and, in fact, the focus of the project discussed here—is by creating a lifestory book (Huizing & Tromp, 2005).

Research on Effects of Life Review

Clinical experience shows that life review may have a positive impact on psychological well-being (Clarke, Hanson, & Ross, 2003; Hansebo & Hihlgren, 2000). Wong and Watt (1991) have demonstrated the types of reminiscence that correlate with successful aging. There is also a growing amount of empirical evidence about the benefit of reminiscence work (Bohlmeijer, 2007; Bohlmeijer & Westerhof, this volume; Cappeliez & Webster, this volume; Haber, 2006; Hanaoka & Okamura, 2004; Hendrix & Haight, 2002).

However, despite an increasing amount of research on the processes of reminiscence and life review among older adults, there is still no satisfactory understanding of why and how the contents of life review or the recollection of past events contributes to the quality of the lifestory, to narrative identity, and to the experience of meaning. The research on reminiscence and life review focuses mainly on their effects on quality of life, or on subjective well-being, but research on the *explanation* of such effects is still in the initial phases (Coleman & O'Hanlon, 2004; Haber, 2006; Haight & Hendrix, 1995; Schroots & van Dongen, 1995). Fry (1995) and others have suggested that the impact of reminiscence on the narrative organization of personal identity may provide an understanding of the working principles of reminiscence and life review. Coleman and O'Hanlon (2004) have added that the quality of the lifestory, and especially the degree of its coherence and integration, may be the clue to understanding the function of life review (p. 97). At this time, however, no studies are available that elaborate these otherwise plausible suggestions.

The lack of a satisfactory explanation turns out to be an obstacle to the implementation of life review. Time and again, working with life history methods or doing life review work is discredited with the suggestion that it is but another way of giving attention to older persons. A demonstration of the working principles of narrative methods may provide arguments, however, concerning the specific contribution that they can make to the well-being of older adults.

RESEARCH QUESTION

This is our challenge: we are convinced that the narrative construction of meaning is an essential factor in how people experience their lives. Remembering, telling and retelling, and, in doing so, reworking autobiographical memories could account for the effects of well-being and, to some degree, of ego-integration. Our central question, therefore, is as follows: What are the effects of the lifestory book method on the construction of meaning in the lifestories of older adults? We understand "the construction of meaning in lifestories" to mean the way that people order events, and assign significance to them, in the telling of their life history (Sommer & Baumeister, 1998).

To support this hypothesis, we conducted research in an eldercare context in which we measured the effects of a life review intervention on the quality of older adults' autobiographical stories. Informed by the theory of Erikson and the suggestions of Coleman and O'Hanlon (2004), as well as of Habermas and Bluck (2000), we assumed that the effects of life review would be apparent in the degree of coherence and integration reflected in the narratives our participants disclosed.

RESEARCH DESIGN AND PROCEDURE

Our research design was experimental in nature. For it, we developed a particular method of life review, called *Open Cards*, that involves a standardized lifestory book (Huizing & Tromp, 2005). Professional (assistant) nurses, who are trained in the method, engage in a series of seven encounters in which they talk with an older person about his or her life, using a set of cards with different questions on them for each of the themes the method contains. Between the sessions, the client, together with a family member, collects photographs and other important documents, plus anything else that deserves a place in the person's lifestory book. We used this method as the intervention in our experimental group (N = 64), whereas for our control group (N = 28), we simply provided equal hours of extra attention. Residents of 12 nursing homes were invited to participate in a research project about the lifestories of older persons. In the letter of invitation, the specific mode of intervention was not mentioned. Participants were randomly distributed among the experimental group and the control group. During the three interview periods for each participant—before (t0), immediately after (t1), and 5 months after (t2)—we attempted to collect three brief autobiographical narratives. In order to test our hypothesis, however, we needed to develop a standardized analytical instrument, discussed in the section that follows.

To obtain the autobiographical narratives, we used an open-ended interview. After participants were informed that the interview would last about 30 minutes, the interviewer commenced with one standardized question: "Would you please tell me your lifestory?" The interviewer interfered only when the narrator came to a standstill. The interventions were kept as minimal and as formal as possible: for instance, repeating the last sentence, asking if there was anything else the person wanted to add, or, if the participant was still unable to continue the narration, asking a general opening question about a theme the participant had already mentioned. We instructed our interviewers to use this last intervention only as a last resort. Our reasoning was that we wanted to determine the competence and structure imposed by participants themselves in their storytelling, and to avoid imposing the structure of the interviewers on the interview process.

ANALYSIS OF MEANING IN NARRATIVE

We regard the interviews as instances of the construction of meaning by the participant. In other words, the meaning constructed is not a static, completed entity. Even in very late life, it is an ongoing process. The story people tell is not a fully developed and final version of their life. Rather, it is meaning that is constructed at that particular moment and is influenced by the interview context itself.

Criteria for Narrative Quality

An essential question for us was how to evaluate differences in the narratives between the three measurement points, and how to value them in terms of quality. The formal categories we sought needed to be related to the issues of life review and narrative as described above. At the same time, they needed to be capable of some degree of objectification and quantification, or of operationalization, to be used in a large sample.

Following Erikson's suggestion about ego-integration, we assumed that life review would lead to an increase in the coherence and integration of the autobiographical narratives. Both of these concepts are well established in the literature as factors that demonstrate the quality of self-narratives. Coherence, in particular, is considered to be the main characteristic of lifestories (Baerger & McAdams, 1999; Barclay, 1996; Brugman, 2000; Goldman, Graesser and van den Broek, 1999; Hermans & Hermans-Jansen, 1995; Linde,

1993; McAdams, 2001). On the one hand, *coherence* refers to the formal aspects of the narrative that make the story into an intelligible whole; on the other hand, it refers to the aspect of content, which makes the story fit together in a semantic sense. *Integration* refers to the way that people actively evaluate the events of their life course within their narrative, preferably in a positive way; how they can consider those events from different perspectives; and the degree to which they can recount intrusive occurrences without losing themselves in fragmentation. That is, the storyteller is able to hold discordant experiences in a concordant whole (de Vries, Suedfeld, Streufert, 1992; Hermans & Hermans-Jansen, 1995; Pennebaker & Stone, 2003; Petzold, 1985).

A Multidimensional Method for Analysis

We based our analyses on Barclay's (1996) model of an autobiographical narrative, which can be summarized in terms of three stages. First, he distinguishes between symbolic organization and formal narrative organization (Fig. 16.1).

Symbolic organization concerns the content of the story and includes the themes, roles of the characters, dramatic form, the way things turn out, the use of imagery and metaphor, and the tone and plot of the story. In turn, *formal organization* refers to the structural aspect of the story: the linguistic means by which the parts of the story are connected to a meaningful whole. This aspect emphasizes grammatical conjunctions, the logical ordering of sentences and episodes, and the story as a whole.

In the second stage, the formal organization is characterized by temporal organization, narrative density, and narrative functions (Fig. 16.2).

Temporal organization refers to the way events and acts are connected in time—that is, the way the narrator perceives and constructs order amid contingency by putting in connections of causality, intentionality, or synchronicity. Narrative density is created by the use of subject–verb clauses

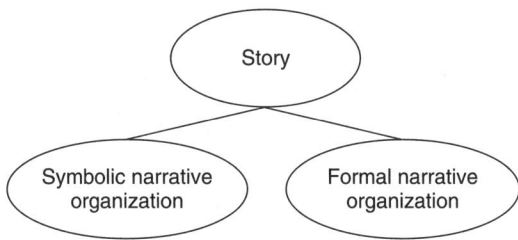

Figure 16.1 Barclay's model of narrative organization.

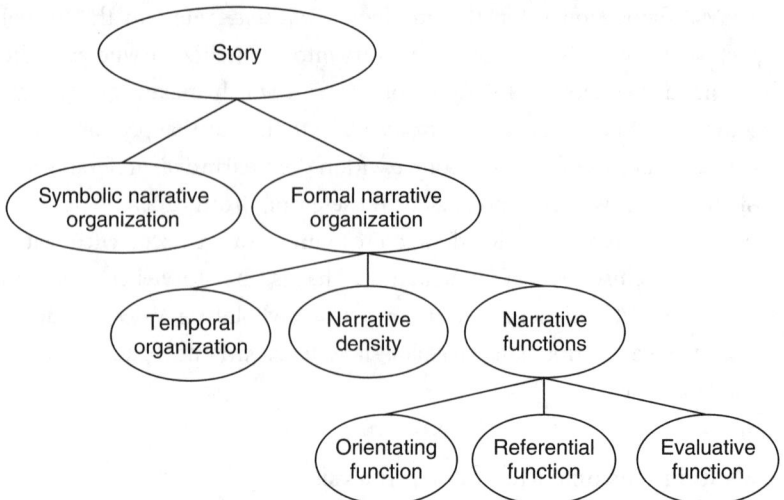

Figure 16.2 Barclay's model of formal narrative organization.

("she went"), assuming that this is in fact the most condensed form of a story. Finally, Barclay distinguishes among three narrative functions. By the *orientating* function, he means the adverbial adjuncts of time and place (where and when). The *referential* function concerns what happened and who did what in what way, while the *evaluative* function is about the way the narrator values what happened or what he or she did. It is Barclay's conviction that these three formal aspects of an autobiographical narrative determine the quality of the story overall.

Finally, in the third stage, Barclay distinguishes three levels in a narrative: the phenomenal, the epiphenomenal, and the metaphenomenal (Fig. 16.3).

For our analysis, we have added a fourth or preliminary level, which indicates the level of fluency in the storytelling. This first level refers to the process of narrating; the second, to the linguistic characteristics of the narrative; and the third, to the episodes and storylines. The fourth level, finally, is concerned with the overarching plot and tone of the narrative.

Subinstruments on Different Levels

Regarding the *narrating process*, we expected to find certain effects on narrative competence, in the sense that respondents would tell their story more fluently after the intervention that involved the life review method. Our belief was that this is linked to the narrative mastery of the narrator and is, therefore, an indication of the coherence as well as the degree of integration,

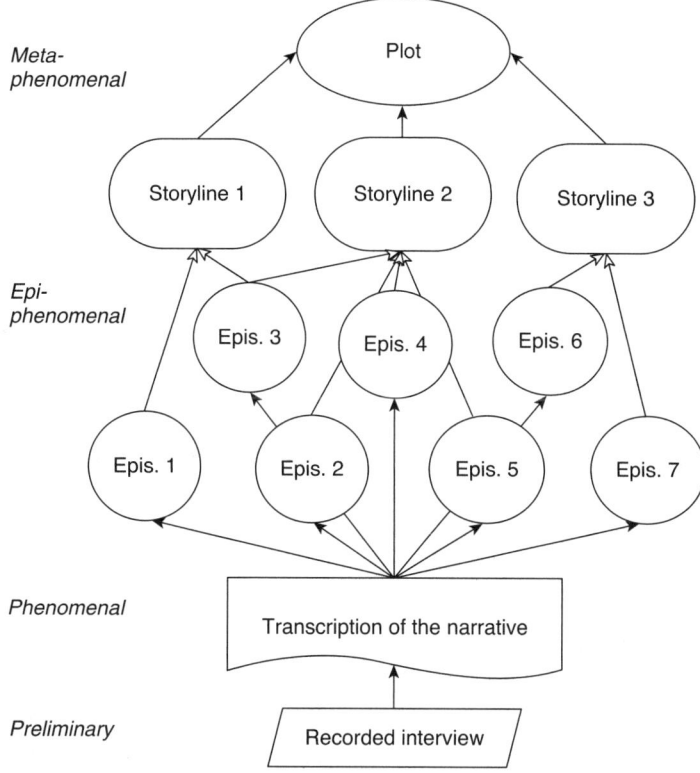

Figure 16.3 Multilayered model of the story.

based on the assumption that coping with uncomfortable or disturbing memories causes a "halting" narrative style (Schütze, 1984). The more the narrator is, so to speak, *together* with his or her story, and the more he or she is able to accept the positive and negative events alike, the more fluent his or her storytelling will be (de Vries et al., 1992).

On the *phenomenal level* we expected to observe an increase in the frequency of terms of causality (referring to temporal organization), subject–verb clauses (narrative density), adjuncts of time and place (orientating function), and explicit evaluations (evaluative function). In accordance with Barclay (1996), we regard such things as manifestations of increasing coherence (Brugman, 2000; Klein, 2003). Special attention is given to the positive evaluations as an indication of integration.

With respect to the *epiphenomenal level,* we expected to find effects on the quality of the episodes, measured by the presence of *episodic characteristics,* as distinguished by Labov and Waletzky (1967)—i.e., abstract, orientation, complicating action, and evaluation or coda. The more complete an episode, the more coherent the story. We further expected that the narrator whose grip on his or her lifestory is challenged would use more words to describe an episode (de Vries, Blando, & Walker, 1995; Janoff-Bulman, 1991). Increasing integration is negatively correlated with decreasing *length of the episodes*. We also thought that the life review would affect the character of *the long storylines*, namely storylines containing three or more episodes. Long storylines can be divided into those referring to a) one of the main aspects of personal identity, b) troubling events that demand coping, and c) traumatic events that cause the episode to become constrained or "stalled." We expected these last ones to diminish, an indication of increasing integration.

On the epiphenomenal level, we expected a change in the type of reminiscence that the narrators employed. This measure was established by using the instrument designed by Wong and Watt (1991; Wong, 1995), whereby the following types or functions of reminiscence are identified: narrative, instrumental, integrative, transmissive, obsessive, and escapist reminiscence. More intensive use of integrative reminiscence correlates with a higher degree of integration, and the same applies for a decrease in the use of obsessive and escapist reminiscence. Finally, we measured the symbolic ordering of the episodes, using the instrument designed by McAdams and colleagues (McAdams, Reynolds, Lewis, Patten, & Bowman, 2001), who distinguish between episodes with a redemption sequence (bad things turning good) and episodes with a contamination sequence (good things turning bad). An increase in the first will provide an indication of an increase in integration.

On the *metaphenomenal level*, we make use of the insights of Janoff-Bulman (1992). Based on her work with victims of trauma, there are three fundamental assumptions that govern self-narratives. It is the challenge of every narrator to construct the lifestory in such a way that the three of them are honored. Many narrators are at pains to solve the conflicts in their story when they are unable to synthesize all three and are tempted to save two of them at the expense of the third. A healthy and adequate lifestory then covers all three fundamental assumptions.

The first assumption is that of the *meaningful order* of the world: the assumption of order and significance that is threatened by chaos and coincidence. Narrators have to tell their story in such a way that their life and their world make sense as a whole, and that the world they live in is just. The second assumption concerns the *benevolence* of the world: the assumption of care and positive intentions in the social and natural context, countered by experiences of evil and neglect. Narrators have to tell their story in such a way that they can put trust in the people and structures they encounter. The third assumption has to do with *self-worth*. Narrators must tell their story in such a way that their individual existence is affirmed and positively valued. The challenge for narrators, then, is to create a meaningful story that fits the criteria of all three of these fundamental assumptions. Every lifestory in our sample was assessed for the way the three were integrated within it. Meaningful order was regarded as an indication of both coherence and integration; the other two—benevolence and self-worth—were seen as indications of integration.

Following this, an assessment of *the order in the story* was made. Chronological and/or thematic order were scored as organized; chaotic or fragmented, as disorganized. We also tried to characterize *the plot*, using the model of Northrop Frye (1990), which was originally designed in the context of literary criticism but has been increasingly used in research with autobiographical narratives (Brugman, 2007; Ganzevoort & Visser, 2007). Frye distinguishes four basic configurations of plot: romantic, comic, tragic, and ironic. For our purposes, we simplified these plots by scoring two aspects: the nature or outcome of the story (good or bad), and the degree to which the narrator, as protagonist of his or her own story, has influence or control over this outcome (active or passive, high or low). Examples of this procedure are romantic (good, active, high), comic (good, passive, low), tragic (bad, passive, low), and ironic (bad, active, low). In our analysis, we usually found a mixture of plot types, and this made us decide to treat the different types as aspects of the plot of the narrative. The plot can thus be a combination of romantic and comic, comic and tragic, and so on (Brugman, 2007). Finally, we analyzed the implicit "spirituality" in the story—i.e. fighting, resignation, acceptance, gratefulness, denial, or staying unaffected. Our special interest here was in acceptance and gratefulness as indicators of integration.

All of the subinstruments incorporated into the multidimensional method for analysis contribute to the formal narrative organization, except for the sequences, the plot, and the implicit "spirituality." A happy ending, one's own contribution to the ending, and acceptance clearly concern the symbolic narrative organization.

Expected Effects

We expected to find an increase in coherence and integration in the brief autobiographical narratives of the experimental group at t1. We expected similar but smaller effects in the control group at t1, because of the reminiscence effect of the measuring instrument. But given the specific and intensive character of the life review intervention and the fact that the lifestory book itself remains available as a physical object, we expected that the values observed in the control group at t2 would be at the t0 level, whereas for the experimental group we anticipated a lasting increase.

RESULTS

Of the 64 participants in the experimental group, only 37 sets of interviews at the three points of measurement were available for analysis. One of them, however, was not usable because of faulty recording. Thus, the results are based on a sample of 36 persons, 30 female and 7 male, with a mean age of 83 years (minimum 80) and an average length of stay in the nursing home of 2.1 years. The main cause of dropping out of the program was the refusal of 16 people to participate after initially pledging their commitment. Many of them told the nurses that, on second thought, they did not like the idea of looking back. The other cases of nonparticipation were due to illness and/or death of the participant or to organizational problems. The control group produced only 13 complete sets to analyze (11 female and 2 male). In this group, those choosing to leave the program dropped out after the first and second interviews. The participants did not see the point of telling their lifestory again (and again) and for this reason ended their participation. The rate of dropout was much higher than we expected, leading us to the conclusion that a) life review is much more intensive and possibly more frightening than we had thought, and b) telling one's lifestory repeatedly without a meaningful context may not be attractive to some older adults.

Most of the lifestories were told in a similar sort of narrative order. The first and usually longest part consisted of a more or less chronological overview of the person's life. In two thirds of the stories, this was followed by a thematic section in which the narrator expanded on certain episodes in more detail or gave lively and illustrative anecdotes related to them. In some cases, the narrator added a completely new theme or episode in the second part, usually an episode of shame, guilt, or trauma. A substantial number of stories ended up with descriptions of what life is like in the nursing home.

Our hypothesis about the effects on the control group is not confirmed. On all the items of our instrument of analysis, we observed a steady decrease from t0 to t1 and t2 (Fig. 16.4).

The results from the experimental group were quite different, however, and led us to distinguish three patterns. The first pattern showed an increase at t1, and after that a decrease (1a), stabilization (1b), or further increase (1c)

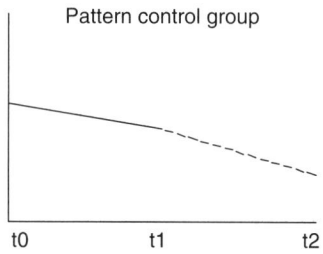

Figure 16.4 General pattern, control group.

at t2 (Fig. 16.5). The second showed stabilization at t1 and then further stabilization (2a) or increase (2b) at t2 (Fig. 16.6). The third looked very much like the pattern for the control group (Fig. 16.7).

Table 16.1 present the results in percentages, all calculated from t0. Only percentages over 5% were counted as an effect. There were no significant differences between male and female participants.

There is a remarkable differentiation in the results. Most of the sub-instruments that indicate coherence show an increase at t1—i.e., immediately after completing the life history book—whereas the majority of the subinstruments that indicate integration show an increase or stabilization at t2—i.e., 5 months after completion (Table 16.2).

The items that indicate both coherence and integration produce the pattern 1b or 1c. An intervention with life review apparently has different effects after a different time span. First, there is an increase in coherence (aspects of the formal narrative organization), an effect that dissipates after awhile, and only after several months is there an effect on integration. A closer look at the items concerned with symbolic organization demonstrates that life review promotes a happy outcome—i.e., redemption sequence, comic plot in favor of tragic plot, and degree of acceptance. There are effects,

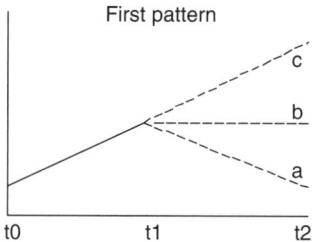

Figure 16.5 First pattern, experimental group.

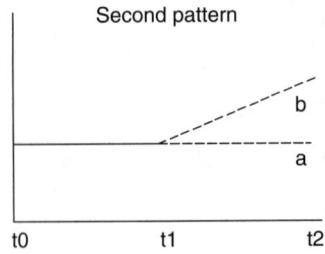

Figure 16.6 Second pattern, experimental group.

therefore, not only on the formal level but on the symbolic level as well, albeit effects that need time to mature.

DISCUSSION

Before we answer the question as to whether these results justify or falsify Erikson's theory about ego-integration, we need to discuss a number of other issues.

Limitations

First, it is important to note that not all participants liked the idea of engaging in life review, even after they gave their approval to participate in the project. This might confirm the insights of other researchers on life review, namely that not every older person has a need for, or is interested in, engaging in a life review (Kenyon, 1996; Merriam, 1993). That would explain the dropping out at the beginning of the project. A closer look at the dropout rate after the first interview—that is, during the life review process—suggests that life review can lead to such emotional pressure that some

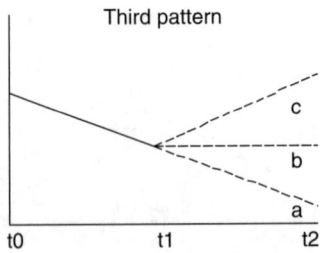

Figure 16.7 Third pattern, experimental group.

Table 16.1 Results of study

Criteria level	Coherence	Pattern	Integration	Pattern
Preliminary	Fluency (normal[a]) (t1[b]: +15%*, t2[a]: +19%*)	1c	Fluency (normal) (t1: +15%, t2: +19%)	1c
Phenomenal	Temporal index (high)(t1: +10%[†]; t2: −5%)	1a		
	Causality index (high)(t1: +6%[†]; t2: +2%)	1b		
	Evaluation index (high)(t1: +21%[‡]; t2: +25%*)	1c	Evaluation index, positive evaluations (high) (t1: +22%[‡]; t2: +31%[‡])	1c
	Total number of words (moderate) (t1: −2%; t2: −12%[†])	2b	Total number of words (moderate) (t1: −2%; t2: −12%)	2b
	Spatial index (normal)	3		
	Proposition index (high)	3		
Epiphenomenal	Episode quality (high) (t1: +6%*; t2: +3%)	1b		
			Length of episodes (moderate) (t1: +1%; t2: −3%)	2a
			Long storylines with coping or jam (moderate) (t1: +1%; t2: −13%)	2b
			Integrative reminiscence (high) (t1: +4%[‡]; t2 + 16%*)	2b
			Obsessive and escapistic reminiscence (t1: −27%; t2: −55%*) (high)	1c

(continued)

Table 16.1 Results of study   (*cont'd*)

Criteria level	Coherence	Pattern	Integration	Pattern
			Redemption sequence (high) (t1: −4%; t2: +12%‡)	2b
Metaphenomenal	Meaningful order (moderate) (t1: +12%*; t2: +15%‡)	1b	Meaningful order (moderate) (t1: +12%*; t2: +15%‡)	1b
	Story order (high) (t1: +28%*; t2: +18%†)	1a		
			Implicit ideology "acceptance" (moderate) (t1: +4%; t2: +10%*)	2b
			Romantic plot aspect (high): (t1: −4%; t2: +6%)	2b
			Comic plot aspect (high) (Com t1: 0%; t2: +19%‡)	2b
			Tragic plot aspect (high) (t1: 0%; t2: −26%*)	2b
			Self-worth (moderate)	3
			Benevolence of the world (moderate)	3

to, before 3 interview periods; t1, immediately after interviews; t2, 5 months after interviews. For definition of pattern codes, see text. N = 36; 30 female, 6 male. ªIndicated here is the value we attached to the instruments (moderate, normal, high). This valuation is based on several assessments: theoretical foundation, validation of the instrument, and reliability (inter-rater score). ᵇAll percentages are calculated from to. Significance is determined by *t*-test: †$p < .10$; ‡$p < .05$; *$p < .01$.

Table 16.2 Effects per pattern

	Coherence	Integration
Pattern 1	8	5
Pattern 2	1	9
Pattern 3	2	4

participants do not want to continue. If this suggestion turns out to be right, then the positive results could be distorted by a degree of selection bias in favor of the participants who benefited from it. Others may have excluded themselves by prematurely quitting the process. It may be, then, that not all older adults like to engage in life review and that the process does not necessarily benefit everyone. Another limitation of the study is that we did not perform statistical analyses on the mutual correlations between the results of the different subinstruments. In this respect, the study should be characterized as exploratory in nature.

Explanations for Central Findings

First, what could account for the appearance of such a remarkable difference between the effects on coherence on the one hand and on integration on the other? In order to explain this, it is useful to distinguish between two different mental processes involved in life review: externalization and internalization (Barclay, 1996; see Fig. 16.8).

Externalization is about remembering and telling the story. It is focused on the presentation of a coherent narrative that is intelligible to the public. It is quite likely that the narrator embeds important episodes in the existing narrative frames with which he or she is familiar. Some degree of narrative smoothing will be used to get the story straight. In the second stage, life review participants are confronted with the story that they told through the feedback that the nurse gives them during the telling, by hearing themselves telling their own story, and by reading or hearing the story that the nurse wrote down. It may well be the case that these confrontations lead to

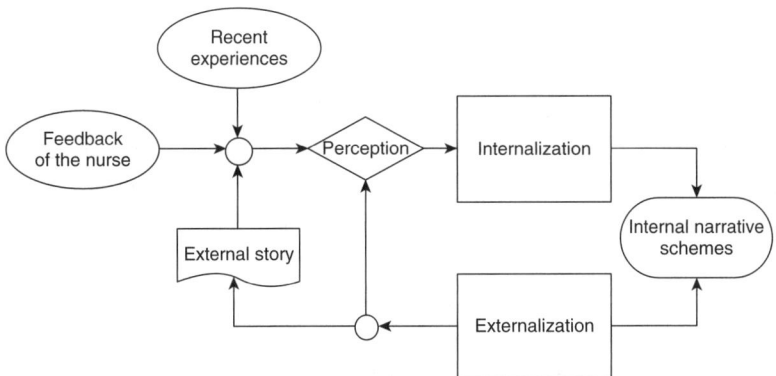

Figure 16.8 Cognitive processes of externalization and internalization. (Adapted from Jahn, 2003, and expanded by the author.)

a process of internalization in which the embedding of the memories in the existing frameworks is no longer the primary concern. Rather, the question is whether these narrative frames are adequate to integrate older and recent experiences (especially experiences of loss) into their ongoing lifestory.

To develop this insight further, the increase in coherence of the story may be connected to the process of externalization, whereas the increase of integration may be connected to the process of internalization. In *internalization*, the existing narrative schemes are evaluated. Apparently, this process needs more time, possibly because the process is closely related to the organization of one's personality.

We must also find an explanation for the steady decrease in the quality of coherence and integration in the control group. A first explanation is that the degree of frailty of some participants would lead us to expect such a decrease. However, although participants experienced frail health, this explanation is not very plausible, because no correlation between health situation and narrative competence has ever been established. Perhaps the decrease can be explained by a diminishment of concentration and intensity caused by the fact that many of the participants in the control group, as they themselves mentioned, did not see the use of telling their life history three times without understanding the reason behind it. It is interesting to note that the fact that they received attention did not actually influence the quality of the lifestory.

Theoretical Implications

At this point, we are ready to answer the question of whether the results of the experimental group are in line with Erikson's theory. At first glance, they seem to support Erikson's insights, inasmuch as both coherence and integration do show an increase, just as we hypothesized. However, the difference in the results on coherence and integration at the two measurement points requires a qualification of this conclusion. The increase in story coherence (the formal organization) seems to be a condition for a more far-reaching effect, namely, a reconsideration of the narrative frames from which the events of the life course derive their meaning (the symbolic organization).

This hypothesis is confirmed by the results for those items referring to symbolic organization (increase in redemption sequence and degree of acceptance, and decrease in tragic plot and favoring of comic plot). In other words, the participants in life review tend to tell their stories in a more hopeful and accepting way, emphasizing the good ending and de-emphasizing their own contribution to this good ending. In the words of Gutman (1976), they tend toward an identity with "passive mastery" and "magical mastery" (cited by Tornstam, 1996, p. 40). It was Tornstam who first suggested that Erikson's theory of ego-integration refers primarily to an integration of the elements in life that constitute a backward-looking integration process within the same overall definition of the world. Instead of this, Tornstam proposed the concept of *gerotranscendence*, which is a more forward and outward-directed process and includes a redefinition of reality. That is, older adults reconsider reality as they have experienced it thus far and then move on to redefine or restory the value of things that did matter to them in the past, such as possessions, activities, social status, superficial relationships, appearance, and even their own identity (Tornstam, 1996, p. 43). Nevertheless, he perceived that a more intensive use of integrative reminiscence was positively correlated with a higher degree of gerotranscendence (Tornstam, 1999).

Perhaps we can take these observations one step beyond the theory of Tornstam. Perhaps the redefining of narrative frames is not exclusively reserved for older persons but also for people who are experiencing major changes in their circumstances (Kenyon, this volume). We should not forget the fact that residents of nursing homes are typically confronted with removal from their own homes, loss of partners, the deaths of friends and acquaintances, and physical and/or mental health problems that are more or less severe. Such transitional experiences put pressure on the perception of their narrative identity. The safe cocoon of the lifestory (Giddens, 1991) begins to tear. Their safe lifestory is unable to integrate the new experiences, unless the perception of what makes a life "a good life" is readjusted and events in the life course are reconsidered in light of this new perspective. This concept is in line with Freeman's theory of "narrative foreclosure," the phenomenon whereby one feels one's lifestory is completed, even though one's life is still going on. If the narrative frames are incapable of providing meaning to new and often disruptive experiences, then the story gets stuck (Freeman, 2000; this volume). The study reported here provides strong evidence that intensive and structural attention to the lifestories of older persons in nursing homes can re-energize the internalizing process and keep the story going (Kenyon, this volume; Noonan, this volume; Ubels, this volume; van den Brandt, this volume).

NOTE

The research project "Effects of Making Life History Books," under the supervision of Prof. Dr. R. Ruard Ganzevoort, was conducted during 2004–2009 by the Protestant Theological University (Kampen) in cooperation with Reliëf, Christian

Association of Healthcare Organizations (Utrecht), and Kaski (Nijmegen). This project was funded by ZonMw (Care Research in the Netherlands, Medical Sciences). A full report of it is available at http://www.zorgvoorhetverhaal.nl.

REFERENCES

Baerger, D., & McAdams, D. (1999). Life story coherence and its relation to psychological well-being. *Narrative Inquiry 9*(1), 69–96.

Barclay, C. (1996). Autobiographical remembering: Narrative constraints on objectified selves. In D. Rubin (Ed.), *Remembering our past: Studies in autobiographical memory* (pp. 94–127). Cambridge, UK: Cambridge University Press.

Bohlmeijer, E. (2007). *Reminiscence and depression in later life.* Amsterdam: Vrije Universiteit.

Brugman, G. (2000). *Wisdom: Source of narrative coherence and eudaimonia. A lifespan perspective.* Delft, The Netherlands: Eburon.

Brugman, G. (2007). Het levensverhaal als constructie [Life as a construction]. In E. Bohlmeijer, L. Mies & G. Westerhof (Eds.), *De betekenis van levensverhalen* [The meaning of life stories], (pp. 41–60). Houten, The Netherlands: Bohn Stafleu Van Loghum.

Clarke, E., Hanson, E., & Ross, H. (2003). Seeing the person behind the patient: Enhancing the care of older people using a biographical approach. *Journal of Clinical Nursing 12,* 697–706.

Coleman, P., & O'Hanlon, A. (2004). *Ageing and development: Theories and research.* New York: Oxford University Press.

de Vries, B., Blando, J., & Walker, L. (1995). An exploratory analysis of the content and structure of the life review. In B. Haight & J. Webster (Eds.), *The art and science of reminiscing: Theory, methods, and applications* (pp. 123–137). Washington, DC: Taylor & Francis.

de Vries, P., Suedfeld, P., & Streufert, S. (1992). Conceptual/integrative complexity. In C. Smith (Ed.), *Motivation and personality: Handbook of content analytic procedures* (pp. 393–400). New York: Cambridge University Press.

Erikson, E. (1963). *Childhood and society.* Harmondsworth, UK: Penguin.

Erikson, E. (1978). Reflections on Dr. Borg's life cycle. In E. Erikson (Ed.), *Adulthood* (pp. 1–31). New York: W. W. Norton.

Erikson, E. (1982). *The life cycle completed.* New York: W. W. Norton.

Freeman, M. (2000). When the story's over: Narrative foreclosure and the possibility of self-renewal. In M. Andrews, S. Slater, C. Squire, & A. Treacher (Eds.), *Lines of narrative: Psychosocial perspectives* (pp. 81–91). London: Routledge.

Fry, P. (1995). A conceptual model of socialization and agentic trait factors that mediate the development of reminiscence styles and their health outcomes. In B. Haight & J. Webster (Eds.), *The art and science of reminiscing: Theory, methods, and applications* (pp. 49–60). Washington, DC: Taylor & Francis.

Frye, N. (1990). *Anatomy of criticism: Four essays.* London: Penguin Books.

Ganzevoort, R., & Visser, J. (2007). *Zorg voor het verhaal. Achtergrond, methode en inhoud van pastorale begeleiding* [Care for the story: Background, method, and content of pastoral counseling]. Zoetermeer, The Netherlands: Meinema.

Giddens, A. (1991). *Modernity and self-identity: Self and society in the late modern age.* Cambridge, UK: Polity Press.

Goldman, S., Graesser, A., & van den Broek, P. (1999). *Narrative comprehension, causality, and coherence.* Mahwah, NJ: Erlbaum.

Gutman, D. (1976). Alternatives to disengagement: The old men of the Highland Druze. In J. Gubrium (Ed.), *Time, roles and self in old age* (pp. 88–108). New York: Human Sciences.

Haber, D. (2006). Life review: Implementation, theory, research, and therapy. *International Journal of Aging and Human Development 63*(2), 153–171.

Habermas, T., & Bluck, S. (2000). Getting a life: The emergence of the life story in adolescence. *Psychological Bulletin 126,* 784–769.

Haight, B., & Haight, B. (2007). *The handbook of structured life review.* Baltimore: Health Professions Press.

Haight, B., & Hendrix, S. (1995). An integrated review of reminiscence. In B. Haight & J. Webster (Eds.), *The art and science of reminiscing: Theory, methods, and applications* (pp. 3–21). Washington, DC: Taylor & Francis.

Hanaoka, H., & Okamura, H. (2004). Study on the effects of life review activities on the quality of life of the elderly: A randomized controlled trial. *Psychotherapy and Psychosomatics 73,* 302–311.

Hansebo, G., & Hihlgren, M. (2000). Patient life stories and current situation as told by carers in nursing home wards. *Clinical Nursing Research 9*(3), 260–279.

Hendrix, S., & Haight, B. (2002). A continued review of reminiscence. In J. Webster & B. Haight (Eds.), *Critical advances in reminiscence work: From theory to application* (pp. 3–29). New York: Springer-Verlag.

Hermans, H., & Hermans-Jansen, E. (1995). *Self-narratives: The construction of meaning in psychotherapy.* New York: Guilford.

Huizing, W., & Tromp, T. (2005). Open kaart. Met ouderen in gesprek over hun levensverhaal [Open cards: Talking with older people about their life]. Utrecht, The Netherlands: Reliëf.

Jahn, M. (2003). "Awake! Open your eyes!": The cognitive logic of external and internal stories. In D. Herman (Ed.), *Narrative theory and cognitive science* (pp. 195–213). Stanford, CA: Center for the Study of Language and Information.

Janoff-Bulman, R. (1991). Understanding people in terms of their assumptive worlds. In D. Ozer, J. Healy, & A. Stewart (Eds.), *Self and emotion* (pp. 99–116). London: Jessica Kingsley Publishers.

Janoff-Bulman, R. (1992). Shattered assumptions: Towards a new psychology of trauma. New York: Free Press.

Kenyon, G. (1996). Ethical issues in ageing and biography. *Ageing and Society, 16*(6), 659–675.

Klein, K. (2003). Narrative construction, cognitive processing, and health. In D. Herman (Ed.), *Narrative theory and cognitive sciences* (pp. 56–84). Stanford, CA: CSLI Publications 158.

Kunz, J., & Soltys, F. (Eds.). (2007). *Transformational reminiscence.* New York: Springer-Verlag.

Labov, W., & Waletzky, J. (1967). Narrative analysis. In J. Helm (Ed.), *Essays on the verbal and visual arts* (pp. 12–44). Seattle, WA: University of Washington Press.

Linde, C. (1993). *Life stories: The creation of coherence.* New York: Oxford University Press.

McAdams, D. (2001). *The person: An integrated introduction to personality psychology.* New York: Harcourt.

McAdams, D., Reynolds, J., Lewis, M., Patten, A., & Bowman, P. (2001). When bad things turn good and good things turn bad: Sequences of redemption and contamination in life narrative and their relation to psychosocial adaptation in midlife adults and in students. *Personality and Social Psychology Bulletin 27*(4), 474–485.

Merriam, S. (1993). Butler's life review: How universal is it? *International Journal of Aging and Human Development 37*(3), 163–175.

Moody, H., & Carroll, D. (1997). The five stages of the soul: Charting the spiritual passages that shape our lives. New York: Anchor Books.

Pennebaker, J., & Stone, L. (2003). Words of wisdom: Language use over the life span. *Journal of Personality and Social Psychology 85*(2), 291–301.

Petzold, H. (1985). Sich selbst im Lebensganzen verstehen lernen. Erlebnisaktivierende Methoden in einem integrativen Ansatz zur Vorbereitung auf das Alter [Learning to understand oneself in terms of a total life: Experience-activating methods for use in an integrated approach to preparing for aging]. In H. Petzold (Ed.), *Mit alten Menschen arbeiten. Bildungsarbeit, Psychotherapie, Soziotherapie* [Working with old people: Education, psychotherapy, social therapy], (pp. 93–122). Munich: Pfeiffer.

Pieteikainen, P., & Johnson, M. (2003). On the origins of psychoanalytic psychohistory. *History of Psychology 6,* 171–194.

Schroots, J. & van Dongen, L. (1995). *Birren's A B C: AutoBiografieCursus* [Autobiography course]. Assen, The Netherlands: Van Gorcum.

Schütze, F. (1984). Kognitive Figuren des autobiografischen Stehgreiferzahlens [Cognitive representations in impromptu autobiographical narratives]. In M. Kohli & G. Robert (Eds.), *Biographie und soziale Wirklichkeit. neue Beitrage und Forschungsperspektiven* [Biography and social reality: New contributions and research perspectives], (Vol. 13, pp. 78–116). Stuttgart: J. B. Metzler.

Sommer, K., & Baumeister, R. (1998). The construction of meaning from life events: Empirical studies of personal narratives. In P. Wong & P. Fry (Eds.), *The human quest for meaning: A handbook of psychological research and clinical application* (pp. 143–161). Mahwah, NJ: Lawrence Erlbaum.

Tornstam, L. (1996). Gerotranscendence: A theory about maturing in old age. *Journal of Aging and Identity 1,* 37–50.

Tornstam, L. (1999). Gerotranscendence and the functions of reminiscence. *Journal of Aging and Identity 4,* 155–166.

Wong, P. (1995). The processes of adaptive reminiscence. In B. Haight & J. Webster (Eds.), *The art and science of reminiscing: Theory, methods, and applications* (pp. 23–35). Washington, DC: Taylor & Francis.

Wong, P., & Watt, L. (1991). What types of reminiscence are associated with successful aging? *Psychology and Aging 6*(2), 272–279.

Seventeen

REMINISCENCE INTERVENTIONS: BRINGING
NARRATIVE GERONTOLOGY INTO PRACTICE

Ernst Bohlmeijer and Gerben Westerhof

As discussed in the Preface, one of the levels of discourse on which the narrative metaphor is particularly effective is that of practice, or intervention. Indeed, narrative functions as the basis of several interventions, a well-known one being reminiscence (Cappeliez & Webster, this volume). In reminiscence, storying later life, and sometimes *re*storying later life, is the central activity. Over the last 10 years great progress has been made in The Netherlands in the development, study, and implementation of reminiscence interventions in health care for older adults. In this chapter, we offer an overview of these developments. First, we present a framework for implementing reminiscence in mental health care for older adults, one based on recent empirical studies; second, we provide two examples of interventions that have been developed within it.

FUNCTIONS OF REMINISCENCE AND
MENTAL HEALTH

In his seminal article, "The Life Review: An Interpretation of Reminiscence in the Aged" (1963), Butler argues that, whereas reminiscence has often been seen as a corollary of cognitive decline, reminiscence in later life fulfils a positive function by helping people come to terms with unresolved conflicts from their past in the face of approaching vulnerability and death. He interprets it as a process of life review that could be functional for older adults from the perspective of mental health. Such a conceptualization inspired a range of empirical studies and practical applications of reminiscence among older adults. However, many of these studies failed to find positive effects on mental health. In order to inform practice, it was concluded, better definitions and better studies of the functions of reminiscence were required (Thornton & Brotchie, 1987; Webster, 1994).

Bluck and Levine (1998) have defined reminiscence as

> the volitional or nonvolitional act or process of recollecting memories of one's self in the past. It may involve the recall of particular or generic episodes that may or may not have been previously forgotten, and that are accompanied by the sense that the remembered episodes are veridical accounts of the original experiences. This recollection from autobiographical memory may be private or shared with others. (p. 188)

This definition draws attention to the fact that memories of our lives can be purposefully recollected, even bringing back those that appeared to be forgotten. Indeed, volitional recall is a cornerstone for reminiscence as an intervention. More importantly, such a definition describes memories as veridical.

At present, it is generally assumed that the process of remembering involves more than just the simple recall of instances from long-term memory. Rather, memories are reconstructed in accordance with existing schemas about the self, and vice versa (Bluck & Levine, 1998; Conway, Singer, & Tagini, 2004; Wilson & Ross, 2003). Insofar as memories are shared with other persons, the retellings of them are also attuned to the social situation at hand (Marsh, 2007; Pasupathi, 2001). This *reconstructive* nature of reminiscence makes it difficult to grasp, yet it also provides a second cornerstone for reminiscence interventions.

In addition, much progress has been made in understanding the different functions of reminiscence (Wong & Watt, 1991; Webster, 1993, 1997) and the relation of reminiscence to mental health (Cappeliez & O'Rourke, 2006; for a review, see Westerhof, Bohlmeijer & Webster, (2010). Overall, current research suggests that reminiscence has both interpersonal and intrapersonal functions. The interpersonal or social function of reminiscence involves the use of it to relay personal experiences and life lessons to others, as well as to connect or reconnect to others. Some studies have shown a relation with happiness. However, no strong relations with psychological well-being or distress have been found. The intrapersonal or self-functions are either positive or negative. Positive self-functions imply the use of memories to discover, clarify, or crystallize our sense of who we are, to cope with present problems, and to reconcile ourselves to our mortality. In some studies, a positive relation with psychological well-being has been found. Negative self-functions imply the use of reminiscence to escape an understimulating environment or a lack of engagement in goal-directed activities, and it can be used to maintain negative thoughts and emotions vis-a-vis self and others. Studies have consistently shown that people who make more use of this function suffer from higher levels of depression and anxiety and experience less satisfaction with their lives. There is thus much evidence that reminiscence can cut two ways—positive and negative (Wong, 1995). When implementing reminiscence as an intervention, it is important to take these findings into account.

A FRAMEWORK FOR IMPLEMENTING REMINISCENCE IN HEALTH CARE

At present, the use of reminiscence and life review in interventions and therapies for older adults is widespread. Reminiscence interventions are used for many different target groups, among them community residents, family members, volunteers, persons with chronic illness, persons with mental illness, rural-dwelling older adults, lesbian and gay older persons, war veterans, migrants, and ethnic minorities. Reminiscence activities range from autobiographical writing to storytelling to instructing younger generations about specific events in the past, conducting oral history interviews, compiling scrapbooks, engaging in artistic expressions, and doing family genealogy, as well as blogging and other Internet applications. Finally, reminiscence programs are used in local neighborhoods, in higher education, and in primary schools; in museums, theatres, and churches; in voluntary organizations and assisted living communities; in nursing homes; in dementia care units; and in mental health institutions.

It has been argued that reminiscence interventions should make use of research findings and scientific theories that link the outcomes of reminiscence with the psychological processes at work in it (Bluck & Levine, 1998; Goldfried & Wolfe, 1996). Furthermore, reminiscence interventions need to take into account factors such as the characteristics of the target group (for example, the context and the level of psychological distress), the goals of the intervention, the skills of the counselors, and relevant developmental theories (Lin, Dai, & Hwang, 2005). What we propose here is that the new insights into *functions* of reminiscence, and their relation to mental health, bring more clarity to the theoretical and practical dimensions of intervention. We also suggest that the three distinct functions of reminiscence—simple reminiscence, life review, and life review therapy—can be seen as the basis for a framework of applying it in various settings. Simple reminiscence corresponds most closely to the use of social reminiscence in interventions, life review to the use of positive functions, and life review therapy to the discouragement of negative functions. In the following discussion we will give a short description of each of these types of interventions, focusing on target groups, goals, activities, and counselors' skills.

Simple reminiscence will meet the need of older adults who are in relatively good mental health and who consider the sharing of autobiographical memories to be a meaningful activity. The main mental health goal of simple reminiscence is to enhance positive feelings and happiness. Examples include reminiscence groups in nursing homes where prompts for positive memories are given (Cook, 1991) and groups that foster intergenerational bonding (Van Kordelaar, Vlak, Kuin, & Westerhof, 2008; Westerhof, this volume). The central activity is positive autobiographical storytelling in line with the social functions of reminiscence. Counselors require basic skills in facilitating the process of spontaneous reminiscence and in promoting social interaction. A life span theory that fits well with this type of reminiscence is the *socioemotional selectivity theory* (Carstensen, 1995, 2006), which proposes two important motives: emotion regulation and information gain. In later life, motivational priorities shift in such a way that the regulation of emotional states becomes more important than information gain. What is important in this theory is that it is not age as such, but the awareness of endings that originates this shift. One important finding of socioemotional selectivity is known as the *positivity effect*, namely, "a developmental pattern that has emerged in which a selective focus on negative stimuli in youth shifts to a relatively stronger focus on positive information in old age" (Carstensen, 2006, p. 1915).

Life review may ideally be directed at people who struggle with meaning in life or who have trouble coping with transitions or adversities in their lives. The goal of life review is to enhance such aspects of mental health as self-acceptance, mastery, and meaning in life (Birren & Cochran, 2001; Bluck & Levine, 1998; Wong, 1995) by stimulating the reminiscence functions of identity and problem solving (and possibly of death preparation). Individual life-review interviews (Haight, 1988) and guided autobiography groups (Birren & Cochran, 2001) are examples of this second type. The activities are more structured in that they focus systematically on the entire life span and elicit an evaluation and integration of both positive and negative memories (Haight & Dias, 1992; Webster & Young, 1988).

Life review assists people in gaining insight into how they have developed throughout their lives and become the persons they are now, as well as in recognizing and articulating what they have learned from positive and negative experiences. It also helps them in remembering their repertoire of successful past coping strategies and the values that have guided them in their lives. Accordingly, counselors need more advanced skills, such as structuring the sessions, asking questions that link memories to current life situations, and helping participants in reframing the meaning of past events. A life span theory that fits well with this type of reminiscence is *continuity theory* (Atchley, 1989, 1993), which holds that the experience of continuity is essential to an individual's mental health and functioning. Atchley distinguishes between two ways of maintaining a sense of continuity. *External continuity* refers to the preservation of one's life circumstances, whereas *internal continuity* concerns the preservation of one's own sense of identity. Both kinds of continuities are challenged when important life events disrupt an individual's life. This can be the case in age-related life events such as retirement or the onset of frailty (Atchley, 1993). To maintain a sense of continuity, individuals "attempt to preserve and maintain existing internal and external structures and they prefer to accomplish this objective by using strategies tied to their past experiences of themselves" (Atchley, 1989, p. 137). The resulting sense of continuity, achieved with the aid of reminiscence, is expected to promote adaptation.

Life review therapy is applied mostly in a therapeutic setting for older persons who are dealing with serious mental health problems, such as depression or anxiety. The goals are to induce self-change and to alleviate symptoms of mental illness. The focus is to reduce bitterness and boredom and to stimulate the positive functions of reminiscence. This requires a more dynamic reminiscence intervention, as reminiscence with mentally ill persons will normally evoke lifestories that express bitterness or dissatisfaction with their current self and life. Intervention protocols must be explicit, though, about how these lifestories can be transformed in the direction of a more positive self-identity. One approach has been to link life review to theories of autobiographical memory in depressed people, focusing in particular on the specific positive memories that depressed individuals have difficulty grasping in everyday life (Steunenberg & Bohlmeijer, this volume). Another approach has been to link life review with other therapeutic frameworks, such as cognitive-behavioral therapy (Cappeliez, 2002; Watt & Cappeliez, 2000) and narrative therapy (Bohlmeijer, Westerhof, & Emmerik-de Jong, 2008). When life review is linked with other therapeutic approaches, counselors will need more advanced skills in applying interventions that have been developed in the context of these other therapies.

The difference between these three main types of reminiscence intervention may not always be clear or strict. In many instances, there will be an overlap between reminiscence and life review; in others, between life review and life review therapy. The framework is mainly an invitation to take into account such factors as the setting, the counselors' skills, and the health and motivations of the clients. In what follows, we give two examples of interventions that have been developed in The Netherlands and that illustrate how reminiscence interventions can help older adults to story and restory later life. The first, *children interviewing their parents*, is an example of (self-help) life review. The second, *looking for meaning in life*, is an example of life review therapy.

LIFE REVIEW AS SELF-HELP

In this project, we were interested in whether life review can also be applied as a form of self-help. Given the natural character of the process, it is our sense that life review interventions can be applied without professional guidance. In addition, we hypothesized that such a review could take the form of life-review interviews between older adults and their adult children. Not only might this promote the mental health of the older adults themselves, but it could also enhance the affective relationship between parents and their children. We believed this would be the case since, in addition to structural–behavioral dimensions, the affective relationship is a key dimension of intergenerational family solidarity (Bengtson, Acock, Allen, Dilworth-Anderson, & Klein, 2005; Dykstra, Liefbroer, Kalmijn, Knijn, & Mulder, 1999; Katz, Lowenstein, Philips, & Daatland, 2005). The quality of parent-child relationships contributes substantially to the psychological well-being of the parent (Li & Seltzer, 2003; Shin & Cooney, 2006; Umberson, 1992).

A manual for conducting life review interviews with parents was developed for their adult children (Bohlmeijer& Cuijpers, 2007). In it, there is an introduction to reminiscence in general and to life review in particular, along with a description of the potential positive effects on older adults. Also described is the overall aim of the interviews, which is to help the parents reflect on and evaluate important events in their own lives and to help them reflect on the meaning of their lives. The second part of the manual gives tips for conducting the interviews, including instructions for posing not only informative questions but also evaluative questions. The third part presents a structure for four interview sessions dealing with youth, adolescence, adult life, and life in general. Examples of questions in the session about youth include the following: What were your parents like? In what important ways have they influenced your life? What do you think about your relationship with them now? Who was the most important person for you in your childhood? What kind of child were you? Can you tell me about some very special moments in your childhood? Can you explain? It was stressed, however, that the participants (the adult children, that is) were free to add any questions that they were interested in, as long as the questions focused on reviewing one's life. Our protocol was based on a life review protocol developed by Barbara Haight (Haight, Michel, & Hendrix, 1998). We studied the effects of this intervention in a pilot randomized, controlled trial (Bohlmeijer, Onrust, Bode, & Cuijpers, 2009) in which a total of 46 older adults participated, 23 of whom were interviewed by their children; the other 23 were asked to wait for 3 months before being interviewed.

Results

Directly after the intervention, we found a significant positive impact on the affective relationship between parents and children and on the mastery of the participating parents—in comparison, that is, with the participating older adults on the wait-list (Bohlmeijer, Onrust, et al., 2009). But what did the interview experience mean to the involved older adults and their children? Following the interviews, we sent the parents a questionnaire with open-ended questions about the impact of the life review interviews. Seventy-two percent of them rated the interviews as "very special and enjoyable," 28% as "reasonably special and enjoyable." Of more interest, though, is the question of whether a process of life review had, in fact, taken place. Processes such as acceptance of one's life, increased self-understanding, resolving conflicts from the past, and finding meaning and coherence in one's life are often discussed as possible outcomes of life review (Tromp, this volume; Wong, 1995; Garland & Garland, 2001). Analyzing their answers to these open-ended questions, we concluded that about 50% of the older adults had been reviewing their lives in some way or other, as exemplified in some of their statements.

An example of increased coherence is as follows: "Looking back upon my life has helped me to categorize my life. I now better see how one thing led to the other. And every time I became aware that this could only be my life." Another participant wrote about how the interviews had a positive impact on her self-identity: "I never used to think highly of myself, which I can relate to my youth and marriage. But I have always worked on it. During the conversations with my daughter I found out that I am quite contented with myself. It surprised me very much and I am very happy about it." And one participant referred to the theme of intergenerational legacy: "The interviews give me a good feeling. Because they have been audiotaped, I think it is reassuring that I can transfer my lifestory to my children and grandchildren." One may assume from this last quotation that such reassurance helps the participant in some way to face her own mortality.

Unexpectedly, the children were even more positive about the interviews, so we decided to evaluate their experiences in a more systematic manner. Six of the children were randomly selected for semistructured interviews. They were all women, with an average age of 45. The aim of these interviews was to explore the meaning of the child–adult interviews for the children themselves. Three main themes guided the process: the meaning of the (child–adult) interviews for the children, the meaning of the interviews for their parents, and the meaning for the relationship between their parents and themselves. These interviews were recorded on tape and then transcribed; the data were analyzed on the basis of grounded theory. In the first step, the interviews were read and all quotations with respect to meaning were coded. This resulted in 32 relevant quotations. In the second step, all the selected quotations were analyzed carefully for similarities. This resulted in six broad categories of meaning that were coded as follows: intimacy, identity, history, harmony, independence, and residue. The same procedure was then repeated in the third step, resulting in a final coding of three categories that reflected the meaning of the interviews for the adult children.

Meaning 1: Historical Understanding

All six respondents indicated that the interviews had resulted in a more complete picture of the lives of their parents. They now had a better understanding of central themes in their parents' lives, as illustrated in the following statements:

> And because he had reflected a lot about his life, one gets a real good picture of how he has lived his life, how he thinks and what has been important for him.

> I never knew that he had had such a strong relationship with his grandmother. That has become clear to me in these interviews. And how he feels that she really deserted him in his youth… . So now I can better understand his anxieties, his sorrow and also a certain anger.

Meaning 2: Solidarity

All respondents mentioned that the interviews had brought them and their parents together and that there was now more trust between them:

> [W]ell,… he is now ringing me up by himself… . He knows that I am there for him.

… And he shows clearly that he likes it when I am coming over… and our trust in the relationship has only grown stronger.

My father has fallen seriously ill and because of the interviews it has become easier to talk about how he really feels.

Meaning 3: Independence

In addition to helping the children derive a better understanding of their parents and to experience an increased closeness to them, the interviews helped the children become more independent. One respondent told how she always did her best to be liked by her parents. Now, however, she was able to distance herself more from them, and she noticed that they saw her now for who she was:

It is a sort of deepening of the solidarity. I have always been close, sometimes too close, to them. But now I feel that I am connected to my parents as an adult woman; we love each other very much, but for a long time their love was based on my behavior, so I felt. They would love me, only if I was sweet. And now I have the feeling that they love me the way I am.

Another respondent mentioned that becoming more independent was related to an increased self-understanding on the basis of the interviews:

What was very confronting now and then… is that I suddenly see very clearly how things in their lives have worked through with us. Our parents did not interfere with our lives but on some level they passed on their own struggles.

The results show that the life review interviews had elements of both reminiscence and life review. One element is the retrieving and sharing of personal memories that enhance the affective relationship and the sense of intergenerational solidarity, an outcome typical of reminiscence. The other element—the life review element—is the structured progress of the interviews and the evaluation of the meaning of memories. It is important to note that the life review interviews will be effective only if both the parent and child are willing and able to invest in the relationship. Although promising, this was admittedly only a small pilot study with many limitations. In the near future, however, we hope to replicate it with a larger sample.

LOOKING FOR MEANING IN LIFE

The second reminiscence-based intervention we will discuss, which is an example of life review therapy, is entitled *Looking for Meaning in Life* (*Op zoek naar zin*] (Fransen, Bohlmeijer, & Quist, 2007). This program is for people aged 55 and over with depressive symptoms. The course consists of

12 meetings that deal with the following topics: one's name, smells from the past, houses one lived in, standards and values, hands, photographs, friendship, the thread of life and turning points, attitude to life and meaningfulness, desires, and identity. At each meeting, sensory recall exercises, creative activities, and group discussions are introduced. We can take, for example, the meeting devoted to "Houses You Lived In." This session is divided into four steps. The participants first make a list of the addresses where they have lived during their lives. Some people will appear to have never moved, whereas others will have moved numerous times. This prompts discussion and the sharing of experiences. Second, participants select a house that they especially liked living in, or a house with special memories. This is followed by an exercise of guided imaginative recall, which brings them back to that one house. In the next step, they are asked to depict the house and a particular part of the house with the aid of colored chalk. Then, in small groups, they exchange their experiences, emotions, and memories. In the last step, each participant relates a memory associated with the house in a circle involving the whole group. This is followed by group discussion about the importance of home and houses in one's life. For those wanting to pursue this further, there are more assignments that they can do at home. These involve reading pieces of text written about houses and writing down associations about their own house, followed by a short piece of prose or a poem. If participants want to proceed still further, there is an exercise that involves placing themselves within the house: "What does the house have to say? What did the house observe during the time that you lived there?"

The other meetings are similar in structure. In the meeting about friendships, for example, the participants make a collage in which they depict important friendships; then in small groups, they share their experiences of friendship. In the meeting about desires, the participants select a picture of a bridge. In front of, on, and beyond the bridge, they write down their associations with the past, the present, and the future. Then they fantasize about how their lives will be in 5 years' time if a number of their dreams and wishes have come true. After this, the participants enact a reunion in which they are that "new person." The meeting concludes with a group discussion about how each participant intends to realize his or her plans in the "right" direction.

The re-creation of feelings and experiences in drawings or poems is an important element of this program. It gives the participants the opportunity to express themselves without first having to verbalize their thoughts. For various reasons, this is an essential component of the course. Expressing images through drawings and collages creates an aesthetic illusion that makes it less threatening to express emotions, thus facilitating the process of reconciliation. Images can act as metaphors. They say something, in a nonrational way, about an internal process. Thus, they transcend the rational, familiar reality and can help the user to discover new possibilities and experiences (see Randall, this volume). Gibson (2004) summarizes these functions of "imaginative recall" succinctly:

> Art gives hope—a hope that transcends the immediate world of experience.
> Creative activity provides a counterbalance to all that is restrictive,
> pedestrian, ordinary and limiting in our lives as we age.... Feeding the world
> of the imagination is as essential as nourishing the physical body. And, if we
> attend to one and not the other, we hasten dreariness and death." (p. xvii)

Based on the experiences of participants in the pilot study, who commented that they missed verbal exchange and would like to learn about applying new insights to problems in the here and now (Bohlmeijer, Valenkamp, Westerhof, Smit, & Cuijpers, 2005), three sessions were replaced. Sessions 4, 8, and 11 were adapted and based on elements of problem-solving therapy. These elements were included in the course that came after the pilot. *Looking for Meaning in Life* has now been rigorously tested in a randomized, controlled trial with 160 older adults. Substantial significant effects on depressive symptomatology were found (Pot, Bohlmeijer, Onrust, & Melenhorst, in press). We also found significant effects on meaning in life; moreover, we were able to show that these effects mediated the effects of depression (Westerhof, Bohlmeijer, Pot, & van Beljou, in press). For the purposes of this chapter, we want to present an illustration—a case study, as it were—of one participant in particular.

A Case Study

Janny signed up for the course *Looking for Meaning in Life* because she still had issues from her past and felt low. Prior to the course, she had an introductory interview with the two course facilitators. During the conversation, she revealed that she was born in 1940 in East Germany. After the war, the area in which she lived was compulsorily returned to Poland. Her father was from East Germany and her mother was Polish. Janny was a late arrival in the family; she has two older sisters. Life was a struggle for the family, both during and after the Second World War. First they lived in German territory, although her mother was Polish. Her father was a prisoner of war in Russia. During that period, life was difficult for the mother and her three daughters. It was a time when many mothers in similar situations starved or drowned both themselves and their children. But Janny's mother was a tough woman who wanted to fight for their survival. During the introductory interview,

Janny described her youth as lacking in love. After the war, the family was reunited in East Germany, where they lived together with several other families in a single house. Their lives were overshadowed by Communism. It was dangerous to express one's own opinions or even to talk. By now, Janny had qualified as a hairdresser. At the age of 17, she decided to flee. As she said herself, "I could not continue to live in a state of imprisonment, in a colony of Russia." Besides, she wanted to earn her parents' respect by showing them that she had the courage to do so. Her parents agreed to let her go, and she was successful in her second attempt to escape to West Germany.

At the first few meetings of the course, Janny spoke very quietly. She said she was ashamed of her German accent. At the initial meeting, the participants were given a pen with a nib, blotting paper, and ink. They were to write down their names and expand on this theme. This assignment typically brings participants back to their schooldays. Initially, Janny had very negative feelings about her maiden name. By using the pen, she sensed once more her mother's disapproval. During the meeting, Janny related that she had negative thoughts about her mother. In the second session, which is about houses, she drew the house in which she grew up, following a creative imaging exercise. Drawing seemed to evoke positive memories for the first time in ages. She remembered the "only compliment she ever received" from an uncle, who said that she was good at drawing. This was after she had drawn a bowl of apples. As a child, Janny was left at home alone for long periods of time. She could do whatever she wanted. She often wrote poems. The drawing now brought back these memories.

At the fourth meeting, the participants were asked to pick out five photographs from albums and to describe these in detail. Janny chose a photo of her mother, in which the woman stood strong and proud. Janny told the group that her mother always wanted to be the center of attention. For the first time, however, there was a sense of acknowledgment that Janny had made it, thanks to her mother. In the meeting about friendships, she presented a collage of her cousin in which nature played a big part. "This friendship meant a lot to me. I was always made to feel welcome, later as well, and we went for a lot of walks in the countryside." Janny was proud of her collage.

In the seventh meeting, about the thread of life and turning points, she drew a black sphere with a kind of arrow pointing to a sun that radiated bright colors. The sun symbolized the West shining its rays on East Germany. She experienced a feeling of triumph: "I had the guts to do that," she said. It was the first time that she had talked about her escape from the former GDR. She had never even spoken about it with her husband and her children.

At the last meeting, which is about identity, the participants were asked to make a trifold about past, present, and future. Janny now talked with enthusiasm and confidence about her model. The trifold contained a heart in different colors with a photo of herself and her grandchildren. "The colors express sorrow and joy. Green has always meant sorrow to me, but also hope. I used red to express love for my grandchildren." The model now hangs in her bedroom.

After completing the course, Janny told us that she had gained self-knowledge and had learned to deal with her past. She would not have managed this, she said, without the creative assignments. "These made the course more intensive for me, and brought up issues that would otherwise have remained undisclosed." By recapturing her memories and feeling them again, Janny realized that that they are not as negative as she had always thought. By being able to accept her mother, she was able to achieve acceptance of her existence and her past. She admitted that, whereas she had previously "camouflaged" many aspects of her life, she has now become more honest.

This short case study shows a process of restorying that is typical of life review therapy. For a long time, Janny had a very negative self-identity, symbolized by the disapproval of her own name. She experienced herself as a victim of a disapproving mother and of a harsh youth in general. As she was able to experience exceptions to this self-story, alternative, less black-and-white stories emerged that helped her find a more authentic and agency-filled identity.

CONCLUSION

Reminiscence and life review are essentially means of creating a "wisdom environment" (Randall & Kenyon, 2001) in which careful listening with an open and curious mind is an essential component. Asking the right questions at the right moment is part of this ability (see also van den Brandt, this volume). This process facilitates people in retrieving important but possibly painful memories and in finding and expressing new stories about these memories that, in turn, provide the possibility of living a more meaningful, active, intimate (i.e., connected), and, possibly, authentic life, as shown in the case of Janny. It may help people at the end of their lives to die in a peaceful and accepting way. In this chapter, we have shown that the listener need not be a professional caregiver. Reminiscence and life review can take place with friends, children, volunteers, and informal caregivers. They can happen spontaneously in the community and in institutions alike.

We have also discussed in this chapter, however, that current empirical evidence on the functions of reminiscence underscores the need for careful planning if reminiscence is implemented as an intervention in the context of health care. The goals, training, and education of the facilitators or counselors, the setting, and the level of psychological distress are all factors that should be taken into account when implementing reminiscence. Here, we have presented a framework that builds upon life span theories and research that examine the relationship between functions of reminiscence and mental health. Reminiscence and life review are not therapies as such, yet may very well have therapeutic effects (see also van den Brandt, this volume; Noonan, this volume; and de Medeiros, this volume.) When reminiscence is applied to older adults experiencing psychological distress, a modality that we call "life review therapy" should be used. An explicit description of the working mechanisms in relation to depression or anxiety is needed (Cappeliez, 2002; see also Steunenberg & Bohlmeijer, this volume). Professional counselors must understand these mechanisms and be able to work with them accordingly.

Research using mixed methods—experimental and hermeneutical— is preferable for showing and understanding the effects of reminiscence interventions. In the current political climate, evidence from experimental studies is needed for the implementation of therapies in mental health care. According to our research, *Looking for Meaning in Life* has now been implemented in 60% of the mental health care institutes in The Netherlands. It has also been adapted for people with chronic psychiatric illnesses. Until recently, no effective interventions were available for these patients. Preliminary evidence suggests that life review is helpful in increasing overall satisfaction with life (Willemse, Depla, & Bohlmeijer, 2009). The program is currently being adapted for older adults in nursing homes. The self-help manual has been published, and over 2000 copies have been sold to date. Other reminiscence and life review interventions have been developed, and the prospects for their implementation are promising. We are hopeful that the implementation of effective, specific life review interventions will contribute to the transformation toward narrative-based health care (Bohlmeijer, Kenyon, & Randall, this volume). As a significant first step, such interventions contribute to the effort of putting narrative gerontology into practice in the form of narrative care.

REFERENCES

Atchley, R. (1989). A continuity theory of normal aging. *Gerontologist, 29*, 183–190.

Atchley, R. (1993). Continuity theory and the evolution of activity in later adulthood. In J. Kelly (Ed.), *Activity and aging: Staying involved in later life* (pp. 5–16). Newbury Park, CA: Sage.

Bengtson, V., Acock, A., Allen, K., Dilworth-Anderson, P., & Klein, D. (2005). *Sourcebook of family theory and research.* Thousand Oaks, CA: Sage.

Birren, J., & Cochran, K. (2001). *Telling the stories of life through guided autobiography groups.* Baltimore: Johns Hopkins University Press.

Bluck, S., & Levine, L. (1998). Reminiscence as autobiographical memory: a catalyst for reminiscence theory development. *Ageing and Society, 18*, 185–208.

Bohlmeijer, E., & Cuijpers, P. (2007). *Handleiding voor life-review interviews* [Guide for life-review interviews]. Utrecht, The Netherlands: Trimbos-Instituut.

Bohlmeijer, E., Onrust, S., Bode, C., & Cuijpers, P. (2009). The effects of self-help life-review on mastery and affective relationships, a randomized controlled trial. Manuscript submitted for publication.

Bohlmeijer, E., Valenkamp, M., Westerhof, G., Smit, F., & Cuijpers, P. (2005). Creative reminiscence as an early intervention for depression: Results of a pilot project. *Aging and Mental Health, 9*, 302–304.

Bohlmeijer, E., Westerhof, G., & Emmerik-de Jong, M. (2008). The effects of integrative reminiscence on meaning in life: Results of a quasi-experimental study. *Aging and Mental Health, 12*(5), 639–646.

Butler, R. (1963). The life-review: An interpretation of reminiscence in the aged. *Psychiatry, 26*, 65–76.

Cappeliez, P. (2002). Cognitive-reminiscence therapy for depressed older adults in day hospital and long-term care. In J. Webster & B. Haight (Eds.), *Critical advances in reminiscence work: From theory to application* (pp. 300–313). New York: Springer-Verlag.

Cappeliez, P., & O'Rourke, N. (2006). Empirical validation of a model of reminiscence and health in later life. *Journals of Gerontology: Psychological Sciences, 61*, 237–244.

Carstensen, L. (1995). Evidence for a life-span theory of socioemotional selectivity. *Current Directions in Psychological Science, 4*, 151–156.

Carstensen, L. (2006). The influence of a sense of time on human development. *Science, 312*, 1913–1915.

Conway, M., Singer, J., & Tagini, A. (2004). The self and autobiographical memory: Correspondence and coherence. *Social Cognition, 22*, 491–529.

Cook, E. (1991). The effects of reminiscence on psychological measures of ego integrity in elderly nursing home residents. *Archives of Psychiatric Nursing, 5*, 292–298.

Dykstra, P., Liefbroer, A., Kalmijn, M., Knijn, G., & Mulder, C. (1999). *Family relationships: The ties that bind. A sociological and demographic research programme 2000–2006.* The Hague, The Netherlands: NIDI.

Fransen, J., Bohlmeijer, E., & Quist, T. (2007). *Op zoek naar zin* [Looking for meaning in life]. Utrecht, The Netherlands: Trimbos-Instituut.

Garland, J., & Garland, C. (2001). *Life review in health and social care: A practitioner's guide*. Hove, UK: Brunner-Routledge.

Gibson, F. (2004). *The past in the present: Using reminiscence in health and social care*. London: Health Professions Press.

Goldfried, M., & Wolfe, B. (1996). Psychotherapy practice and research: Repairing a strained relationship. *American Psychologist, 51*, 1007–1016.

Haight, B. (1988). The therapeutic role of a structured life review process in home-bound elderly subjects. *Journals of Gerontology: Psychological Sciences, 43*, 40–44.

Haight, B., & Dias, J. (1992). Examining key variables in selected reminiscing modalities. *International Psychogeriatrics, 4*, 279–290.

Haight, B., Michel, Y., & Hendrix, S. (1998). Life review: Preventing despair in newly relocated nursing home residents: Short-and long-term effects. *International Journal of Aging and Human Development, 47*, 119–142.

Katz, R., Lowenstein, A., Philips, J., & Daatland, S. (2005). Theorizing intergenerational family relations. In V. Bengtson, A. Acock, K. Allen, P. Dilworth-Anderson, & D. Klein (Eds.), *Sourcebook of family theory and research* (pp. 393–402). Thousand Oaks, CA: Sage.

Li, W., & Seltzer, M. (2003). Parent care, intergenerational relationship quality, and mental health of adult daughters. *Research on Aging, 25*, 484–504.

Lin, Y., Dai, Y., & Hwang, S. (2005). The effect of reminiscence on the elderly population: A systematic review. *Public Health Nursing, 20*, 297–306.

Marsh, E. (2007). Retelling is not the same as recalling: Implications for memory. *Current Directions in Psychological Science, 16*, 16–20.

Pasupathi, M. (2001). The social construction of the personal past and its implications for adult development. *Psychological Bulletin, 127*, 651–672.

Pot, A., Bohlmeijer, E., Onrust, S., & Melenhorst, A. (in press). The effects of the reminiscence program "In search of meaning" on depression: A randomized clinical trial. *Psychogeriatrics*.

Randall, W., & Kenyon, G. (2001). *Ordinary wisdom: Biographical aging and the journey of life*. Westport, CT: Praeger.

Shin, A., & Cooney, T. (2006). Psychological well-being in mid to late life: The role of generativity development and parent-child relationships across the lifespan. *International Journal of Behavioral Development, 30*, 410–421.

Thornton, S., & Brotchie, J. (1987). Reminiscence: A critical review of the empirical literature. *British Journal of Clinical Psychology, 26*, 93–111.

Umberson, D. (1992). Relationships between adult children and their parents: psychological consequences for both generations. *Journal of Marriage and the Family, 54*, 664–674.

Van Kordelaar, K., Vlak, A., Kuin, Y., & Westerhof, G. (2008). *Groen en grijs: Jong en oud met elkaar in gesprek* [Green and gray: Conversations between younger and older adults]. Houten: Bohn Stafleu.

Watt, L., & Cappeliez, P. (2000). Integrative and instrumental reminiscence therapies for depression in older adults: Intervention strategies and treatment effectiveness. *Aging and Mental Health, 4*, 166–177.

Webster, J. (1993). Construction and validation of the Reminiscence Functions Scale. *Journals of Gerontology, 48*, 256–262.

Webster, J. (1994). Predictors of reminiscence: A lifespan perspective. *Canadian Journal on Aging, 13,* 66–78.

Webster, J. (1997). The reminiscence function scale: A replication. *International Journal of Aging and Human Development, 44,* 137–148.

Webster, J., & Young, R. (1988). Process variables of the life review: Counseling implications. *International Journal of Aging, Human Development, 26,* 315–323.

Westerhof, G., Bohlmeijer, E., Pot, A., & van Beljou, I. (in press). The effects of the reminiscence program "In search of meaning" on the experience of personal meaning in life: A randomized clinical trial. *The Gerontologist.*

Westerhof, G., Bohlmeijer, E., & Webster, J. (2010). Reminiscence: Recent progress in conceptual understanding, empirical study and implications for practice. *Ageing & Society, 30*(4), 697–721.

Willemse, B., Depla, M., & Bohlmeijer, E. (2009). The effects of creative reminiscence on life-satisfaction of chronically ill elderly. *Aging & Mental Health, 13,* 736–743.

Wilson, A., & Ross, M. (2003). The identity function of autobiographical memory: Time is on our side. *Memory, 11,* 137–149.

Wong, P. (1995). The processes of adaptive reminiscence. In B. Haight & J. Webster (Eds.), *The art and science of reminiscing: Theory, research, methods, and applications* (pp. 23–35). Philadelphia: Taylor and Francis.

Wong, P., & Watt, L. (1991). What types of reminiscence are associated with successful aging? *Psychology and Aging, 6,* 272–279.

Eighteen

LIFE REVIEW USING AUTOBIOGRAPHICAL RETRIEVAL: A PROTOCOL FOR TRAINING DEPRESSED RESIDENTIAL HOME INHABITANTS IN RECALLING SPECIFIC PERSONAL MEMORIES

Bas Steunenberg and Ernst Bohlmeijer

When I was 14 years old we spent Christmas at the Salvation Army. We were very poor. We had a very good dinner of beans and bacon. It tasted really delicious. I will never forget the taste, smell, and sight of that meal. I went there with my father and my two sisters and three brothers. We sang songs during the Christmas celebration at the Salvation Army. They had a beautiful Christmas tree. They gave mandarins wrapped in red paper that we hung in the tree. I will never forget that Christmas. We were poor at home, my mother had passed away, we were hungry. We were very grateful for receiving the meal of beans and bacon.

This memory was recalled by a depressed woman, 85 years of age, who was living in a residential home in the center of Amsterdam, the city where she had resided all her life. As a participant in the training program ("Dear Memories") discussed later in this chapter, she did not hesitate when asked for her most precious childhood memory but began telling this story right away. As she did, she started smiling, became increasingly enthusiastic, and for a while looked once again like that girl of 14. She even began singing a Christmas song.

FIGHTING DEPRESSION IN OLDER ADULTS: THE SEARCH FOR EFFECTIVE INTERVENTIONS

The incidence of depression among residential and nursing home inhabitants is high. One review (Jongenelis et al., 2003) concluded that the average rate of prevalence in The Netherlands is 43.8% (with a range from 30 to 48.2%), a rate remarkably higher than that among community-dwelling older adults 65 or older, which is about 13.5% (Beekman, Copeland, & Prince 1999). Among the oldest and most vulnerable old, the prevalence of major depression, or depression according to the DSM-IV diagnostic criteria, is 17.6% (6–26%), while that of minor depression (depressive symptoms not meeting the standard for a diagnosis but seriously affecting the balance of daily life) is 25.7% (range 18.1–50%). By contrast, in the general population the prevalence of major and minor depression is 1.7% and 8.5%, respectively. Considering such high rates, there is a need for effective, low-threshold, preventive interventions and psychotherapeutic treatments that are tailored to this population. Despite the fact that psychological interventions have been found effective in the treatment of depression in older adults (Bohlmeijer & Westerhof, this volume; Cuijpers, van Straten, & Smit, 2006), few of these programs have been adapted for nursing home inhabitants in particular. Although treatment has improved, there is still an urgent need for alternative strategies—urgent because more people are living longer and, as a consequence, the number of years spent in ill health increases. This situation in turn leads to an increase in the number of those with depression. Thus there will also be a greater need for effective treatments that are both easy to administer within this population and appropriate to the emotional needs of later life.

LIFE REVIEW: AN EFFECTIVE INTERVENTION FOR TREATING DEPRESSION AND PROMOTING PSYCHOLOGICAL WELL-BEING IN LATER LIFE

Life review as a mode of therapy has been popular since its introduction by psychologist Robert Butler (1963) in the early 1960s. More recently, it is again gaining popularity as an intervention for depressive symptoms, a trend supported by meta-analyses showing it to be potentially effective in enhancing psychological well-being in older adults (Bohlmeijer, Smit, & Cuijpers, 2003; Bohlmeijer, Roemer, Cuijpers, & Smit, 2007). There are three reasons why structured life review is an attractive intervention for residential older adults with depressive symptoms.

First, Cappeliez (2002) has defined life review as a type of reminiscence that consists of a structured evaluation of one's past aimed at the acceptance of negative events and at resolving past conflicts, identifying continuity between past and present, and finding meaning in life. As such, life review is easily linked to a common and recognizable activity that is part of daily life (Webster, 1995), which means that older patients do not have to learn a new vocabulary or framework (Watt & Cappeliez, 2000). In other words, everybody seems capable of practicing this kind of therapy.

A second reason is that moving to a nursing home is a serious life event. Life events, it has been demonstrated, are related to an increase in reminiscence (Korte, Bohlmeijer, Westerhof, & Pot, 2010), since they require adaptation and may challenge existing identities. Insofar as nursing home residents may experience a loss of autonomy as an important part of their identity, reminiscence can help them find continuity in their lives and restore to them a more positive sense of identity. That said, many will not be able to do this sort of "restorying" (Kenyon & Randall, 1997) by themselves. Given that for many older adults, narrative is the primary form by which experience is made meaningful (Sherman & Peak, 1991), a process of structured reminiscence can thus be helpful (Tromp, this volume).

A third reason is that many nursing home residents are approaching death, and for some of them this will initiate a spontaneous process of life review (Merriam, 1993). But again, not everybody, and especially not depressed older adults, will be able to do this by themselves. Structured life review therapy allows people to develop these skills for themselves, accept how their lives have been thus far, and achieve some form of reconciliation and ego-integrity (Erikson, 1959).

This chapter discusses a new life review protocol for nursing home residents who suffer from depression. In line with a recent framework for the implementation of reminiscence with people with depression (Bohlmeijer & Westerhof, this volume), it links life review to a cognitive theory of the mechanisms that underlie depression—in this case, processes that are involved in the retrieval of autobiographical memories. First, we will describe how the autobiographical memory system works, and how it is related to depression and aging. This will be followed by an introduction of the autobiographical training protocol and a discussion of results from a study of its effectiveness.

AUTOBIOGRAPHICAL MEMORY: THEORY AND FUNCTION

According to the "multiple memory systems" perspective (see Tulving, 1995, for a review), long-term memory is composed of at least four systems.

Two of these act at the implicit (or unconscious) level of information processing.

The first system is *procedural memory*, which is essentially learning by experience and is employed primarily in learning motor skills. We do better in a given task, for instance, simply through repetition. No new explicit memories have been formed; rather, we are unconsciously accessing aspects of our previous experiences. The second is the *priming system*, a part of visual memory that allows us to replace information concerning particular objects, places, animals, or people with a sort of mental image of them. The third system, *semantic memory* (also referred to as our knowledge system), is involved in both implicit and explicit memory and concerns facts that are known independent of their context. Fourth, and finally, there is *episodic or autobiographical memory*, which consists of memories of personally experienced events. In fact, this type of memory enables us to travel mentally through time by providing us a direct link to awareness of the course of our life overall. Typically, it implies the processing of emotion. It is engaged specifically in the meaningful reconstruction of our own past (Fink et al., 1996), thus enabling a sense of self-coherence and self-continuity by creating subjectively significant personal past experiences that are embedded in our life history (for a review see Levine, 2004; Tulving, 2002). For example:

> Imagine yourself in the following situation…. . You are thinking back to the day you started working for the very first time. You may remember yourself being a bit nervous, having slept not so well the night before, or being afraid of waking up late, missing the train, or getting stuck in a traffic jam. At work, you remember meeting your new colleagues. You may remember their names and the first impression they made on you. You may remember the building you worked in, your workplace, the work you had to do. You may even remember what kind of weather it was or what clothes you were wearing that first day at the office. And you may even remember what you ate at your first office lunch.

This rather typical example of autographical memory contains episodic details and self-relevant information. Retrieving such a memory is more, therefore, than a matter of objective description, as in the case of a semantic memory: "When is your birthday?" or "What is the first name of your grandchild?". Retrieving it, one consciously experiences the fact that one is remembering a particular event, and the experience includes one's personal perspectives on the event, plus one's self-awareness, emotions, and thoughts, as well as particular perceptual details or images. In short, episodic and self-relevant information are relevant components of autobiographical memory.

Autobiographical memory has been studied in different contexts and in terms of different models. Here, we will be conceptualizing it in terms of the Self Memory System (SMS) proposed by Conway and colleagues, which explains autobiographical memory in relation to the concept of "the self" and its goals (Conway, 2005; Conway & Pleydell-Pearce, 2000; Conway, Singer, & Tagini, 2004). According to this model, autobiographical memory consists of three essential components.

The first component is *the autobiographical memory knowledge base*, a hierarchical structure that contains three levels: "lifestory schemas," "lifetime periods," and "general events." *Lifestory schemas* consist of knowledge concerning one's overall personal history; for instance, concerning "my high school days." The next level contains particular periods that reflect broad goals and activities, such as "holidays in France" and "working at the bank." These *lifetime periods* can be organized both temporally and thematically; moreover, some of them may overlap. For instance, "during my high school days, my parents and I always went on holiday to France." The bottom level of the hierarchy, *general events*, is a category of still more specific experiences that have to do with a particular shared theme, such as "going to my grandparents" and "first-time experiences," or a specific span of time, such as "my trip to Moscow."

The second essential component of autobiographical memory is *the conceptual self*. This consists of abstract knowledge about the self, including nontemporal self-structures like self-images and self-guides (questions such as "Who am I?" and "Who do I want to be?"), along with attitudes, values, and beliefs ("What beliefs do I have, and why?" and "What is important to me?"). Such knowledge helps to define the self, others, and general interactions with others and the world. The conceptual self and the autobiographical memory knowledge base form the basis of autobiographical memory. Together, they are called *the long-term self*. The third component is the *episodic memory system*, or event-specific knowledge. Next to the memory itself, this component includes the various sensory and perceptual details—images, sounds, and smells—that one tries to remember.

For these three components to cooperate with one another in an actual autobiographical memory, an additional component is required: *the working self*. This component links the other three together by means of current goals. It regulates short-term goals, such as catching the train, and is concerned with the processes necessary to attain them. Here, the most important function of memories is that they correspond to the goals that need to be attained. In summary, then, autobiographical memory is a central aspect of human functioning and contributes to one's individual sense of self

(Conway et al., 2004). It also helps one to gain a better sense of one's world, to pursue one's goals in problem-solving situations, and to regulate one's emotions.

Overgeneral Autobiographical Memory

In recent years, there has been considerable interest in the ability to retrieve specific autobiographical memories. It has been widely established, though, that for depressed adults, such memories are difficult to recall. Williams (1996) and colleagues (Williams et al., 2007) have found, for instance, that unlike healthy, nondepressed, "control" participants, depressed participants tend to come up with "overgeneral" memories, especially in response to positive cues. In response to the cue word *happy*, whereas the controls retrieved a specific event (such as "the day we left to go on holiday to Florida"), the depressed individuals often retrieved a summary memory or a categorical memory that did not refer to any event in particular—for example, "when buying a new pair of shoes" (Evans, Williams, O'Loughlin, & Howells, 1992).

The term *specific autobiographical memory* refers to a memory of a personally experienced event that happened at a particular place and lasted less than a day. Failing to retrieve such memories is called "overgeneral memory." Typically, two types of overgeneral memory are distinguished (Williams & Dritschel, 1992). On the one hand, *extended memories* have to do with a single event that lasts longer than one day: for example, "my summer vacation after graduation from high school." On the other hand, *categorical memories* refer to a group of similar events that occurred on repeated occasions, such as "every time I went to my parents."

Williams, Stiles, and Shapiro (1999) have proposed the "affect regulation hypothesis," in which reduced specificity of autobiographical memory is related to difficulties in searching the self-memory system. The proposal is that in order to recall a specific autobiographical memory in response to a given cue word, one's first step is to generate a restricted set of categorical descriptors that the cue word itself constrains. These descriptors are used to search the memory system for memories that pertain to that word. Subsequent sets of descriptors are then generated iteratively, allowing an increasingly refined search of this categorical subset of memories to retrieve specific episodes that comply with the task instructions. When people attempt to retrieve specific events from their past, they first access higher-level, general descriptions, using these as intermediate steps to derive pointers to the lower-level, specific events (Reiser, Black, & Abelson, 1985;

Rubin, 1996). Autobiographical memory can be seen as a hierarchy, with categorical or prolonged memories at the higher level and specific memories at the lower level. Put another way, the enormous number of episodic or specific memories represent the base of a pyramid, with categorical memories at the top. Williams et al. (1999) proposed further that, during memory search, in order to progress beyond the categorical descriptor stage to a more refined interrogation of the specific memory database, one must in some way inhibit unneeded categorical descriptors. Failure to do so leads to the generation of overly general responses (reduced specificity) to cue words. Depressed individuals become engaged, therefore, in a cycle of rumination with even more categorical memories being activated. This tendency of depressed patients to retrieve categorical autobiographical memories Williams (1996) has called the "mnemonic interlock." Another possible explanation for overgeneral memory, however, is the relatively poor executive or attentional control of depressed individuals in the face of a cognitively demanding task (Dalgleish et al., 2007). In other words, a clear empirical link between overgeneral memory and executive control, as proposed by the affect regulation hypothesis, has yet to be established.

Overgeneral memory seems to interfere with normal human functioning in everyday life. In particular, individuals with an overgeneral-memory retrieval style have trouble with problem solving, they recover less well from therapy, and they seem more vulnerable to psychopathology (Williams et al., 2007). They find it difficult to retrieve specific memories about similar past experiences, which in turn may hinder successful interpersonal contact and interaction with their environment. Such people experience difficulties in making prospective plans, in solving day-to-day problems, and in directing their lives toward the specific aims they would like to achieve (Goddard, Dritschel, & Burton, 1996; Williams et al., 1999). Moreover, they have difficulty imagining specific events that might happen in the future (Williams et al., 2007).

Autobiographical Memory and Depression

The course of depression appears to be influenced by overgeneral memory (Brittlebank, Scott, Williams, & Ferrier, 1993; Dalgleish, Spinks, Yiend, & Kuyken, 2001). Several studies have demonstrated that clients who have recovered from depression are still less specific in their recollections than individuals who have never been depressed (Williams and Dritschel, 1992). Difficulty in retrieving specific autobiographical memories may therefore hinder progress in psychotherapy and, as such, may influence the outcome of depression. Although overgeneral memory was originally described as a stable characteristic (Brittlebank et al., 1993), it may, in fact, be open to change. Williams, Teasdale, Segal, and Soulsby (2000) found that, compared with a group of controls, depressed patients who received 8 weeks of mindfulness-based cognitive therapy showed a reduction in overgeneral memories.

Autobiographical Memory and Aging

There are only few studies of the effects of aging on autobiographical memory in older adults. It is well established that working memory is lower in later life (Lezak, 1995). According to the theories proposed by Williams (1996) and Conway and Pleydell-Pearce (2000), older adults should therefore have more difficulty than younger ones in retrieving specific autobiographical memories. Episodic memory recall seems, in general, to be more vulnerable than semantic memory to the processes of normal aging (Greene, Hodges, & Baddeley, 1995; Helkala, Laulumaa, Soininen, & Riekkinnen, 1989; Laukka, Jones, Small, Fratiglioni, & Backman, 2004; Piolino, Desgranges, Benali, & Eustache, 2002; Piolino et al., 2003). The fact that episodic autobiographical memory is affected by age-related processes is also compatible with the finding that in older adults, most autobiographical recollections refer to personal past episodes that occurred during early adulthood—i.e., the so-called reminiscence bump (Rybash & Monaghan, 1999; Schroots, van Dijkum, & Assink, 2004).

Frombolt, Larsen, and Larsen (1995) have observed that, in free recall, depressed older adults retrieve less detailed memories than do nondepressed ones. However, in a systematic review of literature on this topic from 1986 to 2005, Birch and Davidson (2007) identified no studies that compared older and younger adults in terms of specificity of memory performance, nor any that compared depressed and nondepressed older adults. In investigating the topic themselves, Birch and Davidson found that nondepressed older adults do not retrieve significantly more categorical memories than depressed ones. This is in contrast with studies that have compared depressed and nondepressed younger adults (Goddard, Dritschel & Burton, 1996, 2001). One possible explanation is that nondepressed older adults retrieve more categorical memories than do their nondepressed younger counterparts. As a consequence, the difference between depressed and nondepressed older adults may be relatively small. In our own study with older adults, the number of specific memories retrieved was unrelated to age, response latency, or depression scores. However, a significant association was found between the number of specific or categorical memories that participants recalled and their test scores on working memory, which might seem to provide evidence for a link between aging, working memory and the number of memories (specific or categorical) retrieved. Still, although working memory capacity explained the considerable variance in the number of specific memories retrieved, it did not fully account for reduced memory specificity. Despite not having lower working memory scores, the depressed participants retrieved fewer specific memories than did the controls, while older adults with a better functioning working memory retrieved more specific ones.

All of this indicates the important role of emotional factors, and not simply cognitive factors, in explaining the relationship between depressed feelings and overgeneral autobiographical memory in later life.

OUR PROTOCOL

On the basis of research conducted on the specificity of autobiographical memory and its relation to depression, Serrano, Latorre, Gatz, and Montanes (2004) developed a structured life review intervention for older adults with depressive symptomatology. Their approach was to provide participants with practice in recalling specific autobiographical memories. The life review protocol consists of an autobiographical retrieval practice that runs for 4 weeks and each week focuses on a particular life period: childhood, adolescence, adulthood, and, finally, life in general. For each period, 14 questions were prepared, based on the work of Haight and Webster (1995), to prompt specific memories. Sample questions include the following:

- What is the most pleasant situation that you remember from your childhood?
- What did your mother or father do one day when you were a child that astonished you?
- During adolescence, what moment do you remember as special because it was the first kiss you received, or because you shared something special with a person you were in love with?
- Tell me about a day when you were an adolescent and you did something out of the ordinary.
- Tell me about a time that you remember experiencing the most pride at work.
- Did someone close to you or someone you knew recuperate from a grave illness?

- If everything in your life were to happen exactly the same, what moment would you like to relive?
- What do you consider to be the most important thing you have done in your life?

Participants were explicitly encouraged to retrieve positive memories in response to the positively stated questions. Intervention sessions were tape-recorded. Adapting the protocol for use in The Netherlands, we rephrased several questions, introduced sessions more elaborately, and developed more specific guidelines for counselors (Bohlmeijer & Steunenberg, 2009).

Application and Therapeutic Skills

There are no exclusion criteria for our protocol. Anybody can begin it, with one exception. We are unable, as yet, to test its effectiveness with older adults who are cognitively impaired, although we hope to in the near future. Of course, participants should have a sufficient mastery of the language spoken during the training—in our case, Dutch. They should be able to communicate verbally and have no hearing impairments (although we once performed the training with a deaf participant who read all the questions out loud). And those with speaking problems due to seizures might need to be excluded as well. Also important is the motivation of the participant. Before starting the intervention, the therapist should be sure of the participant's willingness to complete the four sessions and to speak about personal, private memories. In other words, a positive attitude toward reminiscence per se is a possible prerequisite for effective implementation.

The main challenge for the facilitator or counselor is to get the memory to be as specific as possible. One poses the question from the protocol, asks if the participant understands its meaning, and, should the event recalled seem a bit general, requests more information and more specific details, by asking such questions as, "When did this happen?" "Where?" "Who was there?" "Did it happen only once?" "What kind of weather was it?" "Can you describe the location in more detail?" "How did the food taste?" "How did it smell?" "Can you describe how that machine worked?" "Can you describe how you felt?"

Any question is allowed that elicits more specific details about a given memory. Especially in the first session, one needs to help respondents by asking for such details. In doing so, the participant develops a better understanding of what is meant by "specific" memories. It is also important to give participants positive feedback on how well they are doing and on how specific the memories are that they recall. This is important in making the training a success. As the training progresses, participants get increasingly accustomed to this procedure and more competent in recalling specific memories on their own.

What does one do, however, if the participant does not respond? After 20 or 30 seconds, one might ask the question again. If a respondent answers that no memory can be retrieved, one may try by means of explanatory questions to get to a memory. For example, one might ask, "During your childhood, did you have friends that you played with very often?" If the respondent says "no," then one can perhaps ask, "Did you play with children from your class or from your neighborhood?" In other words, one does not simply accept a "no" answer. However, if after one or two of these follow-up questions the participant still does not recall a memory, then one should shift to the next question.

It is important to stay positive. The protocol is aimed at the recollection of specific *positive* events. Of course, participants may retrieve negative emotional events as well. If so, then it is important to give some attention to such events and let the participant talk about them, but not to let them take over, instead to try and get back to positive memories as soon as possible, albeit with respect for the feelings of the participant. It is also important to be an active listener and inquisitive, and not to hesitate to ask for more details. And it is important to give compliments, to tell participants how well they are doing. One is allowed, for example, to give one's personal feelings about a given memory, such as "What a beautiful memory! I am touched by it." But one should guard against giving an opinion about the stories told or about summarizing with remarks, for instance, that the participant has had "a nice life." The participant is depressed and might well think the other way around. In making such remarks one runs the risk that the participant will want to stop or will start recalling negative memories to prove that his or her life was, in fact, not that nice at all. Lastly, it is important to attend to the participant's level of anxiety or energy and to stop when he or she grows tired or asks for a break.

Assessment and Effectiveness

To assess the ability to retrieve a specific memory under timed conditions in response to a cue word, we used the Autobiographical Memory Test (AMT) (Williams & Broadbent, 1986). In administering it, respondents are asked to retrieve a specific memory related to a personality trait such as *creative*, *friendly*, or *guilty*. A specific memory is defined as a discrete episode, lasting no longer than a single day, that happened to the participant. If the memory happened on a number of occasions, then it is coded as general. The cue words are presented to respondents on cards in a fixed order and the respondents have to read each word out loud. There are two sets of such words, each consisting of five positive words and five negative. Examples include *friendly* (positive [P]), *guilty* (negative [N]), *rude* (N), *helpful* (P), *jealous* (N), and *intelligent* (P).

To ensure that our participants understood the instructions we provided examples. If the cue word was *proud,* for example, then they might say, "I was really proud last Wednesday when my daughter gave birth to my first grandchild." This would be a specific personal memory because it refers to a particular event on a particular day when they displayed the trait. If, instead, the participant said, "I always get proud when I see my grandchildren," then the answer was not coded as a *specific* memory, since it does not refer to any event in particular but rather to visits of family members in general. The respondents were instructed to think of a specific personal memory—a time when they displayed the trait in question—and were asked to answer as quickly as possible. Answering time was recorded with a stopwatch. Each memory was rated as either general or specific. Because the total number of stimulus words was 10, the maximum score for either category was also 10. In other words, if a respondent had a score of 10, it is possible that all memories were coded as specific or as categorical/general. Codes given to the memories were rated by the interviewers and were controlled by the coordinating researcher.

In the first half of 2007, the boards of directors of 14 residential homes for older adults in Amsterdam and the surrounding area were approached about participating in this study, and all agreed. All residents of the homes received a letter notifying them of the study. In order to participate, however, participants had to be 65 years of age or older, display a clinically significant level of depressive symptoms, and have normal cognitive functioning. Residents who had a diagnosis of dementia and were cognitively impaired were not asked to participate (selection was conducted by the staff of the residential home). Excluded were those with psychotic symptoms or behavior, no ability to communicate verbally, impaired hearing, or insufficient mastery of the Dutch language. In total, 110 (12.7%) residents were included. Enrollment took place between March 2007 and April 2008.

Our main finding of this study was that the level of depressive symptoms in a nursing home sample significantly decreased after receiving the autobiographical retrieval practice "Dear Memories" (Steunenberg, Bohlmeijer, van Straten, & Cuijpers, 2010). A medium to large effect size was found. The life review process involves emotional processing of events from the individual's past. The protocol focuses on bringing up specific positive memories or pleasant events. The results showed that those residents receiving this retrieval practice experienced an improved mood state and decreased feelings of depression. Participants reported a higher number of specific memories on the test after completing the four sessions of the intervention; this effect size was also moderate. Results showed that the protocol appeared to be more effective for participants with the diagnosis of major depression or with depressive symptoms than for those with minor depression. Of those with minor depression at the outset, 36% experienced worsened symptoms *after* the intervention and they were diagnosed with major depression at the post-measurement stage. Such results suggest, then, that the protocol might be less suited for people with minor depression.

SUMMARY AND CONCLUSION

A central assumption in narrative gerontology is that identity development is a life-long process and that identity is grounded in narrative structures. Age-graded losses and life events may challenge meaning in life and positive identity in later life. Reminiscence is one way of finding continuity and restoring a positive identity (Watt and Wong, 1991). Memories are the building blocks of our lifestories. The way our autobiographical memory works is therefore of crucial importance for interventions that aim at restorying. There is ample evidence that depression is associated with difficulties in retrieving specific positive memories. Indeed, depression may be seen as a condition in which negative memories have (temporarily) won the competition with positive memories in the limited spaces of easily retrievable memories (Brewin, Reynolds, & Tata, 1999). How is one able to maintain a positive, agency-filled identity if one cannot remember precious, once-in-a-lifetime events? Assisting older adults in retrieving memories of these special moments is important in facilitating restorying in later life. The immediate availability of a reservoir of specific positive memories may be a good buffer against depression and may help older adults to find integrity. If one can say, "my life has not been so bad after all," as one might well say when the dark clouds of depression are rising, then it may be easier to accept both oneself and one's life.

In this chapter, we have presented an intervention that facilitates the retrieval of specific positive memories. Its main advantages are that it is short, requires no new language, and can be practiced by any professional capable of careful listening and structured questioning, as difficult as this can sometimes be. In addition, we presented results from a study offering evidence that overgeneral memory in depression can indeed be modified and that enhancing the specificity of such memory is useful in treating the symptoms of depression in older adults, especially among nursing home residents. If we can succeed in time traveling with older adults to special moments in their past, then, as suggested in the example cited at the beginning, we can enable them to give themselves a great gift in their last years of life.

REFERENCES

Beekman, A., Copeland, J., & Prince, M. (1999). Review of community prevalence of depression in later life. *British Journal of Psychiatry, 174,* 307–311.

Birch, L., & Davidson, K. (2007). Specificity of autobiographical memory in depressed older adults and its relationship with working memory and IQ. *British Journal of Clinical Psychology, 46,* 175–186.

Bohlmeijer, E., Smit, F., & Cuijpers, P. (2003). Effects of reminiscence and life review on late-life depression: A meta-analysis. *International Journal of Geriatric Psychiatry, 18,* 1088–1094.

Bohlmeijer, E., Roemer, M., Cuijpers, P., & Smit, F. (2007). The effects of life-review on psychological well-being in older adults: a meta-analysis. *Aging and Mental Health, 11,* 291–300.

Bohlmeijer, E., & Steunenberg, B. (2009). Dear Memories: A protocol for individual life-review therapy based on autobiographical memory training in depressed residential home elderly. Vrije University, Amsterdam.

Brewin, C., Reynolds, M., & Tata, P. (1999). Autobiographical memory processes and the course of depression. *Journal of Abnormal Psychology, 108*(3), 511–517.

Brittlebank, A., Scott, J., Williams, J., & Ferrier, I. (1993). Autobiographical memory in depression: State or trait marker? *British Journal of Psychiatry, 162,* 118–121.

Butler, R. (1963). The life review: An interpretation of reminiscence in the aged. *Psychiatry, 26,* 65–76.

Cappeliez, P. (2002). Cognitive-reminiscence therapy for depressed older adults in day hospital and long-term care. In J. Webster & B. Haight (Eds.), *Critical advances in reminiscence work* (pp. 300–313). New York: Springer.

Conway, M. (2005). Memory and the self. *Journal of Memory and Language, 53,* 594–628.

Conway, M., & Pleydell-Pearce, C. (2000). The construction of autobiographical memories in the self-memory system. *Psychological Review, 107,* 261–288.

Conway, M., Singer, J., & Tagini, A. (2004). The self and autobiographical memory: Correspondence and coherence. *Social Cognition, 22,* 491–529.

Cuijpers, P., van Straten, A., & Smit, F. (2006). Psychological treatment of late life depression: A meta-analysis of randomized controlled trials. *Acta Psychiatrica Scandinavica, 115,* 434–441.

Dalgleish, T., Perkins, H., Williams, J., Golden, A., Barnard, P., Au-Yeung, C., Murphy, V., Elward, R., Tchanturia, K., & Watkins, E. (2007). Reduced specificity of autobiographical memory and depression: The role of executive processes. *Journal of Experimental Psychology: General, 136,* 23–42.

Dalgleish, T., Spinks, H., Yiend, J., & Kuyken, W. (2001). Autobiographical memory style in seasonal affective disorder and its relationships to future symptom remission. *Journal of Abnormal Psychology, 110*, 335–340.

Erikson, E. (1959). *Identity and the life cycle.* New York: International University Press.

Evans, J., Williams, J., O'Loughlin, S., & Howells, K. (1992). Autobiographical memory and problem-solving strategies of parasuicide patients. *Psychological Medicine, 22*, 399–405.

Fink, G., Markowitsch, H., Reinkemeier, M., Bruckbauer, T., Kessler, J., & Heiss, W. (1996). Cerebral representation of one's own past: neural networks involved in autobiographical memory. *Journal of Neuroscience, 16*, 4275–4282.

Frombolt, P., Larsen, P., & Larsen, S. (1995). Effects of late onset depression and recovery on autobiographical memory. *Journal of Gerontology, 50B*, 74–81.

Goddard, L., Dritschel, B., & Burton, A. (1996). The role of autobiographical memory in social problem-solving and depression. *Journal of Abnormal Psychology, 105*, 609–616.

Goddard, L., Dritschel, B., & Burton, A. (2001). The effects of specific retrieval instruction on social problem-solving in depression. *British Journal of Clinical Psychology, 40*, 297–308.

Greene, J., Hodges, J., & Baddeley, A. (1995). Autobiographical memory and executive functioning in early dementia of Alzheimer type. *Neuropsychologia, 33*, 1647–1670.

Haight, B., & Webster, J. (Eds.). (1995). *The art and science of reminiscing: Theory, research methods, and applications.* Bristol, PA: Taylor and Francis.

Helkala, E., Laulumaa, V., Soininen, H., & Riekkinen, P. (1989). Different error pattern of episodic and semantic memory in Alzheimer's disease with dementia. *Neuropsychologica, 27*, 1241–1248.

Jongenelis, K., Pot, A., Eisses, A., Beekman, A., Kluiter, H., van Tilburg, W., & Ribbe, M. (2003). Depression among older nursing home patients: A review. *Tijdschrift voor Gerontologie en Geriatrie, 34*, 52–59.

Kenyon, G., & Randall, W. (1997). *Restorying our lives: Personal growth through autobiographical reflection.* Westport, CT: Praeger.

Korte, J., Bohlmeijer, E., Westerhof, G., & Pot, A. (2010). The relations between life-events, reminiscence functions and mental health in older adults with psychological problems. Manuscript submitted for publication.

Laukka, E., Jones, S., Small, B., Fratiglioni, L., & Backman, L. (2004). Similar patterns of cognitive deficits in the preclinical phases of vascular dementia and Alzheimer's disease. *Journal of the International Neuropsychological Society, 10*, 382–391.

Levine, B. (2004). Autobiographical memory and the self in the time: Brain lesion effects, functional neuroanatomy, and lifespan development. *Brain Cognition, 55*, 54–68.

Lezak, M. (1995). *Neuropsychological assessment* (3rd ed.). New York: Oxford University Press.

Merriam, S. (1993). Butler's life review: How universal is it? *International Journal of Aging and Human Development, 37*, 163–175.

Piolino, P., Desgranges, B., Benali, K., & Eustache, F. (2002). Episodic and semantic remote memory in aging. *Memory, 10*, 239–257.

Piolono, P., Desgranges, B., Belliard, S., Matuszewski, V., Lalevee, C., De la Sayette, V., & Eustache, F. (2003). Autobiographical memory and autonoetic consciousness: Triple dissociation in neurodegenerative disease. *Brain, 126*, 2203–2219.

Reiser, B., Black, J., and Abelson, R. (1985). Knowledge structures in the organization and retrieval of autobiographical memories. *Cognitive* Psychology, *17*, 80–137.

Rubin, D. (1996). *Remembering our past: Studies in autobiographical memory.* New York: Cambridge University Press.

Rybash, J., & Monoghan, B. (1999). Episodic and semantic contributions to older adults' autobiographical recall. *Journal of General Psychology, 126*, 85–96.

Schroots, J., van Dijkum, C., & Assink, M. (2004). Autobiographical memory from a life span perspective. *International Journal of Aging and Human Development, 58*, 69–85.

Serrano, J., Latorre, J., Gatz, M., & Montanes, J. (2004). Life review therapy using autobiographical retrieval practice for older adults with depressive symptomatology. *Psychology and Aging, 2*, 272–277.

Sherman, E., & Peak, T. (1991). Patterns of reminiscence and the assessment of late life adjustment. *Journal of Gerontological Social Work, 16*, 59–74.

Steunenberg, B., Bohlmeijer, E., van Straten, A., & Cuijpers, P. (2010). The effectiveness of life review therapy using autobiographical memory retrieval in a depressed residential home population: A randomized controlled trial. Manuscript submitted for publication.

Tulving, E. (1995). Organization of memory: Quo vadis? In M. Gazziniga (Ed.), *The cognitive neurosciences* (pp. 839–847). Cambridge, MA: MIT Press.

Tulving, E. (2002). Episodic memory: From mind to brain. *Annual Review of Psychology, 53*, 1–25.

Watt, L., & Cappeliez, P. (2000). Integrative and instrumental reminiscence therapies for depression in older adults: Intervention strategies and treatment effectiveness. *Aging and Mental Health, 4*, 166–177.

Watt, L., & Wong, P. (1991). A taxonomy of reminiscence and therapeutic implications. *Journal of Gerontological Social Work, (1)*1/2, 6–56.

Webster, J. (1995). Adult age differences in reminiscence functions. In B. Haight & J. Webster (Eds.), *The art and science of reminiscing: Theory, research, methods, and application* (pp. 89–102). Bristol, PA: Taylor and Francis.

Williams, J. (1996). Depression and the specificity of autobiographical memory. In D. Rubin (Ed.), *Remembering our past: Studies in autobiographical memory* (pp. 244–267). New York: Cambridge University Press.

Williams, J., Barnhofer, T., Crane, C., Herman, D., Raes, F., Watkins, E., & Dalgleish, T. (2007). Autobiographical memory specificity and emotional disorder. *Psychological Bulletin, 133*, 122–148.

Williams, J., & Broadbent, K. (1986). Autobiographical memory in attempted suicide patients. *Journal of Abnormal Psychology, 95*, 144–149.

Williams, J., & Dritschel, B. (1992). Categoric and extended autobiographical memories. In M. Conway, H. Rubin, W. Spinnler, & W. Wagenaar (Eds.),

Theoretical perspectives on autobiographical memory (pp. 391–409). Dordrecht, The Netherlands: Kluwer Academic Publishers.

Williams, J., Stiles, W., & Shapiro, D. (1999). Cognitive mechanisms in the avoidance of painful and dangerous thoughts: Elaborating the assimilation model. *Cognitive Therapy and Research, 23,* 285–306.

Williams, J., Teasdale, J., Segal, Z., & Soulsby, J. (2000). Mindfulness-based cognitive therapy reduces overgeneral autobiographical memory in formerly depressed patients. *Journal of Abnormal Psychology, 109,* 150–155.

Nineteen

"GREEN AND GRAY": AN EDUCATIONAL PROGRAM TO ENHANCE CONTACT BETWEEN YOUNGER AND OLDER ADULTS BY MEANS OF LIFESTORIES

Gerben J. Westerhof

One of the most important functions of lifestories is to enhance social relations. Sharing them is an important means of developing and maintaining social contacts. Stimulating their exchange may thus be used in interventions aimed at increasing mutual understanding among different social groups. Beyond the family, younger and older adults often have few contacts with each other. They tend to rely on mutual stereotypes in their interactions, particularly professional interactions in the fields of social work and health care. This chapter discusses an educational program called "Green and Gray" that uses lifestories to improve relations between younger and older adults and is developed specifically for use in middle and higher education in health care and social work alike.

NEEDS ASSESSMENT

Age Segregation

Social gerontologists have argued that our society is age segregated, i.e., organized according to different age groups that have little contact with one another (Hagestad & Uhlenberg, 2005). A key reason for this separation is that age per se has become a major criterion in the division of labor within our society. Kohli (1985) even argues that the life course has become an institution of its own, divided into the tripartite structure of education—work—retirement. This means that chronological age is used as a central feature of laws and regulations that define the rights and responsibilities of individuals. Cross-cultural research has shown that, in industrialized as compared to nonindustrialized societies, age alone is indeed a significant basis for positioning people (Keith et al., 1994).

Although recent years have seen an increasing flexibility in societal arrangements concerning the life course in general, their effects on the segregation of age groups are still very tangible in everyday life. Children and younger people spend most of their days in daycare centers or at school, and middle-aged adults are at work, whereas older people are largely excluded from these domains. In particular, in a country like The Netherlands with an obligatory retirement age, the participation of older adults in the labor force is very low. In 2006, only 2.6% of those over 65 were working (CBS, 2009). Although lifelong learning has become an important subject of social policies, a study by Künemund & Kolland in 2007 reported that fewer than 5% of Dutch adults over 60 had attended an educational or training course in the preceding month. When older adults attend educational courses, they often visit age-segregated universities and classes for older adults.

As a consequence, byproduct, and catalyst of age grading in the labor force, age has come to play an important role in the cultural and political fields as well. In the highly scattered media landscape in The Netherlands, there are broadcasting companies for younger people (BNN) and for older people (MAX), as well as magazines for younger people (e.g., *Flair*) and for seniors (e.g., *Plus Magazine*—actually the largest magazine in The Netherlands, with a monthly circulation of 300,000). Leisure activities are similarly directed toward different age groups, such as the youth orchestra versus senior fitness, or youth travel tours versus senior travel tours. There are even political organizations that promote the particular interests of different age groups, such as younger workers in the trade unions and older citizens' associations. Social policies have resulted in a spatial segregation as well, as illustrated by student dormitories versus nursing homes. In short, younger and older people lead lives that seldom touch one another.

This conclusion gets further support from studies on social networks. In a representative study of the Dutch older population who live independently, we found that only 1.5% of adults aged 65 and older mentioned a non-kin person below the age of 25 among their eight most important social relations (van Kordelaar, Vlak, Kuin, & Westerhof, 2008). In the Eurobarometer study, Walker and Maltby (1997) reported that almost two out of three Dutch older adults have little or no contact with people younger than 25. Hagestad and Uhlenberg (2005) used the Amsterdam Longitudinal Aging Study to show the age segregation in social networks of Dutch older adults. They compared the actual network composition to a hypothesized network composition based on the age distribution of the Dutch population. They found that persons over 65 had 50 times less non-kin persons under 25 in their networks than would be expected.

Stereotypes

An important consequence of the economical, cultural, political, spatial, and social segregation between age groups is that it contributes to mutual stereotyping on the basis of age (Hagestad & Uhlenberg, 2005; Westerhof & Tulle, 2007). Although stereotypes about younger groups exist as well, here we will focus on stereotypes about older persons. Fiske, Cuddy, Glick and Xu (2002) have proposed a general model for stereotype content, arguing that there are universal dimensions in the content of stereotypes about different social groups, just as there are universal processes at work in stereotyping processes. The authors propose that the two most important dimensions are warmth and competence. Their research shows that stereotypes about different social groups vary systematically along these two dimensions. Most importantly, stereotypes often have a mixed content—for example, being high on warmth and low on competence. Cuddy and Fiske (2002) found that older people as a stereotyped group show exactly this profile: "doddering but dear." Versteegh and Westerhof (2007) replicated this finding in a Dutch study. Their findings match those from a meta-analysis done by Kite and Johnson (1988), who found that older adults were judged more negatively than younger adults on the dimensions of physical attractiveness and competence, whereas no differences in stereotypes were found on the dimensions of personality and desirability of contact.

Groups seen as warm but incompetent are also seen as having low status and not being competitive (Fiske et al., 2002). This mixed stereotype may trigger paternalistic behavior (Fiske et al., 2002). Studies on interactions between younger and older adults have typically found such behavior in the form of patronizing speech (Ryan, Hummert, & Boich, 1995), displaced baby talk (Caporael & Culbertson, 1986), or "elderspeak" (Kemper & Harden, 1999). This kind of communicative style is characterized by a high pitch, strong intonation, loud voice, the use of concrete and familiar words, an easy grammar, and a directive and childish way of speaking—for example, the use of *we* when referring to an individual. Nonverbally, it is signaled by frowning, little eye contact, raised eyebrows, hands on hips, and abrupt gestures. Williams and Nussbaum (2001) describe this communication style as "over-accommodative": the behavior is guided more by the younger person's expectations about older persons in general than by the needs of the particular older person involved.

The stereotype activation model describes how stereotypes about older persons in general are applied in everyday social interaction with them (Hummert, 1994), depending on characteristics of the interlocutor (e.g., age and previous intergenerational experiences); the older person him- or herself (e.g., physique and personal appearance); and the salience of age in the situation at hand (e.g., competition between younger and older job applicants or an age-homogenous environment like nursing homes). The activation of stereotypes in specific interactions may result in communicative patterns that "can be counterproductive in both the long and short term, in that they can reproduce negative attitudes toward aging as well as inhibit successful aging" (Giles et al., 1992, p. 271).

In narrative terms, one might say that older adults are at risk of becoming "storyotyped" by younger adults (Randall, 1995, p. 57). Rather than co-authoring the stories of older persons by listening to and valuing them, younger people may co-opt their stories or even destroy them. By more or less consciously insisting that *their* version of old age is *the* version of old age, the narrative development of older people may be seriously delimited. For example, Gubrium and Holstein (1999) found that nursing homes affect the way people think and talk about the aging person. In analyzing conversations in nursing homes, they found that most conversations included "body talk." They concluded that residents are often seen by the nursing staff as bodies instead of persons.

Professional Settings

As a result of the aging of society, professionals in the fields of social work and health care will increasingly encounter older adults. According to the criteria of the stereotype activation model, professional settings may be especially prone to the negative effects of stereotyping. The often younger professionals have to deal mainly with dependent or frail older persons in age-salient settings that easily confirm existing stereotypes. Studies have indeed shown that health care professionals have even more negative stereotypes about older adults than those of the general population (Anderson & Wiscott, 2004; Beullens, Marcoen, Jaspaert, & Pelemans, 1997; Pasupathi & Löckenhoff, 2002), although studies on social workers are somewhat mixed (Allen, Cherry, & Palmore, 2009; Anderson & Wiscott, 2004). Such stereotypes may have harmful effects on the delivery of care and social support to older persons.

Studies on long-term care, for instance, have shown that patronizing behavior is widely practiced in nursing homes. Sachweh (1998), studying German nursing homes, found high-pitched and exaggerated intonation in almost half of the conversations and the use of *we* in nearly two out of three conversations between nursing staff and residents (see Marks, this volume). Margaret Baltes (1995) found that among institutionalized persons the need for assistance with personal care was rewarded with high levels of interaction, whereas displays of independence in personal care and social behaviors were largely ignored. This eventually resulted in a vicious cycle of dependency and led her to conclude that dependency is also a result of social processes and not just of biological ones.

Studies have also shown that stereotypes compromise the communication between medical doctors and their older patients. Pasupathi and Löckenhoff (2002, p. 210) conclude the following about the medical field: "Taken together, there is substantial evidence that physicians treat older patients differently from younger patients. Specifically, this differential treatment involves the potential for misinterpretation of symptoms and inappropriate treatment, is reflected in less open and receptive communication practices, and results in poor concordance between patient and physician about what has been accomplished in the interview."

In a similar vein, the American Psychological Association (APA, 2004) mentions that both negative and positive stereotypes about older persons can contribute to biases in the diagnosis, prevention, and treatment of psychological problems in older adults. Complaints such as anxiety, depression, fatigue, or confusion may be misinterpreted as belonging to old age. Beliefs that older adults are too old to change or that treatments may not work for older adults may result in suboptimal treatment. Lastly, one's own discomfort with aging and paternalistic behaviors may compromise the therapeutic relationship.

Summary of Assessment

Given these possibly negative effects of stereotyping in professional settings, it is important to combat stereotypes among professionals who will be working with older adults. This is stated explicitly, for example, in the guidelines for psychological practice with older adults that have been developed by the APA (2004, p. 237): "Psychologists are encouraged to recognize how their attitudes and beliefs about aging and about older individuals may be relevant to their assessment and treatment of older adults, and to seek consultation or further education about these issues when indicated."

Many professional organizations have recently argued that social work, health care, and the empowerment of older people should be centered on the needs of older persons themselves, rather than on the needs of providers and organizations. Hence, more person-centered interventions have been developed, including those based on lifestories (for examples, see Tromp; Ubels; and Steunenberg & Bohlmeijer, this volume). This change in focus is related to more general societal developments. For example, the autonomy, choice, and individual responsibility of older adults play an increasingly prominent role in the mass media and in social policies. This has led to new understandings of old age as a period of continued societal participation, autonomy, and consumption (Gilleard & Higgs, 2000).

These shifting discourses call for professionals who are well trained in detecting the needs of older adults. It is therefore important to include the person-centered lifestory approach early in the education of professionals who will be working with older adults. Given the fact that most younger adults have little contact with older adults and that students will mainly encounter older persons with physical and social problems, it is important to bring them in close contact with older "normally aging" persons. The educational program "Green and Gray" was developed specifically for this purpose.

"GREEN AND GRAY": THE PROGRAM

Development of the Program

The educational program "Green and Gray" was developed at the Center for Psychogerontology of Radboud University in Nijmegen, The Netherlands, with financial support from the Stichting Sluyterman van Loo, a private funding agency for projects for older persons.

We started with a series of interviews with 25 older adults between the ages of 65 and 75. The interviews focused on the lifestories of older adults in relation to their retirement and the social and cultural changes they experienced during their lives. Elsewhere we have reported extensively on the outcomes of this study (van Kordelaar & Westerhof, 2007; Westerhof, 2009, 2010). In the context of this chapter, it is important to mention that despite the rather varied attitudes toward retirement and cultural change, a general theme in the lifestories was that older adults experienced little contact with the younger generation outside of their own family. Furthermore, they generally felt that society belongs to the young rather than to their own age group. Many expressed an interest in more contact—and more *meaningful* contact—with the younger generation. This interview-based study corroborated the needs assessment discussed in the previous section from the point of view of older persons.

Program Content

The main goal of the educational program was to improve contact between both age groups and to develop a more personal and less stereotypical approach to the other generation. For younger students, a further goal was to gain experience in organizing and supervising a counseling group with older adults and, for older adults, to integrate the past with the present.

For decades, social psychologists have studied the effects of intergroup contact to reduce intergroup prejudice. A recent meta-analytic review examined 515 studies testing the hypothesis that contact is related to decreased prejudice between groups (Pettigrew & Tropp, 2006). Ninety-four percent of the studies showed a negative relation between contact and prejudice, and the average correlation across all studies was around −.21. The effects generalized to the out-group as a whole and to other situations and were found not only in more classic studies on racial and ethnic groups but also in studies involving other groups such as those based on gender and age. Although structured programs provided stronger effects, even contact as such produced an increased liking for the out-group, simply as a consequence of exposure to it. The authors closed with a call for new insights into the factors responsible for combating prejudice.

In our program we used lifestories to enhance contact between younger and older persons and to reduce stereotypical out-group perceptions. Lifestories are seen as devices to construe and disclose one's identity (McAdams, 2008). They provide personalized rather than stereotypical information about the person. All assignments and exercises were designed, therefore, in such a way that they asked for personal lifestories and not for general attitudes and opinions. General guidelines were formulated to increase openness, trust, perspective taking, and curiosity in the stories of other group members. Lastly, all group members were assigned equal status in that both the younger students and the older adults brought in their personal stories.

The workbook consists of a general theoretical introduction to life-course development that outlines the specifics of age differences related to generation and life phase (van Kordelaar et al., 2008). Next, a general manual describes the organization of courses and general guidelines for all of the discussion sessions. The main part of the book consists of 14 themes that were chosen to solicit lifestories and stimulate their exchange. Each theme has a short introduction, preparatory assignments to be done at home, and exercises for discussion in the group. These themes were derived from theoretical insights about life-course development. Furthermore, they were included because they provide participants the opportunity to express their own personal characteristics, the themes are interesting to people of different ages, and they elicit discussions about the similarities and differences between age groups. The group discussion stimulated comparisons between the past and the present, between different life phases, and between being young in the past and being young in the present, with equal emphasis on differences and similarities. The following themes were formulated.

The first group addresses three themes related to time and age: stereotypes, present life-phase, and life course. The second group addresses four themes related to changes in the macrocontext of society at large: Dutch society, values and norms, traditions, and taboos. The third group addresses three themes related to the mesocontext of social networks: parenting, family relations, and friendships. The fourth and last group addresses four themes related to the individual: life choices, the art of living, meaning in life, and identity.

The program was developed for a group exchange between three to five students and three to five older persons. It should consist of a preparatory meeting in which participants first get to know one another and discuss the content and goals of the course. During this meeting, they are to agree on the number of times they will meet and on the number and choice of themes they will prepare and discuss. The guidelines specify that a course should cover at least four themes to enable the development of mutual trust and intimacy. To make the program more easily applicable in educational settings, we have since adapted it so that it can be used in a setting of one student to one older adult.

Process Evaluation

After developing the program content, we tested it in four separate groups. These groups differed in terms of the students involved. Two groups had Masters students in psychogerontology, a third involved students in higher education, and the fourth consisted of students in middle vocational education. Both the third and the fourth groups were studying in the field of health care. Older persons were recruited through a local social work institution (Stichting Welzijn Ouderen Nijmegen), a nursing home (Oud Burgeren

Gasthuis), and an assisted living facility (Nijevelt). In this way, the program could be tested with students at different educational levels and with older people who varied in their level of health and independence.

The two developers of the program, Karen van Kordelaar and Astrid Vlak, observed and supervised these four pilot groups. They improved the general guidelines, the assignments, and the exercises on the basis of their direct experiences of the group. Furthermore, each group session was followed by a thorough evaluation by the participants. After every session, the participants graded the theme and made suggestions for improvement. On average, the themes were rated 7.9 on a scale from 0 to 10. One theme that was rated less well (the original theme talents was rated 6.5) was reformulated after discussion with the participants into the theme of parenting.

At the end of the program, participants were asked about their experiences. These data show a number of common themes. First, participants were positive about participating in the group. They emphasized the openness within it enabling them to learn from and about the other generation. "The group was even nicer, more interesting, and more instructive than I had expected," said one younger participant. "It was less formal than I expected. There was a surprising openness about feelings from the side of the older as well as the younger persons," explained an older participant. The alternation between individual home assignments and group discussions was valued as well, with participants finding it useful to prepare themselves for the group discussion. An older participant commented, "The home assignments forced me to reflect on the theme. They were good because I am inclined to stay in my own world—that gives me a sense of safety—but now the texts forced me to think." "The home assignments make you well prepared. Sometimes the group discussion made me think differently than I did when making the home assignments," explained a younger participant. Participants were dedicated to preparing their homework and attending the group meetings, although the older participants, particularly those in the assisted living facility, had to occasionally miss sessions for health reasons.

The participants agreed that the groups succeeded in bringing young and old more closely together and in providing a unique opportunity to get into contact with the other age group, outside one's own family. An older participant said, for example, "I have really learned something out of this group. I have actually noticed that I am more in line with the younger people than with my own peers. Of course, I learn from my children and grandchildren, but you discuss different things with them than with this group." In a similar vein, all participants agreed that the conversations had contributed to a revision of their images of the other age group. After the group, they explained that they saw more similarities between the age groups as well as more individual differences within each age group.

CONCLUSION

The needs assessment presented here has shown that there is a lack of contact between age groups and a related reliance on stereotypes whenever younger and older adults do communicate. As a result, older persons do not always get the chance to tell their own story in everyday conversations. Even when they can tell their story, it may remain unheard or become compromised, thereby limiting their further development.

Although professional settings may be at particular risk for stereotypical approaches to older adults, many organizations have taken up new understandings of later life and now ask for more person-centered care and support and for the empowerment of older adults. We therefore developed an educational program that targets less stereotypical conversations and a more person-oriented approach in the next generation of professionals. Lifestories are the main active ingredient of this educational program, which offers the opportunity to share personal stories in an open context that provides equal status and mutual trust. The qualitative evaluation of the process showed that the group indeed provides a positive setting for sharing lifestories. At least from the perspective of the participants themselves, it fulfilled its goal of developing a more personal and less stereotypical approach to the other generation.

This program offers a number of ways of helping future professionals to facilitate contact with older clients and explore their needs for care, support, and empowerment. It will therefore contribute to developing a stronger narrative competence that enables future professionals to co-author the lives of their older clients.

REFERENCES

Allen, P., Cherry, K., & Palmore, E. (2009). Self-reported ageism in social work practitioners and students. *Journal of Gerontological Social Work*, 52, 124–134.

American Psychological Association (APA). (2004). Guidelines for psychological practice with older adults. *American Psychologist*, 59, 236–260.

Anderson, D., & Wiscott, R. (2004). Comparing social work and non-social work students' attitudes about aging. *Journal of Gerontological Social Work*, 42, 21–36.

Baltes, M. (1995). Dependency in old age: Gains and losses. *Current Directions in Psychological Science*, 4, 14–19.

Beullens, J., Marcoen, A., Jaspaert, H., & Pelemans, W. (1997). Het beeld van ouderen bij geneeskundestudenten en de invloed van het medisch onderwijs. [The image of older people with medical students and the impact of medical education]. *Tijdschrift voor Gerontologie en Geriatrie, 28*, 178–183.

Caporael, L., & Culbertson, G. (1986). Verbal response modes of baby talk and other speech at institutions for the aged. *Language and Communication, 6*, 99–112.

CBS. (2009). Work participation according to age group. Retrieved September 9, 2009, from www.statline.cbs

Cuddy, A., & Fiske, S. (2002). Doddering but dear: Process, content, and function in stereotyping of older persons. In T. Nelson (Ed.), *Ageism: Stereotyping and prejudice against older persons* (pp. 3–26). Cambridge, MA: MIT Press.

Fiske, S., Cuddy, A., Glick, P., Xu, J. (2002). A model of (often mixed) stereotype content: Competence and warmth respectively follow from perceived status and competition. *Journal of Personality and Social Psychology, 82*, 878–902.

Giles, H., Coupland, N., Coupland, J., Williams, A., et al. (1992). Intergenerational talk and communication with older people. *International Journal of Aging & Human Development, 34*(4), 271–297.

Gilleard, C., & Higgs, P. (2000). *Cultures of ageing: Self, citizen and the body.* Harlow, UK: Prentice Hall.

Gubrium, J., & Holstein, J. (1999). The nursing home as a discursive anchor for the ageing body. *Ageing and Society, 19*, 519–538.

Hagestad, G., & Uhlenberg, P. (2005). The social separation of old and young: A root of ageism. *Journal of Social Issues, 61*, 343–360.

Hummert, M. (1994). Stereotypes of the elderly and patronizing speech. In M. Hummer, J. Wiemann, & J. Nussbaum (Eds.), *Interpersonal communication in older adulthood* (pp. 162–184). Thousand Oaks, CA: Sage.

Keith, J., Fry, C., Glascock, A., Ikels, C., Dickerson-Putnam, J., Harpending, H., & Draper, P. (1994). *The aging experience: Diversity and commonality across cultures.* Thousand Oaks, CA: Sage.

Kemper, S., & Harden, T. (1999). Experimentally disentangling what's beneficial about elderspeak from what's not. *Psychology and Aging, 14*, 656–670.

Kite, M., & Johnson, B. (1988). Attitudes towards older and younger adults: A meta-analysis. *Psychology and Aging, 3*, 233–244.

Kohli, M. (1985). Die Institutionalisierung des Lebenslaufs [The institutionalization of the life course]. *Kölner Zeitschrift für Soziologie und Sozialpsychologie, 37*, 1–29.

Künemund, H., & Kolland, F. (2007). Work and retirement. In J. Bond, S. Peace, F. Dittmann-Kohli, & G. Westerhof (Eds.), *Ageing in society* (3rd ed., pp. 167–185). London: Sage.

McAdams, D. (2008). Personal narratives and the life story. In O. John, R. Robins, & L. Pervin (Eds.), *Handbook of personality: Theory and research* (3rd ed., pp. 241–261). New York: Guilford Press.

Pasupathi, M., & Löckenhoff, C. (2002). Ageist behavior. In T. Nelson (Ed.), *Ageism: Stereotyping and prejudice against older persons* (pp. 201–247). Cambridge, MA: MIT Press.

Pettigrew, T., & Tropp, L. (2006). A meta-analytic test of intergroup contact theory. *Journal of Personality and Social Psychology, 90*, 751–783.

Randall, W. (1995). *The stories we are: An essay on self-creation.* Toronto: University of Toronto Press.

Ryan, E., Hummert, M., & Boich, L. (1995). Communication predicaments of aging: Patronizing behavior toward older adults. *Journal of Language and Social Psychology, 14*, 144–166.

Sachweh, S. (1998). Granny darling's nappies: Secondary babytalk in German nursing homes for the aged. *Journal of Applied Communication Research, 26*, 52–65.

van Kordelaar, K., Vlak, A., Kuin, Y., & Westerhof, G. (2008). *Groen en grijs: Jong en oud met elkaar in gesprek* [Green and gray: Conversations between younger and older adults]. Houten, The Netherlands: Bohn Stafleu van Loghum.

van Kordelaar, K., & Westerhof, G. (2007). De stille generatie aan het woord [The silent generation speaks out]. In E. Bohlmeijer, L. Mies, & G. Westerhof. (Eds.). *De betekenis van levensverhalen* [The meaning of lifestories] (pp. 219–228). Houten, The Netherlands: Bohn Stafleu van Loghum.

Versteegh, E., & Westerhof, G. (2007). Wederzijdse stereotypen van jongeren en ouderen en hun relatie met zelfbeeld en zelfwaardering [Mutual stereotypes of younger and older adults and their relation with self-concept and self-esteem]. *Tijdschrift voor Gerontologie en Geriatrie, 38*, 28–36.

Walker, A., & Maltby, T. (1997). *Ageing Europe.* Buckingham, UK: Open University Press.

Westerhof, G. (2009). Identity construction in the third age: The role of self-narratives. In H. Hartung & R. Maierhofer (Eds.), *Narratives of lives: Mediating age* (pp. 55–69). Münster, Germany: LIT.

Westerhof, G. (2010). "During my life so much has changed that it looks like a new world to me": A narrative perspective on identity formation in times of cultural change. *Journal of Aging Studies, 24*(1), 12–19.

Westerhof, G., & Tulle, E. (2007). Meanings of ageing and old age: Discursive contexts, social attitudes and personal identities. In J. Bond, S. Peace, F. Dittmann-Kohli, & G. Westerhof (Eds.), *Ageing in society* (3rd ed., pp. 235–254). London: Sage.

Williams, A., & Nussbaum, J. (2001). *Intergenerational communication across the life span.* Mahwah, NJ: Lawrence Erlbaum.

Twenty

IMPLEMENTATION OF NARRATIVE CARE IN THE NETHERLANDS: COORDINATING MANAGEMENT, INSTITUTIONAL, AND PERSONAL NARRATIVES

Gerdienke M. Ubels

> I'm getting older, there's nothing I can do about that. It's not always fun, but death is part of life. My son then tells me I should count my blessings. "Oh, what a load of rubbish," is what I would like to say to him.
> —Anonymous client (Nivel, 2005)

> I find it hard to accept that I can't fix my clients' problems. And it's only when I can really let go of this feeling that my client will feel I have truly connected with his story.
> —Anonymous caregiver (Expertisenetwerk, 2009)

> Narrative attention (dialogue) is not a goal in itself and it goes beyond hospitality. It's not something new and it's not an extra degree. It's about respecting each other in a different way. It's what already goes on between people. I stimulate it by setting the example. I can't make it explicit, or I'll lose it. It's about identity and respect. There is no vision without that source.
> —Anonymous manager (Programma, 2008)

In this chapter, I will describe how we try to stimulate the implementation of insights from narrative gerontology in eldercare in The Netherlands. The focus is on the implications of these insights from the perspective of a national association of care organizations. That is, I will explore the barriers and facilitating factors involved in bringing narrative gerontology into practice and developing a sustainable quality of care.

BACKGROUND

ActiZ is the Dutch national association of residential and home care organizations for older adults. The 425 members of ActiZ (ranging from small to big companies) provide over 90% of all eldercare in The Netherlands. Of a total Dutch population of 16.5 million, 12.5% is over 65 years of age (2008). This will increase to almost 20% in 2025. ActiZ serves primarily as a lobby agent for residential and home care organizations and represents the employers' interests. Besides negotiating the financial framework with the government, ActiZ also conducts negotiations with the workers' unions. Last but not least, however, is the organization's developmental task and challenge: how to better our performance as care organizations and to answer the different (and sometimes seemingly divergent) demands that politics, society, and clients make of us.

In order to do that, innovative concepts of eldercare need to be developed. As one of the staff members of ActiZ, my particular agenda is exploring a theoretical basis and the practical means of promoting and enhancing the spiritual and mental well-being of older adults and incorporating this agenda in our national quality-improvement program. How can we do this? What is the key to giving care that matters, care that is really effective and sustainable?

Narrative gerontology offers a focus on the psychological core of care: the inescapable human way of life, of not just *having* but rather *being* a lifestory (Kenyon, Clark, & de Vries, 2001; Kenyon & Randall, 1997). Storytelling is not just something some of us happen to like; it is what we most fundamentally are. Care should therefore take this storying of life as a starting point.

What emerges in the constant telling of our stories are the "slow questions" (Kunneman, 2005). These are existential and moral questions that cannot be easily answered, that won't go away, that pose themselves time and again whenever life takes a turn, when we realize that we are growing older, when we take care of others, and when we have to rely on caregivers. They are the questions that deal with love and loss, with faith and fear, with time and truth.

How do we deal with these questions? We deal with them by telling (our) stories. And in telling them, in choosing which stories to tell and how to tell them, we create a space and time to live in, a universe that accepts us; we create meaning. Further, by choosing or accepting the public (listeners), we create community. In that sense, human beings story their world. When it comes to care, caregivers are first and foremost "characters" within these storied worlds of their clients.

THREE BASIC PROPOSITIONS

Narrative care is core care (Bohlmeijer, Kenyon, & Randall, this volume), and in this way narrative gerontology opens up a fundamental new avenue by attaining a radical change of perspective. Narrative care as core care suddenly makes us see that we don't have to try and *add something to* the way we care for frail older adults. All we need to do is to *change the way we look at* what we do when we operate in care organizations. It is not an extra; it is the very heart of the matter. This realization translates into the following three propositions:

1. In eldercare, recognizing, respecting, and sustaining the personal identity of older adults has to be seen as the core of the caring business. Narrative gerontology focuses on both the narrative structure of this personal identity and the consequent need for biographical attentiveness.
2. The focus on narrative in eldercare has a reciprocal perspective; it doesn't stop with the care receiver. In helping their clients to story their world, caregivers are also investing and extracting personal biographical energy, which in turn reflects on and influences their way of giving care.
3. Care organizations are (the) societal structures where caregivers and care-receivers meet and co-create quality of life and work. Care organizations can, therefore, also be seen as narrative communities.

These three propositions are the starting point of this chapter. Building on the scientific explorations and findings of the editors of this volume (Bohlmeijer, Kenyon, & Randall, this volume), my focus is on the question of how to incorporate these findings in the day-to-day business that care organizations conduct. How can we get narrative gerontology into practice? Even if we can rely on evidence, we still face the hard question of how to make the narrative perspective acceptable to managers, in an environment that is strongly governed by incentives other than narrative-centered care.

Of course, even without or before calling themselves narrative gerontologists, there are lots of people who feel strongly that attentive care for older person should make room for lifestories, slow questions, and life review. "Co-narrators" can certainly be found among those who care for older adults, and it is a joy to work together in this way. However, it is quite another story to convince less enthusiastic individuals and institutions to have these insights reflected at the policy level.

Central to my approach is the fact that the interrelation between the three propositions is essential: one proposition cannot work without the other. One can choose any of the three as a starting point, but it's vital that one never lose sight of their interconnectedness. Lasting effects will only occur when all three dimensions are properly linked with each other; we have to somehow coordinate the narratives of clients, professionals, and management. All of their respective narratives count; they all add up to quality of life, care, and work, and are at the heart of the matter. These narratives are thus essential managerial items—assets as well as goals. However, we need to ask what constitutes quality for the organization and how narrative gerontology can help the organization to improve its performance in this regard. In The Netherlands, we have sought to address these questions through the recently founded Quality Framework for Responsible Care.

QUALITY OF CARE AND ACCOUNTABLE CARE

Dutch law requires health care professionals to provide "responsible" care. In 2008, this concept was defined and made measurable by means of a set of performance indicators and standardized assessment methods known as the "Quality Framework for Responsible Care." Since September 2008, this system has allowed information about the performance of care providers in the residential and home care sectors to be published on a special Web site (www.kiesbeter.nl) and in annual social responsibility reports, thus establishing transparency and accountability. The Framework is founded on the concept of quality of life and focuses on four domains: living conditions, social participation, mental well-being, and physical well-being (Quality Framework, 2008).

In a long and sometimes agonizing process with this Framework, we have succeeded in setting up a national program called "Accountable Care" that measures outcome of care rather than output of care. Central to this concept is the fact that we haven't set absolute national standards about the content of care. We haven't decided, for example, how many times Mrs. Johnson should be allowed to take a shower, because we don't know that; only Mrs. Johnson knows that. So we have chosen to develop a standard for her caregiver within the boundaries of her specific condition and, while not ignoring the caregiver's professional knowledge and responsibility, to negotiate a way in which Mrs. Johnson can take a shower as often as she wants. Further, we would ask Mrs. Johnson if she is content with her physical well-being.

Because this is the fundamental approach, we have to measure the quality of care that is thus produced in two complementary ways. The first consists of a statistical registration of performance indicators on, among other variables, decubitus (bed sores), polypharmacy, and depression scales. The second measurement consists of a biannual Client Quality Index, in which we do not measure client *satisfaction* but rather the client's *experienced quality of care*. It is interesting to note that when asked about satisfaction, most respondents tend to claim a socially approved level of satisfaction (also because it is hard to admit to dissatisfaction with one's quality of life). However, when asked about experienced quality, people can give a more detached and therefore more honest account of their findings. These two registrations together make up a national survey in which all of the care organizations are rated. We do not measure them against an objective standard; we measure them against their clients' wishes. And we measure them against each other (with the use of a validated case mix).

The creation of the Quality Framework represents a milestone in the achievement of a common aim: to improve the quality of health care services in The Netherlands still further. It enables providers to demonstrate their abilities and accomplishments, with full transparency as an important condition. Every patient is entitled to good and responsible care. Patients' own opinions, therefore, play a significant role within the Quality Framework. Knowing that their services will be subject to open review encourages care providers to discuss patient requirements more thoroughly and to do even more to ensure satisfaction (Quality Framework, 2008).

With this Framework we have set very clear standards. They are relative standards and they put the client first: Mrs Johnson, with her specific problems and wishes, with her own specific way of life, with her own lifestory. We simply have to take a narrative approach to her situation to be able to make the best arrangement for her, within the given financial circumstances.

Further, because of this national survey, the board of directors will ultimately be held accountable for the fact that Mrs. Johnson does or doesn't feel sustained in her quality of life. Client orientation, therefore, can no longer be just a (more or less unattainable) moral ideal or a superficial marketing tool; it is a managerial target. Management will be held responsible for the way in which their organization does or does not succeed in realizing measurable quality of life for their clients, as much as it will be held responsible for the effective deployment of the available resources.

To achieve success in this way, first, much emphasis must be placed on the dialogue between caregivers and clients—that is, on what the clients want and need and in which domains of life, and on what will really sustain their quality of life, given their condition. Second, professional workers must be able to relate to their clients' situation and lifestory and be able to reflect on how their own attitude and input affects their clients' well-being. Finally, the organization needs to view itself as the facilitating structure that enables clients and workers to encounter each other and co-create quality of life and work. These three conclusions lead us back to the three propositions about narrative gerontology. They also form the basis of our "stimulation program."

ENHANCING NARRATIVE CARE

The Program for Accountable Care is well suited to fostering an emphasis on quality of care and narrative. As the national association of home and residential care organizations, we cannot order our members about and tell them how they should conduct their business. We do try, however, to create conditions in which they can be successful and to provide them with relevant knowledge and tools. We present the narrative perspective to them as a crucial source of vision, tools, and empowerment for enhancing the quality of their performance as care providers. With it, we stress the fact that narrative interventions are much less expensive than many other forms of intervention. This point is generally felt to be plausible but is not always easy to prove. Thus, we attempt to facilitate research and evaluative methods that take a broad perspective, such as social return on investment (SROI). We also stress the importance of the so-called economic paradox: even when narrative interventions imply or depend on higher-qualified personnel, they nonetheless repay themselves by being more effective in reducing costs in other aspects of care. In our stimulation program, we focus on the three layers or characters involved in this story: clients, professionals, and management/organization.

Clients: Lifestories (Methods and Evidence)

When we really listen to the needs of clients, it is almost certain that more attention is needed for "biographical" care. But in what form and to what effect? While ActiZ doesn't conduct research on its own, we choose to actively support research projects in this field. By co-reading and co-editing project studies, we further the development of methods and tools. We actively invite our members to participate in research and pilot projects, thereby promoting and recommending narrative methods and helping create evidence as we go along.

We receive help in this endeavor through the annual measurement of factors under Accountable Care, which provides quantitative and qualitative data on the mental well-being of clients. Every care provider inevitably receives an annual report on how their clients are doing in this area, and they need to decide whether and how to follow up on this information.

At that point, we suggest to the care providers the use of narrative interventions. We make sure that, along with more traditional mental health interventions, they can find evidence-based narrative methods and tools. This in itself can form the starting point for learning about the importance of biographical care. To support this effort, we have started more or less close partnerships with institutions for scientific research and implementation, for whom we serve as a gateway to the daily practice of care organizations.

Depression Prevention

An obvious and uncontroversial direction for narrative care is the recent emphasis on depression prevention. This is a recognizable phenomenon for all parties involved, thus it can serve as a very useful first step. ActiZ has chosen to actively encourage the development of effective methods for prevention of depression in older adults, specifically for those in residential care, whose span of control is limited because of either health impairments or age. In theory, standard evidence-based methods for adults apply to these individuals but often require too much mastery and activity. Precisely because older adults in residential care lack these abilities, they are more prone to depression than other older adults. Consciously or unconsciously, many people, as well as caregivers, tend to think that depression is simply part of getting old and being dependent on care and that it cannot be prevented. However, research has shown this not to be the case. Depression can be prevented and should receive significant attention in older adults, who for specific reasons are highly at risk to develop it.

By stimulating research projects that try to establish evidence for age-adjusted methods, ActiZ draws attention to the specific vulnerability of this target group. We help facilitate scientists and care organizations to develop practice-based scientific evidence on narrative interventions for older adults.

"Mapping My Life"

"Mapping My Life" (Tromp & Huizing, 2007) is a narrative method for life-history books and was developed as a means to evaluate the effects of narrative interventions in professional care of older adults. Elsewhere in this volume, the method and research results are presented by Thijs Tromp. His research sheds a most interesting light on the question of when and for whom a narrative life review intervention is appropriate.

ActiZ supported the development of this narrative intervention by co-reading and co-editing the research on it. By actively promoting and recommending the method, we hope to help clarify when and how the use of life history methods is appropriate. We also pay attention to the effects of use of this method on the care organization. That is, the method does not necessarily seem to involve a caregiver but is also (or even more so) effective with the participation of a volunteer. In so far as this is the case, it opens up new and highly promising ways of involving volunteers in care organizations.

"Searching for Meaning"

"Searching for Meaning" (Franssen & Bohlmeijer, 2003) is a narrative intervention for depression prevention developed for older adults in the 50+ age category. It involves group sessions and homework that encourage participants to revive and engage in (former) activities and personal sources of positive energy (see Bohlmeijer & Westerhof, this volume). As it draws on physical and cognitive activity, it is too demanding for most of the clients in residential care. ActiZ has stimulated and contributed to the funding of a research project that enables the Trimbos Institute (Netherlands Institute of Mental Health and Addiction) to develop an adjusted version of the intervention and establish evidence on its effectiveness.

National Partnership Depression Prevention

As background to these activities, ActiZ participates in the National Partnership on Depression Prevention, founded by the Dutch government in 2007. It consists of some 20 organizations that are all involved on a national level. Funded by the government, the Partnership tries to set the agenda for depression prevention and encourage cooperation of the parties involved. Within it, ActiZ strongly promotes attention to older adults, a group that is easily overlooked in this area.

Professionals: Working Stories (Narrative Skills and Attitude toward Narrative)

When the client is the standard, caregivers need to be fully equipped to determine the personal standard of each client. As clients and caregivers present themselves and meet each other as lifestories in a biographical encounter (Randall & Kenyon, 2001), much attention needs to be paid to the narrative skills of caregivers so that they can use these skills to best meet their clients' needs.

Caregivers also story their own world and their identity, and this fact needs to be recognized. Taking care of others is a demanding job; it takes a lot to confront and balance the daily personal experiences of being claimed by people in need, having to set priorities, and trying to relate to clients' lifestories, even in the smallest way imaginable. Precisely because of the demands of giving care, it is important to acknowledge that the quality of the caring relationship is highly influenced by the way in which caregivers reflect on their way of dealing with this as human beings.

In eldercare, this particular side of the job has been increasingly neglected. Is this because care for older adults is seen as a matter of heading toward the end of life? Is this context basically seen as the aftermath of life itself—and therefore not worthy of real attention, because there seems to be nothing much to be gained? Or is it because growing old and perhaps dependent on care is something we know could—or rather *will*—happen to many of us, and is therefore something we do not wish to consider seriously? Is eldercare too much of a confrontation with our own future frailty? Or is it because there are simply too many people growing old and we are blinded by the thought that we need to reduce costs?

I think the lack of respect for eldercare stems from all of these reasons, although policy makers will only admit to the last one mentioned. Nevertheless, this scenario actually strengthens the point I am trying to make. Improving narrative skills is a much-overlooked source for sustainable quality improvement, precisely from the workers' point of view. It can help them in performing their job and it may help keep them on the job as they restory (Kenyon & Randall, 1997) their own personal and professional lives.

ActiZ encourages and participates in different programs that focus on improving the narrative skills of caregivers. In meeting their clients, they are often confronted by their own slow questions. Because of the lack of attention to this, it usually takes the form of privately worrying about frustrating situations or just nagging at the coffee bar about difficult clients. Much could be won by investing in the development of narrative skills of caregivers (Noonan, this volume; van den Brandt-van Heek, this volume).

Moral Deliberation

Methods of moral deliberation are also much needed. In contrast to what is often heard on this issue, care workers do not so much need to be taught how to engage in ethical discourse (though they do need coaching); they simply need to be allowed to engage in narrative care as a legitimate and essential part of their job—that is, as core care. Moral deliberation is not difficult: it is what we all do, in all aspects of our lives. As a part of professionally giving care to older adults, however, it is denied and therefore becomes problematic. For example, a caregiver working with the client mentioned previously, Mrs. Johnson, might ask, "Why is talking to Mrs. Johnson so difficult? Why can't I bear to see the pain on her face? Why do I always want to hurry when I see her son approaching?"

Since the quality of the caring relationship is essential for both care receiver and caregiver, ActiZ strongly promotes the attention given to simple methods of feedback between colleagues. Interventions are encouraged that are unobtrusive but effective, especially those that focus on the sense of well-being on the job. We think it essential to encourage professionals to share and develop sensitivity and practices with regard to ultimate questions, be they their own or those of their clients. To this end, we participate as a partner in a national network of organizations that focuses on the importance of existential questions for older adults.

Expert Network for Existential Questions and Older Adults

This national network aims at combining and strengthening the impact of some of the (national) organizations that try to enhance the mental well-being of older adults. Besides Vilans (Centre of Excellence in Long Term Social Care in the Netherlands) and ActiZ, the Network includes universities, client organizations, and organizations for professionals and community workers. We find common ground in the convictions that mental well-being is essential to the quality of life of and care for older adults and that professionals in care organizations and community workers need to be attentive to this aspect of life. By joining forces, the Network has succeeded in getting the commitment of the government and of some capital funds. Together they now fund a 3-year program in which the Network focuses on starting local and regional initiatives, supporting training programs for care and community professionals and volunteers, and exploring financial and structural conditions.

The network named itself "Network" because its main goal is to get people to exchange their knowledge, expertise, and inspiration on the subject. Many people are already involved and they all try to connect with each other. Much could be gained by not only pooling their knowledge but also bringing together people who in many cases are rather lonely in their quest to provide better eldercare. Networking is thus a very useful and well-suited form of connecting. The main tool of the network is a Web site (www. netwerklevensvragen.nl) that serves as home base for a growing Web community. The Web site is a source of knowledge and a database and serves as a meeting point. A Wiki is also being developed. Other results of the Network after 1 year include the following:

1. Coordination and agenda setting by participating organizations
2. Creation of a Web site and Web community
3. Creation of a database of materials and methods for training programs
4. Development of a description of best practices of local cooperation
5. A symposium on financial and organizational aspects
6. Creation of a digital newsletter (e-zine)

Organization: Management Stories

When the product that care organizations produce can ultimately be described as a caring relation between storying individuals, then the narrative quality of an organization becomes a managerial target and not just some (unattainable) moral ideal. Managers need to find ways to relate the narrative experiences of clients and workers to the financial and statistical language they use to account for their business results. They also need to find ways to keep track of their own story while conducting their business.

Because of the widespread feeling of tension and disconnection between the work floor and management, ActiZ helped facilitate Professor Harry Kunneman, professor of social and political theory, in carrying out a survey among caregivers in home care organizations. He pointedly laid open the gap between the values they expressed and the managerial view of the world. In this analysis, he applied the metaphors of lampposts and campfires, thus identifying the divergent narratives of caregivers and management: the harsh, unaccommodating, and impersonal light of lampposts is in stark contrast to the cosy glow of campfires, around which people gather and tell their stories (Kunneman & Slob, 2007).

It is of no use only to complain about this miscommunication between management and the caregivers; we have to find ways to connect the two parties. We tried, therefore, to design a number of pilot projects for the purpose of developing a dialogical managerial intervention. Through a tool called "Reflect-on" (Kunneman & Slob, 2007), the members of a management team are invited to explore and express the way they feel about their work, the questions and issues they encounter, and the values that are at stake. In group discussion, they are then led to counter these findings with those of their colleagues. At this point they are invited to formulate their (managerial) aims and criteria in a language that also connects to the values expressed by their workers. However, thus far, it has proven difficult to find participants for these pilot projects. The strain on management seems to be too intense to allow themselves the time and energy for such a project. Even if managers are interested in the matter, they don't easily feel free to give it priority. They have a business to run; there are targets to be met.

However, in another related scientific project, Lena van Gastel has not encountered any problems in finding CEOs to participate (Van Gastel & Luijkx, 2008). This study is a qualitative responsive research project in which she investigated the way care organizations manage the changing societal and legislative structures. Research questions include what the CEOs see to be their business, who they relate to as their societal partners, and how they reflect on the development of their responsibilities within this changing arena. In other words, the question concerns how they story themselves as CEOs. When invited, CEOs are immediately very supportive of the project. They seem to be positively relieved to be able to tell their story. As this research focuses completely on their own slow questions as CEOs (and not necessarily on the relation of their questions to those of their personnel), this eagerness is not surprising. This outcome strengthens our conviction that it is essential to start with personal stories and slow questions, whatever quality improvement one is trying to establish.

COORDINATING THE NARRATIVES: DIALOGUE PROGRAM

Because we have been both working on the three earlier mentioned propositions and attempting to implement the narrative perspective in care organizations, we were pleased when, in 2008, the Dutch government decided it wanted to make a qualitative contribution to stimulating the "human scale" in care organizations, for caregivers as well as clients. Undersecretary Bussemaker decided to fund a 3-year program "to stimulate the dialogue." She even set a quantified goal: within 2 years, 100 organizations should have made a move toward "dialogue" in their practice. Vilans (Centre of Excellence in Long-Term Social Care in The Netherlands) was chosen to carry out the program. ActiZ is closely involved as partner in the steering committee, as are STING (the national association for professional caregivers) and LOC (the national organization for clients' councils in health care).

With this financial backing from the government, Vilans has been able to work out a national program and strategy to encourage care organizations to invest in narrative issues. This has been a difficult process, however. What exactly can one do "to stimulate the dialogue?" What is the meaning of *dialogue* in this sense—who needs to be stimulated, and with what? As is so often the case with anything to do with narrative, the people involved all "get it" and recognize each other's good intentions. They're all on the same mission: they share a fundamental enthusiasm and know they're doing something good. They all get it in their own way, however, with their own examples, convictions, and hang-ups.

Precisely because narrative is such a fundamental dimension to all that matters in care, and because it combines focus on the client, professionalism, and organizational development, it is very hard to get clear and simple about which elements to choose, why they are supposed to work, and how this could be validated. It is even more difficult to see how and where the exact stimulation needs to be administered—that is, which organizational nerve reacts to which stimulus, and to what effect. Moreover, such a project also touches on some shaky ground: in order to make itself understandable, there is a danger of trying to fully instrumentalize the power of narrative, an outcome that would be disastrous.

It was decided to first make a theoretical exploration of the matter, then to find and investigate best practices, discern from these best practices both the helpful elements and what seems to block the dialogue, and from there try to connect with the 100 organizations to help them implement or improve their dialogue—not as an end in itself but as a means to help them in their specific quality or organizational improvement projects. Whatever the organizations are trying to do in this field, improving their dialogue will prove to be a fundamental asset toward attaining their goal. They've already set their targets. Dialogue can offer them clear vision of and tools for how to reach those targets (Programma, 2008).

Why Dialogue?

Dialogue is a container concept. It applies to the different settings in which we need to invest: clients, professionals, management, and organization. Everybody knows and appreciates the value of a good dialogue. The program has made a conscious effort to stress the dialogue component as a skill and as a result. Thus, the narrative theory supporting it is not stressed, but instead, improvement of a skill. In this way, the program takes up on the urgent advice given by Rita Charon when referring to teaching narrative medicine: "Don't tell people to be better people, but hand them the skills" (Charon, 2008). Dialogue as a skill in the program is described as being connected to such dimensions as active listening, being respectful, showing empathy, being aware of body language, postponing judgment, not striving to reach an agreement or solution, and ensuring privacy. These qualities thus reflect the mission statement of the Program in Narrative Medicine, founded by Charon at Columbia University (Columbia University, 2010).

Best Practices

There is no such thing as *the* best practice. Nonetheless, the program has focused on finding the working ingredients of good practice—that is, why and how it works, according to clients, professionals, and management. The findings (Vilans, 2009) are as follows:

1. *Vision and culture.* An organization needs a clear vision (and preferably a motto to reflect it) of how to treat the client. This vision finds its way through education of the workforce. Also needed is open communication within the organization, whereby management, professionals, and clients (and their families) are encouraged to express their wishes and feelings. All of this is based on conducting the business in such a way that clear choices are made about how to use the available resources.

2. *Learning and change.* A care organization needs to be a learning organization that enables professionals to develop themselves, reflect on their experiences, and make necessary changes. Dialogue presupposes an organizational culture that is focused on innovation, learning, and flexibility. However, a certain amount of stability and continuity is also necessary.

3. *Space and trust.* Professionals need a working climate of trust and respect. They need to be able to carry out their responsibilities and reflect on their experiences.

4. *Management by example.* There needs to be a clear focus on tending to the care relationship. Management plays an important role in stimulating dialogue, mostly by setting the example (Vilans, 2009).

When we look at these four elements, it is clear that much of this material is not easily transferrable. It is about people, identity, history, culture, atmosphere, environment. There is no easy way to transfer all of this to any one organization, no easy answer or simple trick. It all has to be experienced and discovered by the people involved. The program, therefore, puts great effort into finding the right people and providing them with a toolkit and tailor-made coaching. The toolkit includes a quick overview (combining the three perspectives of clients, caregivers, and management), workshops, checklists, and various other tools for initiating the dialogue. Tailor-made coaching is also offered.

How to Find Participants

Probably the most difficult question is how to create interest within organizations that are not yet interested (otherwise they probably wouldn't be in need of help). It's no use just to invite them to "invest in dialogue"—how could that be a matter of priority? We have to go and find them where they are—not denigrate or blame them for their situation, but help them take stock, become their ally, and go forward together. We have found that the best way to do this is to make connections with other issues at stake, issues that are of immediate importance to organizations, in both professional and managerial ways. The Quality Framework for Responsible Care is just such an issue. Out of the annual results arise goals for the organization that deal with improvement of quality of care.

The Dialogue Program states and shows that to reach these goals, investing in narrative skills is important. What the program offers is fine-tuned coaching and development of narrative tools and methods, aimed at the individual goals and conditions of the organization. The program doesn't sell narrative on its own merits or as a goal in itself; it makes people aware of the power of narrative. In doing so, a shift in culture may be established, in which narrative care as core care becomes the obvious standard of care.

TOUGH QUESTIONS

Creating a shift in culture or awareness is never easy, and it's always a long-term matter. While we are finding out how to implement the insights of narrative gerontology, we are also encountering some tough questions about politics, societal development, and human awareness. These questions seem to create most of the barriers that we encounter.

End of the Welfare State

In the first decade of the twenty-first century, Europe is nearing the end of the welfare state as it was developed in the second half of the twentieth century. Demographic development, economic opportunities, environmental issues, and political views on these issues all touch on one statement: we can't keep it up any longer. This implies and calls forth a whole new range of political discussion, in which, as always, the central issue is how we function as a society: what to share and what to arrange collectively on the one hand, what to leave to personal initiative on the other. In this debate, care organizations as such have the image of being almost luxurious results of what is now considered unrealistic thinking. This view ignores the fact that (in northwestern Europe anyway) care organizations were founded and funded primarily by religious institutions and were taken over by the government after the Second World War. It was then decided that this form of care and support was a right for every member of society and that the sufficient supply of such support would strengthen society in the future.

Memory of these values is short when we mainly hear about the laziness caused by the welfare state, pampered civilians, and the obvious need for a more individualistic approach in which everybody has to fend for themselves. As this line of thinking gains momentum, however, we have to be aware that it reinforces the plea for compliance and cost-effectiveness. Yet precisely because of this focus, the sustainable quality of the narrative approach is of immense importance and should be stressed and proven.

(NOT) DEALING WITH "SLOW QUESTIONS"

Living and working in a care organization gives rise to the slow questions. It is exactly where and when we do not want to deal with these questions, whether they are questions of clients, workers, or management, that problems concerning quality of care arise. Not wanting to deal with such questions is a deeply shared human psychological feature. Not dealing with them, however, only makes them more persistent, and perhaps that's what we're experiencing right now.

The resistance to addressing these questions is what freezes us up and blocks any development toward an open and free narrative community. In some ways, care organizations can suffer from narrative foreclosure (Freeman, this volume) and not be able to keep developing their story, whatever the circumstances. The only way to change this is to slowly and gently try and embark on this path—to see what it means to take our own questions seriously, to see how taking this path enlightens the struggle we see in others, and to find out the degree to which it enables us to fully function in our given place. We are the organization, we determine the climate, we envision the future. I'm getting into the Obama mode here, short of saying, "Yes we can!" He has a point, though, and we need that point in care organizations as well. We need spirit, finding something to believe in, being restored to the story we are, and taking the responsibility to let this story develop.

CONCLUSION

In this chapter I have described the way in which ActiZ tries to stimulate the implementation of narrative care in eldercare in The Netherlands. By promoting narrative care as core care, we stress the three basic propositions that provide the focal point for clients, caregivers, and organizations. These three propositions are manifestations of the fact that people are storying beings. Effective and sustainable care should take this as a starting point.

In trying to foster use of narrative care, we find we can make good use of the Quality Assurance Framework for Responsible Care, which puts emphasis on the measurement of relative standards and the findings of Client Quality Indices. Stimulation of narrative care involves direct support to and promotion of methods, research projects, and training programs. The main point, however, as stressed by ActiZ is that the interconnectedness of the three propositions is essential to the chances of success:

1. Attention to the lifestories of clients cannot do without sufficient room for reflection by caregivers.
2. Such consideration of the personal and professional dynamics in giving care cannot flourish without their having effects on the self-understanding of the care organization as such.
3. Dialogue, therefore, is a crucial tool and asset in conducting the business of being a care organization.

We need to know more about how people story themselves (either as care receivers or as caregivers), what slow questions keep rising to the surface, and how the care organization as a societal structure can facilitate this narrative community and thus co-create a "wisdom environment" (Randall & Kenyon, 2001).

These questions are seemingly hard to explore, but once narrative care is conceived not as an extra demand but rather as the heart of the matter, they point to a very effective way to enhance the quality, effectiveness, and sustainability of eldercare. Narrative care is not pushing care to some new, expensive horizon. Rather, it is a process of becoming increasingly clear about what it is that defines real quality of life, care, and work.

Coordinating the narratives takes place in small ways. It starts with finding the right people and helping them to deal with the slow questions that go with their position. Narrative care is not an extra, so it is vital not to present it as if it were an extra. It is the heart of good care, and its effectiveness can be shown in quality measurements. So, basically, it is good business instinct to invest in narrative skills. By making full use of the potential we have as human beings, we find that we do not need anything we do not already have. We need only to be determined to listen closely to the stories we hear from others and utter ourselves. Without these stories, we wouldn't be here, whether we are clients, caregivers, or managers. To slightly misquote William Shakespeare (1623/2009), we are "such [narrative] stuff as care organizations are made of."

REFERENCES

Charon, R. (2008, May). Keynote speech, Narrative Matters Conference, Toronto, Canada.

Columbia University (2010). *The Program in Narrative Medicine.* Retrieved February 20, 2010, from http://www.narrativemedicine.org/

Expertisenetwerk Levensvragen en Ouderen. [Expert Network for Existential Questions and the Elderly]. (2009). *Kwalitatief onderzoek* [Qualitative survey]. Utrecht, The Netherlands: Vilans.

Franssen J., & Bohlmeijer E. (2003). *Op zoek naar zin* [Searching for meaning in life]. Utrecht, The Netherlands: Trimbos.

Kenyon, G., Clark. P., & de Vries, B. (2001). *Narrative gerontology: Theory, research and practice.* New York: Springer.

Kenyon, G., & Randall, W. (1997). *Restorying our lives: Personal growth through autobiographical reflection.* Westport, CT: Praeger.

Kunneman, H. (2005). *Voorbij het dikke ik. Bouwstenen voor een kritisch humanisme* [Beyond the big ego: Building bricks for a critical humanism]. Utrecht, The Netherlands: Humanistics University Press.

Kunneman, H., & Slob, M. (2007). *Thuiszorg in Transitie. Een onderzoek naar de gevolgen van het recente overheidsbeleid voor centrale waarden in de thuiszorg* [Homecare in transition: Investigating the effects of recent government politics on central values in homecare]. Bunnik, The Netherlands: LSBK.

Nivel. (2005). *Verantwoorde zorg en kwaliteit van leven bij cliënten in verpleeg- en verzorgingshuizen: een kwalitatief onderzoek* [Accountable care and quality of life with clients in residential care: A qualitative investigation]. Utrecht, The Netherlands: Nivel.

Programma Het Goede Gesprek (2008). [Dialogue Programme]. *Expert meeting.* Utrecht, The Netherlands: Vilans.

Quality Framework for Responsible Residential and Domiciliary Care (VV&T) Steering Committee (2008). *De toon gezet, één taal voor kwaliteit.* [The tone is set: A common language for quality]. Utrecht, The Netherlands: ActiZ. Available in English at www.biomedcentral.com/content/supplementary/1472-6963-10-95-S2. PDF

Randall, W., & Kenyon, G. (2001). *Ordinary wisdom: Biographical aging and the journey of life.* Westport, CT: Praeger.

Shakespeare, W. (2009). *The Tempest.* A. Quiller-Couch & J. D. Wilson (Eds.). Cambridge, UK: Cambridge University Press. (Original work published 1623)

Tromp T., & Huizing, W. (2007). *Mijn leven in kaart. Met ouderen in gesprek over hun levensverhaal* (Mapping my life: Making life history books with elderly people). Houten, The Netherlands: BSL.

Van Gastel, L., & Luijkx, K. (2008). Besturen in de zorg: Verantwoordelijkheden in Beraad [CEOs in care: Counseling responsibilities]. *Opinieblad voor beslissers in de ouderenzorg* [Magazine for Eldercare], *4*(6), 30–31.

Vilans (2009). *Het Goede Gesprek, dialoog als basishouding in de zorg* [Can I talk to you? Dialogue as caring attitude]. Utrecht, The Netherlands: Vilans.

Twenty One

ASKING THE RIGHT QUESTIONS: ENABLING

PERSONS WITH DEMENTIA TO SPEAK

FOR THEMSELVES

Marie-Elise van den Brandt-van Heek

As a psychologist who works with frail older adults, one of the things I focus on is the way residents, their relatives, and staff members interact. In this interaction, older adults often talk about their memories. According to Erik Erikson (1997), this is an important activity in the last stages of life. By talking about your life, you can look back and be proud of most of the choices you have made. It is a way to make peace with yourself and your accomplishments. Talking about your life provides insight into how you have become the person you are today. Because we can learn from other people's mistakes, older adults have something to give to the younger generation. They accept help from the younger generation but, at the same time, share their wisdom by telling the stories of their lives. These are all reasons why it is important to provide older persons with opportunities to talk about their lives. It is no different for people with dementia. Caregivers stimulate patients with dementia to tell stories by using photos, objects, and all kinds of other things. Most of the time this works quite well. However, in many cases the conversation stops, the older person feeling ashamed because he or she does not know the answers. The person may feel like a schoolchild who has failed a test. In this chapter, I propose trying an alternative way of asking questions.

METHOD

My method emphasizes the importance of avoiding questions that confront dementia patients with their flaws. Through this method, called "Living and Working with a Story," patients are stimulated to tell their lifestories. Staff members then use what they learn from the stories to provide individual, personalized care. The method is outlined in my book, *My Life in Fragments* (van den Brandt-van Heek & Huizing, 2009), which is written for a broad audience such as professionals, volunteers, and relatives. The basic principle is that it is significant that people, with or without dementia, tell their own stories. Although family members are important in the telling of these stories, the most important factor concerns the way residents themselves speak about the way they feel. Their well-being depends on the way they are stimulated to tell us who they are.

WELL-BEING AND DEMENTIA

Knowing how residents feel about the choices they have made during their lives provides insight into both their preferences and their identity. Caregivers can use this information in their daily care tasks. People with dementia often forget parts of their lives. One of the horrors of dementia is the loss of one's identity, since other people have to make decisions for the person with dementia. Knowing someone's lifestory enables caregivers to understand patients better and support them in expressing their own identity.

Asserting the identity of persons with dementia and giving them sufficient opportunity to talk improves their well-being. Talking with dementia sufferers requires great sensitivity. As a result of the dementia, they sometimes see the world and themselves from a totally different perspective; they cannot help it. Thus, we have to listen carefully and connect with the world as they experience it. In The Netherlands, we often divide dementia into stages of self-perception, outlined below.

The "Threatened Me"

Persons with dementia feel there is something wrong, because they can no longer get a complete grip on the world. Facts about their life become blurred, and questions can make them feel insecure and fearful. Their perception of time changes; they do not know what year it is and how old they are. They cannot remember things that happened not so long ago. All their energy is put into denying thoughts about the future. They are constantly trying to hide their decaying autonomy and identity. This effort makes them tired, irritated, and defensive, and they may accuse others of doing them wrong. This is an extremely distressing stage for them and their caregivers. At first, they do not know that dementia is the cause of all this tension. After that, both the patient and caregiver have to get used to the idea that the future is not what they had expected. The relationship and the well-being of the patient and their caregiver are threatened.

The "Lost Me"

Persons who suffer from dementia are lost in time and in their thoughts. They struggle to get in touch with reality without the help of their caregivers. Patients do not know how old they are and may think, for example, that they are still a 56-year-old who has to go to work. A healthy person sees someone who is almost 90 years old. It can be very hard for a daughter, son, or spouse to cope with these situations. For instance, it is difficult to accept that your mother is worried about her husband because he has not come home yet. She thinks she is 63 and happily married, whereas you know that your father passed away many years ago. How do you cope with that? What do you tell your mother? You seem to be losing touch with one another.

The "Hidden-and-Succumbed Me"

As the process of the dementia continues, the gap between the real world and the world perceived by the patient keeps growing wider. In the last stage of the dementia, contact becomes rare. The interaction between the patient and his or her caregivers consists of enjoying pleasant moments in the present time. This can be achieved through such activities as looking at children playing, tasting ice cream together, or enjoying music. The use of words is no longer an option, but, among other things, the caregiver can hold the patient's hands or stimulate other senses through massage (touch) or food (taste).

THE BASIC PHILOSOPHY

As long as the patient possesses the ability to use language, the method "Living and Working with a Story" can facilitate communication. When the dementia progresses, the method can be used to continue to enhance the well-being of patients. Because caregivers will have helped the person with dementia in earlier stages to tell them what he or she feels, they will know the patient's likes and dislikes and can provide care that fits the patient's personal wishes. This method focuses on the first stages of dementia.

People with Dementia Speak for Themselves

In nursing homes, people live together in groups. They have little privacy and may share bedrooms at night and living rooms during the day. They are constantly surrounded by people they have not chosen. Because of the dementia, they cannot decide what help they need, so staff members will discuss their type of care with family members. If the care-home management thinks lifestories are important, they will often ask families to write them down. But even the most loving daughter cannot tell the exact emotional impact of her mother's recent life events. Stories about her mother's childhood are secondhand, thus she can hardly be expected to produce an accurate representation of the impact of these events. Therefore, the basic principle of our method, based on respect, is to start with listening to patients and hearing what they themselves have to say about their identity and feelings.

The Constraints of Dementia

Dementia limits people in telling a chronological story, though they can relate fragments of their lives. When having a conversation with dementia patients, we need to adapt to their capabilities and meet their problems. Apart from particular conversation techniques and a good deal of empathy, we need to keep in mind that the way patients perceive themselves can be totally different from the way we see them. Their ability to use language may be limited, they may not be able to concentrate, and all kinds of emotional thoughts may distract them. We have to compensate for the effects of dementia in a conversation.

Basic Needs Stay the Same

While dementia changes many things, everyone wants somebody to listen to them without being judged or feeling tested. This implies that the conversational partner of dementia patients focuses on equality. The story's accuracy is not the main concern; the emotions that accompany the story are important. Letting patients tell their story without judging them emphasizes that their opinions are valued, that they themselves are valued. This is a strong tool in improving the quality of life and well-being of the frail older adult.

WELL-BEING AND STORYTELLING

Conversations with people suffering from dementia often take place in groups. Most of the time, an object is used to stimulate memories—for example, a paraffin stove. It doesn't matter if one's thoughts wander off. Looking at the object, one sees what other people are talking about and can join in again. For years, there was a tendency to try and keep dementia patients in touch with the present time. All of the questions that staff members asked referred to knowledge instead of opinions or emotions. Examples of this kind of question are, "Do you know what this is?"; "What can you do with this object?"; "Did you have one yourself?".

Storytelling and Knowledge

Knowledge-based questions often confront patients with serious challenges. They have to reproduce facts from their memory. When they realize they are not capable of answering these questions, they withdraw. Hearing the question, "Did you have one yourself?" may be confusing. If a patient perceives him- or herself as a 30-year-old person, he or she still *owns* a kerosene stove. It is frightening to hear the young nurse implying that there is no kerosene stove to return to after this meeting. How will he or she cook dinner for the children?

Storytelling: Opinions and Emotions

Asking dementia patients for knowledge can be frightening to them. To enhance the well-being of residents, confrontation with their shortcomings must be avoided. Instead, it is important to focus on their strengths: sharing wisdom based on life experiences. The dementia does not allow older persons to reflect on a whole life span, compare different events, and judge them. But patients can relate fragments of their lives, share their opinions, and talk about choices they would make. They can advise us if we ask them if it would be wise to marry or have seven children. They can tell us how to decorate the room when asked what they like about the current furniture.

AIDS TO ASKING THE RIGHT QUESTIONS

The method "Living and Working with a Story" has been developed in homes for older adults and focuses on the way conversations are initiated by staff members. Residents are neither tested nor asked to talk about things considered to be (common) knowledge. This may seem the obvious way to interact, but in listening to conversations, most of the time residents are asked about what they know. In order to learn how to ask the right questions, staff members at local nursing homes took part in a course and practiced this new way of interacting with the aid of theme books. Although there has been no scientific research on the method, it has received several prizes and ample media attention. The book *My Life in Fragments* (van den Brandt-van Heek & Huizing, 2009), which presents the method to a wider audience, includes background information about dementia and focuses on the consequences for emotional life. It also contains approximately 60 picture theme cards with example questions that focus on opinions instead of knowledge. The book also provides information on the making of lifestory books.

Lifestory Books and Theme Books

The right-hand page of a lifestory book or theme book is intended for the person with dementia. It contains one picture and a keyword. We use only one picture on every page to avoid confusion. People who suffer from dementia have problems concentrating. If more pictures are used, chances are that persons with dementia will start telling a story related to one picture, but then during the conversation, their attention will drift to another one. It would be impossible for the conversation partner to know which part of the story relates to which picture. When using only one picture, both parties will be talking about the same image.

The left hand page is meant for the conversation partner. In a lifestory book, it contains a summary of the stories the patients themselves have told in previous conversations with regard to the picture. In a theme book, it contains a short text in which the picture is introduced, followed by questions to start the conversation. These questions do not concentrate on knowledge about the event in the picture but instead focus on opinions and emotions in connection with the image on the right-hand page.

Focus on Opinions and Emotions

Most important to the method are theme conversations, in which questions about opinions and emotions are asked. Conversations can take place individually or in groups. A memory can be triggered by hearing a story or seeing a picture. Because both senses are stimulated, chances are that persons with dementia can tap into their memories more easily. The picture serves as a focal point for patients. Should their thoughts wander off, one look at the picture will remind them what the conversation was about. It also serves as a focal point for the conversation partner, because it contains questions that focus on emotions and opinions. This helps to suppress any tendency to use questions about knowledge.

Knowledge

The tendency to use knowledge-based questions is understandable. Our society focuses on sharing knowledge. Listening to group conversations in homes, one often hears questions like the following: "Did you ever have a stove like this?"; "Do you know how to make stew?"; "What is the purpose of the pan in the picture?" (see Fig. 21.1). The words *did you have* in the first

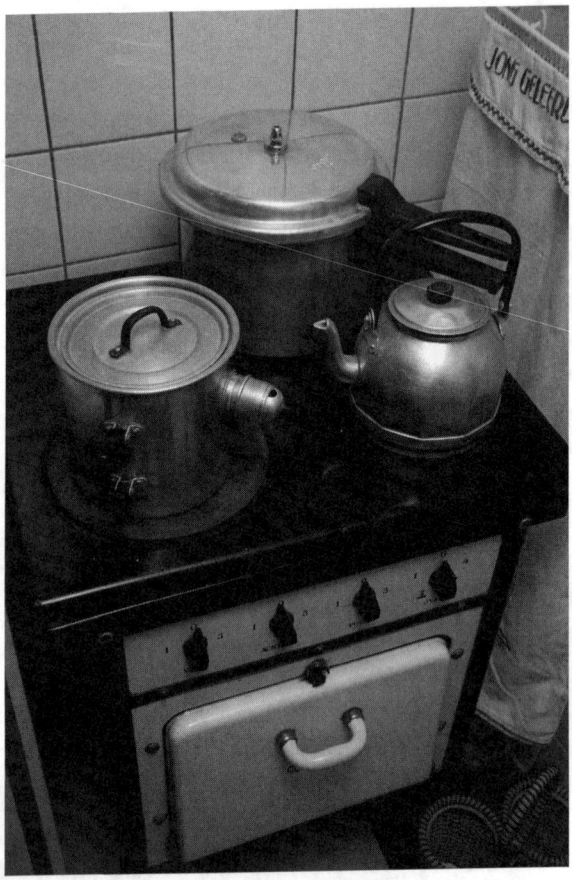

Figure 21.1 Pots and pans on the stove. Photo by Michael van Heek at the Remembering Museum Humanitas in Rotterdam, The Netherlands.

question imply that the patient does not have a stove at the moment. This may severely distress persons with dementia. As mentioned earlier, if they think they are 35 years old, they probably believe they are going home after this conversation to prepare dinner for their children.

All of the above questions refer to knowledge, which confronts patients with their flaws (loss of quick access to their memories). In contrast, as we will discuss next, in my method only questions that focus on opinions and feelings are used. At first glance, this does not seem difficult, but it is quite a challenge to think of 10 questions referring to a picture that do not require knowledge.

Opinions and Emotions

In the method "My Life in Fragments," there is a picture of a stove with pots and pans on it on the front of a theme card; it is also on the right-hand page of a theme book in the method "Living and Working with a Story." Sometimes with a picture a keyword is added, such as *stove* or *cooking* for the picture of pots and pans. For the conversation partner using this method, a short text is added to give some historical-background information, such as "a woman was supposed to become a housewife after marriage and there were no electrical aids like vacuum cleaners to keep the house clean." Another piece of text is meant to be read to the person with dementia. This text tells the person all there is to know about the picture. Then a list of questions is given, all focusing on opinions and emotions, instead of knowledge, for example:

- Do you like to cook?
- Is it hard to think of a different thing to cook every day?
- Are you a picky eater or do you fancy almost anything?
- Do you think this stove is a practical one?
- A kettle can be used to boil water for tea or coffee. Do you prefer tea or coffee?
- Is a low-fat diet important for you?
- Do you think cooking is just for women (or can men cook as well)?
- How do you feel about the statement that women can only become housewives?
- There is an oven in this picture for baking. Do you like to bake cakes?
- Is it your opinion that a homemade pie tastes better than a pie you buy in a store?
- Cooking under high pressure is a fast way to cook. Do you think this influences the taste of the things you cook?
- What would be a good way to learn how to cook?

- How do you feel about using canned vegetables? Do you prefer fresh ones?
- Do you like to invite dinner guests?
- What do you think about...?

TIPS FOR CONVERSATIONS WITH PERSONS WITH DEMENTIA

Both the theme cards and the theme books assist participants in conversations with persons with dementia. Avoiding test situations where questions about knowledge are asked helps to create an atmosphere of equality and respect for the wisdom of the older person. The most important tips may be summarized as follows: be careful with time references—use the present tense, and ask for opinions and emotions instead of knowledge. Other tips for using this method are to connect with the perception of the person with dementia, avoid test situations, use short sentences, avoid leading questions, try not to judge, and be patient.

Connect with the perception of the dementing person

People with dementia are older, but they often think that they are adolescents or children. This misconception can be related to the phase of the dementia, but it may also vary throughout the day. Instead of focusing on their physical appearance, it is better to concentrate on the way they see themselves. When persons with dementia think they are 30 years old, we have to understand that in their experience, there are few household appliances. They live in a world in which women quit their jobs when they marry and cars are rare.

Avoid test situations

In a normal conversation, the roles switch continually. One moment the caregiver is the story listener; the next moment, the storyteller (Kenyon & Randall, 1997). The caregiver and patient complement each other in conversations by reacting to each other's stories. People who suffer from dementia will hesitate to initiate a story. We encourage and enable them to tell stories by asking the right questions. The theme cards and books can help the caregiver do this correctly.

Use short sentences

Using and understanding language takes a lot of energy when one suffers from dementia. It thus helps to use short sentences and uncomplicated terms, without sounding childish.

Avoid leading questions

The way we ask questions can imply that we expect a certain answer. Dementia patients rely on others for almost everything, so they tend to agree with their caregivers. Therefore, it is important to talk only about neutral subjects and ask questions that allow patients to give their personal opinion. For example, do not ask, "Don't you think this is a lovely dog?", but instead ask, "Do you think this dog is good or mean?".

Try not to judge

Dementia tends to diminish the capacity to judge if something is socially desirable. Residents can say things they would not have said if they were mentally healthy. Of course, you do not want to be insulted, but if you ask for an honest opinion, do not correct the other person immediately. Equality and trust are important in a friendly conversation.

Be patient

When you ask someone a question, an effort is required to answer it. One has to remember the question, remember the subject of the conversation, think about the answer, and find the right words to phrase the answer. It takes time to do all of this. Sometimes it takes awhile before the question has reached the mind of persons with dementia. If you start talking before they can absorb the question, the process of thinking is disturbed, and all is lost.

NOT A "TRICK"

When you ask the right questions and truly listen, people feel noted. Residents can escape the role of passively accepting help from others and embrace the role of the wise old man or woman who gives advice to a younger generation. Asking the right questions is not a "trick" to be learned from the theme cards; it is a way of looking at older people and having respect for their lifestories.

Daily Care

What a caregiver has heard about the dementia patient's preferences can be directly used in daily care. "Living and Working with a Story" is a cyclical process in which conversations with residents are both starting and evaluation points. In these conversations, staff members learn how residents perceive themselves, what they think is important in life. This knowledge can be used to bolster the identity of residents in daily care. In The Netherlands, we use a plan of action to register the daily care (Ubels, this volume). One of the goals of this plan concerns the well-being of residents. Actions related to this goal include determining what the residents like (or do not like) to talk about, their lifestyle (for example, do they want to take a shower every day and then eat breakfast, or do they prefer to eat first and then get dressed?), and what can be done to make residents happy (for example, putting on their favorite music or taking them to a quiet place). The most important evaluation criteria are provided by the residents themselves. They should be frequently asked their opinions about the care they receive, and if they enjoy the activities in which they take part.

Visualized Stories

After hearing stories told by residents, caregivers can make them visible. These visualized stories trigger others to ask the residents to talk more about their lives. The visualized stories become like theme cards themselves, and the storytelling continues. *My Life in Fragments* shows many ways to make stories visible and recommends taking into account the problems that dementia can bring. One of the recommendations is mentioned above: it is best to show the resident only one picture and keyword at a time. The picture is not surrounded by decorations (pretty flowers or decorative drawings), as this would be distracting. The story itself is represented on the left-hand page for the caregiver to read. It is not important that residents tell the "right" story. It is important that they talk about the feelings they experience while looking at the picture.

It is not essential to make a book out of the stories; there are many other ways to visualize stories. Objects can be placed in a box. Residents can then see the object and hear a story about it, as well as touch the object to trigger their memory. When residents forget the names of their family members, use a family tree or calendar with photos and names (Fig. 21.2). In the morning, when the caregiver enters the room to help residents get dressed, he or she may remark on the pictures on the calendar. It is much nicer for residents to start the day with a conversation about one of their relatives, who looks just like them, than to start their day with a caregiver who is starting to undress them. Residents may still not recognize the caregiver, but this person knows about their family and is interested in their opinion about them, so it must be all right. These are only a few examples of visualizing stories. Essentially, the visualized story is a new trigger to start a conversation.

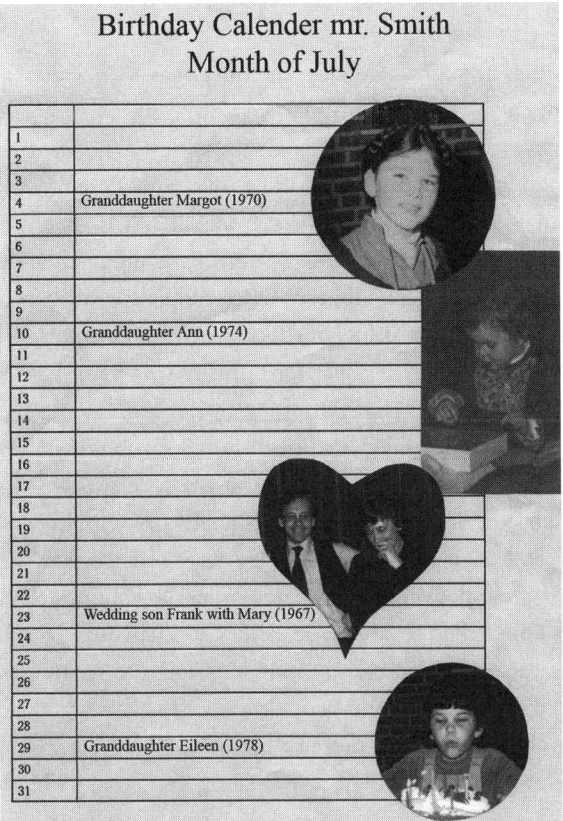

Figure 21.2 Example of monthly birthday chart showing photos of family members.

Privacy and Fading Memory

When memories fade, the visualized story must change. If residents do not remember parts of their life anymore, pictures of those parts will not trigger them to talk. Caregivers will then have to consider removing the pictures. It can be hard for family members to be confronted with the inescapable process of dementia. With the removal of every picture, the lifestory book gets shorter and the identity of the family members become less and less defined.

The residents themselves cannot decide when the time is right to remove pictures. Family members have to make that decision for them. When visualizing a story, it is best to decide in advance who will be in charge of this process. Designating, in advance, who is allowed to make changes or who receives the book when the resident passes away can prevent future problems.

THE FUTURE

Residents, their families, and staff members have been very enthusiastic about the method "Living and Working with a Story". They are convinced that it improves the well-being of residents, as well as the professional satisfaction of staff members, and that it assists relatives in keeping the conversation with their frail family members going. It has been established that the well-being of older people with minor depression can be improved by talking about their lives (Tromp, 2009). Residents who suffer from dementia are often depressed by their loss of control. It would be interesting to study the effects of using the right questions on the well-being of residents and their caregivers.

We have also shared residents' stories in public exhibitions (See Appendix). Residents and their relatives were proud of their stories. Residents got to know each other. An important outcome of this activity was that some residents were more accepted by others because their "strange" behavior was explained by their lifestories. Staff members learned many new things about the residents that they could use in daily care. It would be interesting to repeat the same exhibition in other nursing homes to see if the same social and psychological results could be achieved.

Residents were proud of these creations and interested and surprised by the stories of other residents. By reading each other's lifestories, they understood how these stories shaped a person's personality. A sense of understanding was developed. For example, when they read the lifestory of a resident with schizophrenia, he was perceived in a different way. As an artist, he made beautiful paintings. These days he is not so frightening, because everybody knows artists are a little eccentric sometimes. It is encouraging to see this man leaving his apartment more often to participate in activities. Another example is that of a lady with dementia. She still frustrates others when she knocks on all the doors at night. But now they know she spent a good part of her life collecting money for charities. Knowing more about each other improves mutual understanding and helps people with eccentric behavior patterns to integrate into the culture of the nursing home. It certainly is a way to improve the quality of life of frail older adults.

APPENDIX

Exhibition "Wie ben ik?" ("Who Am I?")

People with severe dementia were asked to paint a self-portrait. During the painting sessions, they talked about what they were painting. The portraits and a summary of these conversations were exhibited (Fig. 21.3). Most of the residents recognized their own portrait or the summary when it was read out loud. They were proud that so many people had come to listen to their stories and view their paintings. Families and staff were fascinated by the way the residents rendered the essence of their identity.

Exhibition "Uit het leven gegrepen" ("Snapshots of Life")

Residents were asked to tell about their lives. The answers to the following questions were used to create the "snapshots" (Fig. 21.4):

- What do you find important in life?
- What do you want to mean to other people?
- What makes you happy?

These questions represent the following:

- The strength of older people: giving the wisdom of life to the next generation.

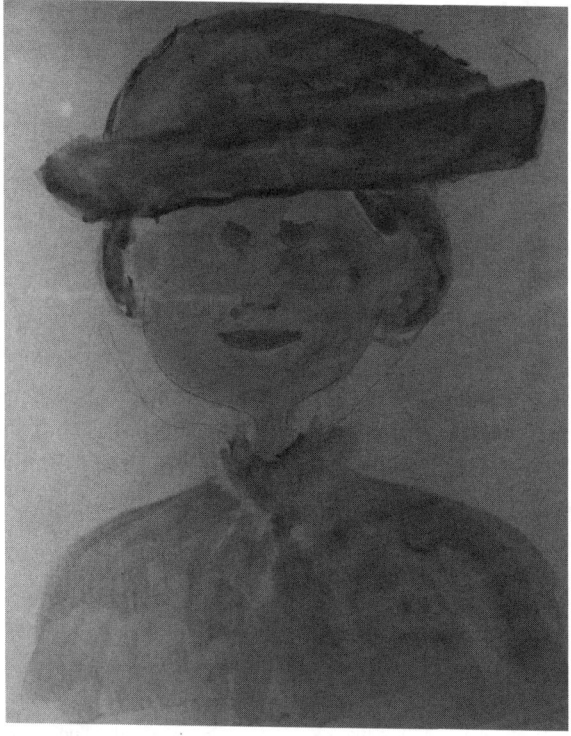

Figure 21.3 Self-portrait from "Who Am I" exhibition.

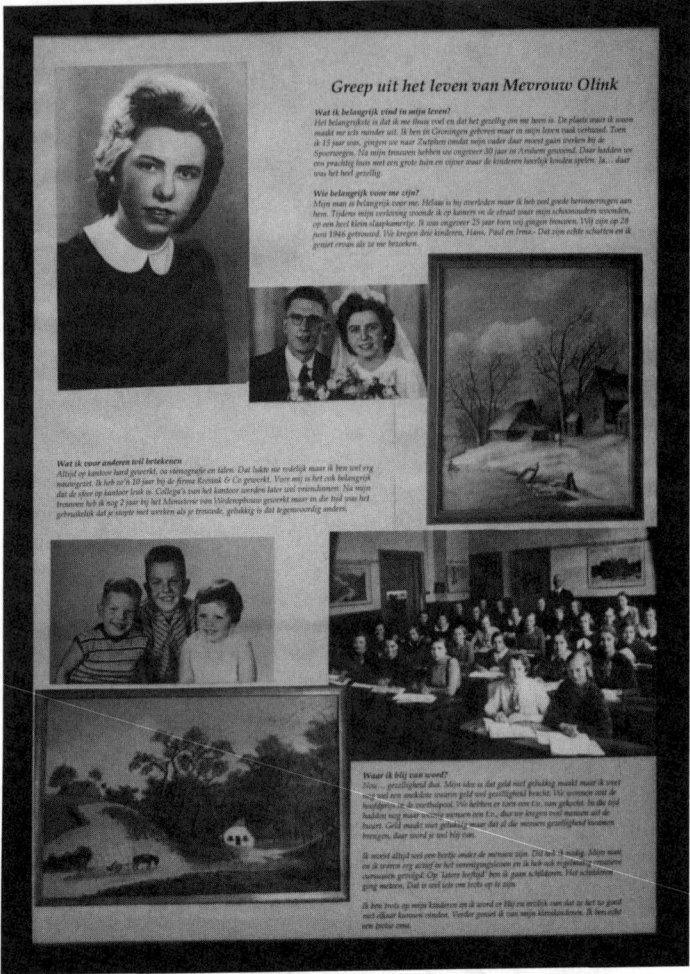

Figure 21.4 From "Snapshots of Life" exhibition.

- Playing an active role instead of passively receiving care.
- Making people happy is the main goal of care giving, improving the quality of life.

REFERENCES

Erikson, E. (1997). *The life cycle completed*. New York,: W. W. Norton.

Kenyon, G., & Randall, W. (1997). *Restorying our lives: Personal growth through autobiographical reflection*. Westport, CT: Praeger.

Tromp, T. (2009, 15 May). De zin van het ouder worden [The effect of aging]. Presentation at Bijdrage aan studiedag existentiële gerontologie [Existential

Gerontology Seminar]. Beroepsvereniging van Sociaal Gerontologen [Professional Association of Social Gerontologists]. Protestantse Theologische Universiteit, Kampen, The Netherlands.

van den Brandt-van Heek, M.-E., & Huizing, W. (2009). *Mijn leven in fragmenten* [My life in fragments]. Houten, The Netherlands: Bohn Stafleu van Loghum.

Twenty Two

THE RIPPLE EFFECT: A STORY OF THE

TRANSFORMATIONAL NATURE

OF NARRATIVE CARE

Daphne Noonan

Day-to-day activities are often taken for granted as natural or instinctive. Unless incapable of completing such a routine task, we may never, for example, pose the question, "Why do I know how to brush my teeth?" To do so would inevitably require a much more complex explanation about learned behavior, body mechanics, and the like. So it is with narratives, or stories. Our ability to think and *be* in narrative terms is so natural, so common, that we rarely pause to consider it. And if we do, we fumble uncomfortably with the realization that this is uncharted territory. "We are not very good," suggests Bruner (2002), "at grasping how story explicitly transfigures the commonplace" (p. 4). Could it be that this seemingly trivial, ordinary process known as narrative is actually the epitome of significance (see also Ubels, this volume; van den Brandt-van Heek, this volume)? What is more, could a narrative approach be the key to effecting deep, transformational change in a variety of contexts? I believe that it is, and in what follows, I will walk the reader through the development of a program of "narrative care" in a long-term care home, from the program's inception, through the challenges met along the way, to its effects on both the institution itself and the community beyond.

"CELEBRATING OUR STORIES"

In the fall of 2006, my mind was opened to narrative gerontology through a course I took at St Thomas University. From that point on, I found it hard to "put the lid" on my narrative spirit. I began relating the concepts of story and narrative to numerous aspects of my life, in particular, to my work in the department of therapeutic recreation of a large, local nursing home. The idea of starting a narrative program at York Care Centre had been on my wish list for quite a while, but I was timid to ask for the time and resources to plan it on a formal basis. I assumed such a project would not appear as valuable as other, more clinical, more measurable programs. However, along with other passionate colleagues, I continued to exercise narrative techniques with residents and families on an informal basis, all the while attempting to weave narrative themes into conversations with my colleagues and with people in our wider community.

Finally, a door opened in late spring of 2007 when our executive director attended a national leadership conference in Ontario. During the event, he witnessed a large, leading-edge care home in Montreal (one we strive to model ourselves on in many ways) receive an award for excellence in leadership in long-term care. The award was granted for a biography program that the recipients had developed with their residents. In fact, the program had been woven into the very fabric of their home, so they told him, and had changed the atmosphere of the institution as a whole.

Upon his return, our director questioned me about the possibility of developing a similar program in our own care home. Having gleaned an insight into the transformational nature of narrative, he was hopeful we could use such an initiative to enhance the lives of our residents, too, and at the same time improve our organization's culture. With wholehearted agreement, I partnered with another colleague, Jana Jones, and together we began planning a narrative program at York Care Centre. Thus, "Celebrating Our Stories" was born.

BUILDING A FOUNDATION

After approximately 8 months of careful research, reflection, and conversation on existing programs and possible techniques, as well as the unique nature of our context at York Care Centre, the goals of our program emerged: first, to honor our residents' rich histories and experience by listening to and recording their stories; and second, to challenge assumptions about aging—in particular, about aging in a long-term care home—by allowing staff, volunteers, and everyone associated with our institution to see our residents in a truly holistic sense.

Having both been immersed in the world of narrative during our respective studies, my colleague and I sensed immediately the positive effects such a program could bring—to our residents, to their families and friends, to our staff and volunteers, and to the environment of our workplace in general. When one begins viewing others from a different perspective, such as a narrative perspective, the effect, I often jest, is like starting an avalanche or opening a can of worms. The effects cannot be reversed. We knew instinctively that as people in our community began to experience the narrative phenomenon, they would see one another in a different light and, in turn, their approaches to interacting with one another would change as well.

The question remained, though, how we were going to develop our program in such a way as to facilitate not only a quaint appreciation for narrative in others but also the adoption of a narrative perspective as a way of being in the world. As Randall (2001) observes, "one does not so much teach a narrative perspective… as tempt people to try it on for size." However, "once they overcome their awkwardness, and even guilt… at thinking about themselves," he says, "they become energized" (p. 43). They have an "aha" moment. To have a similar moment, we felt, people in our community needed to experience narrative firsthand for it to effect deep change. With this as our mantra, then, we settled on two non-negotiable factors that have become the foundation of our program. First, whenever possible, our residents would be directly involved in the writing of their stories, and in the absence of that as a possibility, their closest loved ones would be their voice. Second, interested members of the York Care Centre community would be trained by us as "biographers" and work interactively with residents and their loved ones to record their stories.

Although recognizing that this kind of collaborative approach would ultimately require some investment of extra time and resources, we remained firm in our plan because we felt such an approach reflected the very core of our program: relationships. Indeed, our hope has been that an emphasis on the process, as much as on the finished product, would allow the forming of new relationships, the revisiting or nurturing of old ones, and the changing of existing ones as not just our biographers, but also spectators of the program began viewing our residents from different perspectives.

To appreciate the influential effects that "Celebrating Our Stories" has had on our community, it is important to understand the scope of the program fully. Its basic details (the result of many months of careful, deliberate planning) can be outlined as follows:

- New "classes" of (four to six) biographies are launched every 4 months, with each class involving a different mix of staff and volunteers.
- Biographers receive a half-day of training and, as needed, ongoing support. Training includes experiential exercises related to narrative, a review of the recording tool chosen[1], interviewing and editing skills, and a small lecture on ethical considerations and the emotional side of the interview experience.
- Once the recording of each story is completed, biographers work with the program coordinators to pull from it highlights and photographs to create a 15- to 20-minute DVD slide show tribute.
- Each month, one or two residents are honored at a "narrative ceremony," to which they can invite family and friends to view their biography. Staff and volunteers are encouraged to attend as well. Attendance at these ceremonies has, in fact, grown considerably over time, to an average of over 50 participants per month.
- Observing a minimum of two DVD tributes per year has been made a workplace education requirement for all staff. If they are not able to attend a ceremony, they can access the DVDs in our library.

THE RIPPLE EFFECT

At the end of our first full year of "Celebrating Our Stories," we had completed 18 biographies, including eight special stories done by grade 11 students from a local high school. The program has exceeded, and continues to exceed, our hopes and aspirations. At times we have been quite overwhelmed by its impact, not only on our residents and their loved ones but also on members of our York Care Centre community and of the larger community around us. It has had what we are now calling a "ripple effect" that is felt at several levels, beginning with the residents at the Centre and radiating outward through the families, the biographers, the York Care Centre community, and eventually to the community of the wider region (see Fig. 22.1).

Common to every one of these circles are three themes: meaning-making and growth, connectedness, and empowerment. Indeed, they have been

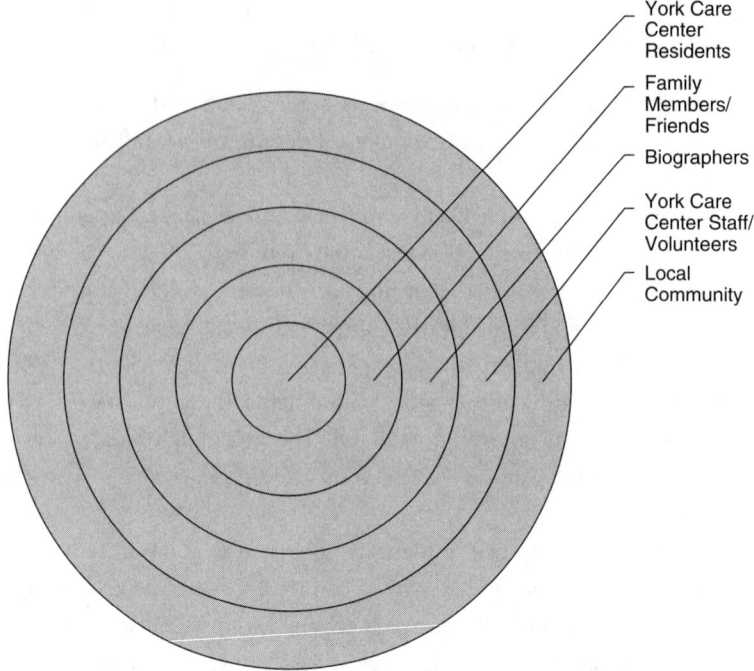

York Care
Center
Residents

Family
Members/
Friends

Biographers

York Care
Center Staff/
Volunteers

Local
Community

Figure 22.1 The ripple effect.

exhibited with an intensity that is sometimes beyond what we could ever have predicted. What follows is a collection of impressions, stories, and quotations that illustrate these themes and the far-reaching effects that "Celebrating Our Stories" has had.

Meaning-Making and Growth

Always at the core of our stories are our wonderful residents. In them, we have witnessed some of the most profound meaning-making taking place through their participation in the program. More than one has used the process to revisit and work through painful pieces of their past: alcoholism, the deaths of children and spouses, broken relationships with parents. In such instances, the biography experience was the first time they had spoken openly about these difficult times. One resident expressed contentment at having talked about and reflected on his relationship with his mother, and from the biographer's perspective, he was visibly able to put it to rest and move on in his story. Another expressed gratitude for the opportunity to tell "Hazel and Tom's Love Story" through his biography. About a month into the program, he lost his beloved wife, but in the months that followed, we saw him actively use the life review process to help him with his grief. Finally, we have "Verna," who, when asked what writing her biography had meant to her, replied, "I realized I did some good."

Family members also experienced meaning-making through the telling of their loved ones' stories. For virtually all of the family members and friends who were involved in some capacity, we could literally see healing taking place amid the process. Many expressed gratitude that it had allowed them to see their loved one as a whole being once again. One family member encapsulated this sentiment perfectly when she said: "The past 8 months have been all about my grandmother's physical condition and ailments, and about being admitted to a 'nursing home,' with all of the emotion that comes with that. This program has allowed us to remember and recognize my Gram again." Another shining example of this ability for family members to heal and to make meaning from reviewing their loved one's life came from the daughter of a male resident who passed away soon after his story had been completed:

> I feel privileged to be a part of this program, and to be able to share my father's life with so many people. Father had a saying, if he respected another man, he would say they were "a man among men." Well, in doing this book I got to know my father as a person, and realized that he was 'the man among men' to all who knew him. I feel so blessed to be his child.

Yet another example of meaning-making within at least some families who participated in the program was their awakening to the value of their own personal stories. After their loved one's story was completed, some went on to continue the story of their family by contacting others in different areas of the province and the world. One family managed to trace its roots back to the Scotland in the 1700s. The experience began to cultivate an appreciation for life as part of a story.

The biographers who worked with residents and their families to record the life stories experienced a profound form of growth, in several ways. Many have been inspired to begin telling their own stories and to connect with members of their family to further this process. During a period when caring for a family member in palliative care, one individual turned for comfort to her journal and to the writing of her story. Others began working with parents and grandparents to ensure that their family legacy was being recorded.

Those of us on staff who volunteered to be biographers have grown not only as individuals, but as professionals as well, each of us changed for the better with a new perspective on our working lives. One biographer, a registered nurse, expressed this new perspective candidly and eloquently as she reflected on her experience working with a 95-year-old resident:

> As a registered nurse, I do not always have the opportunity to know and to understand residents beyond their medical conditions and daily living needs. Working on "Celebrating Our Stories" allowed me to show an interest in helping create a permanent record of their legacy. It is true that we live in a time where our seniors often disappear from the society that they gave so much to. Every person should have the opportunity to bring their history, their legacy, and their knowledge to life and preserve their contribution to society and culture. This program has been a rewarding and exciting opportunity for me to connect to the residents I interact with on a daily basis.

Within our York Care Centre community, we have seen evidence of growth among those who have attended the monthly narrative ceremonies. Many have become ignited to take part in the program, craving the same impact that they witnessed happening in those more directly involved. As a result, several new biographers have come forward. After being inspired by our narrative DVDs, a number of people have also gone on to complete life-stories with their parents and grandparents. Among those who speak about the program, whether informally or publicly, there has developed a sense of camaraderie and ease, of "being in it together," and of doing truly important work. Such an atmosphere has cultivated growth in interpersonal relationships within our workplace overall.

Connectedness

The program has connected people in various ways: with one another, with places and times, and with different disciplines. As for our residents, we have seen a true connection to times and places that are dear to their hearts. Many were extremely descriptive in their accounts, including smells, sounds, and scenes from important events in their past. Their ability to retrieve such details illustrates firsthand how narrative transcends time and place. Virtually all of those interviewed commented on how happy they felt to have gotten close to those special memories again. Here is a beautiful example from one of our male residents who was interviewed by a high school student:

> The thing I remember most about my mother was her cooking. She loved to cook. I can remember the smells of the wood stove and the bread and cookies baking. My father was a hard worker. I remember his singing and the snowshoes he used to make.

Residents who actively participated in the telling of their stories also developed special and intense relationships with their biographers. They waited anxiously for each meeting and exuded excitement about sharing their legacy in such a heartfelt fashion. When I think about the relationships that formed between our residents and their biographers, whatever the biographers' ages, I am reminded of MacKeracher's (2004, p. 184) observation that a narrative exchange permits a "soul-to-soul" connection.

For the family members, we have seen relationships with one another blossom to a new level. In one example, a mother and daughter working on their loved one's biography spent Tuesday evenings "sleeping over" for a period of several months as they worked on the story. Both individuals and other family members commented to me on various occasions that working on the project allowed a special bond to form between mother and daughter.

Throughout the project we have also observed an intense connection between the families and the biographers. In at least two instances, this connection was poignantly illustrated at the time of the death of a resident whose biography had been completed. In both cases, I had been the biographer. On seeing me for the first time after the resident had died, the family displayed an almost desperate desire to cling to me. I had the impression that they felt I truly understood what they were experiencing at that moment. These connections were some of the most profound experiences I have ever had. The feeling that I had been responsible for giving something to these individuals that, after the loss of their loved one, carried so much meaning for them is difficult to articulate. Following the deaths of these and other residents who completed their biographies, we have also (after a certain length of time) had conversations with the family members. During these conversations, we have begun to see a new level of the ripple effect, when the family members indicate that, with the loss of their loved one, both the experience of doing the biography and the finished product have taken on a whole new dimension. Indeed, the project continued to feed them and help them through the dying and grieving process, and kept them feeling strongly connected to their loved one.

For the biographers, the effects were very similar to those on the residents and their family. All of the biographers felt connected to history through their residents' storytelling. Said one of the student biographers from Leo Hayes High School, "When looking at older people now, I think of the life they had, working hard, their parents making enough money to put food on the table. It was way harder back then than it is now." Nearly every biographer expressed the same soul-to-soul connection as that experienced by the residents and their families. To sum up, these relationships *run deep* for those actively involved in the process; they become, in fact, sacred.

For the greater York Care Centre community, connectedness has taken different forms. The most powerful form is characterized by a changed perspective, an ability to look at each person whom we care for as an individual. Members of our community have developed an ability to see the residents beyond the "now" of everyday life. As one staff member has said, "It gives a better insight of the person as to who they were, and not just 'Sue' in the Broda chair [a type of wheelchair]." Another family member, who observed one of the first narrative presentations, sent me an E-mail as soon as she returned home:

> Just got home from the WONDERFUL presentations you guys put together.
> I can't imagine how much this project will impact families and staff. It was
> really moving and I did not know either resident very well, just saw them as
> I passed by. My friend and I both said we will look at them now and not just
> see a person in a wheelchair.

There have been countless testimonies such as these, all passionately illustrating the changing perspectives of each person who observes a resident's lifestory. In two profound examples, after seeing the biographies, staff were able to change their approach to direct care with residents who exhibit aggressive behaviors. The labels commonly used in the culture of long-term care—labels like "the demanding resident" or "the aggressive one"—seem to have diminished and, in some cases, even fallen away.

"Celebrating Our Stories" has also created a connection between York Care Centre and the community at large. Leo Hayes High School, for example, is now forever linked with our institution through the success of our shared initiative. In June 2008, in fact, the school proudly accepted the Premier's Award for Excellence in Education for their work with us on the project, a high honor indeed. We have also seen an increased desire for collaboration being expressed by staff at other nursing homes in our province, as well as nationally, who want to launch similar initiatives. People from all walks of life—social work, acute care, palliative care, pastoral care, and other fields—are talking and learning together about the transformative impact of a narrative approach.

EMPOWERMENT

One rather lovely and somewhat unexpected outcome we have observed at every level of our ripple effect has been empowerment. For our residents, this has been demonstrated by their delight in "showing off" their stories, often after having begun the process declaring, "I probably won't have much to say." One resident who rarely shows excitement can be found carrying her lifestory book around with her in her walker, proudly displaying it to visitors and friends. Another resident dutifully keeps a small notepad next to her bed to record her thoughts as they come to her in the middle of the night. These notes have become treasures, characterized by her quick wit and sense of humor. In one instance, she describes herself as "the best dessert maker EVER!" One 95-year-old male resident, having begun by saying that he had not had very much formal education, finished by recognizing that he had, in fact, accomplished a very successful career: running a large family farm through hard work, intelligence, and dedication. Through his story, he came to see himself as a cornerstone of his community—and rightly so, as he had helped to build it. Finally, a resident with no children of her own and very few surviving family members expressed happiness over being able to leave a legacy behind her: "This book... that will let them know about me."

For the families, the greatest form of empowerment that the program has created is the feeling that they are participating actively in their loved one's care. They realize that they are critical resources in the process. And when they see the finished product, there is always such a sense of accomplishment, where previously there had been a sense of helplessness as far as their loved one was concerned. More than a few family members have also stepped outside their personal comfort zones to speak in front of large groups to educate others about the effects of our program because they believe in it and value it so much.

From our biographers, we have seen an unshakable confidence emerge when it comes to their ability to care for others. Whether staff, volunteers, or high school students, in their own ways they have become confident in their ability to relate to others on a truly human level, as illustrated by the following comments:

> Being a part of "Celebrating our Stories" has been one of the most rewarding things I've ever done. As soon as I was introduced to the world of narrative, I immediately wanted to incorporate it into every aspect of my life in a deeper and more meaningful way. Having the opportunity to share this program with a resident really meant a lot to me. By assisting someone in writing their biography, we are ensuring that their story is not lost, and I was honored to be a part of it. Seeing the expressions on her face as she watched the story of her life unfold reaffirmed that we are doing the right thing with this program.... Each time a biography is completed, we are unearthing another unique treasure. ("Celebrating Our Stories" co-chair and biographer)
>
> (I experienced) a lot of emotional things. I now realize that life was harder in the past. I got to meet new people. I feel more comfortable talking to people and asking questions. (Leo Hayes, high school student biographer)

> Residents are people. They were young once, had careers, families, faith. It changes the way you look at a person. (York Care Centre biographer)

In the York Care Centre community as a whole, we have seen a sense of pride at being a part of such an important story. We often hear comments about how the program is affecting perceptions of what it means to be living in a nursing home, and how proud people are to be involved in our community. "It has made me very proud to be a part of the York Care Centre family," said one staff member. Another expressed pride about giving such a gift to the residents:

> This has been the most refreshing idea in a long while. It is an activity that includes the residents' families. I am sure in many occasions it helps them realize how special their loved one is and how much of a fulfilling life he or she has had. It also involves the frontline caregivers, allowing them to see the residents in a different light. Finally, it involves all nursing home employees, making us feel wonderful working in a long-term care environment. It puts more focus on the human side of care giving and [we] certainly need more of this. (York Care Centre, Director of Finance)

Along the way, and even now with the momentum that has been established, our program has not been without its challenges, as is true of any initiative of this nature. To others wanting to embark on similar narrative adventures, I would suggest the following guidelines:

1. *Love it.* Our program could not have progressed beyond its initial stages without the innate conviction of the two co-coordinators that it could change our culture for the better. This love for and belief in our program came in handy when we were feeling tired of "propagandizing" narrative to sometimes cynical onlookers.
2. *Go slowly.* Time must be given at the outset to discerning which type of narrative initiative will work in your context, generating a buzz about it, and building a solid base of support. Successful completion of these tasks before beginning the formal program is crucial; once the process begins, most of your energy should focus on refining the program, not on continually convincing others of its validity.
3. *Be dedicated.* Our motto, although it has meant sacrifice, has been "say no to nothing." Narrative care has a sneaky way of becoming infectious if people receive a little encouragement. As was the case in our partnership with Leo Hayes High School, taking on an extra initiative may just work out to mean an even bigger ripple effect for your program.

4. *Enjoy it.* At times, the co-coordinator and I have been so close to the process that we have lost a little of our energy and desire for it. At such times, we have taken a moment to review a biography or two or look back over our journey and to be proud (again) of all that has happened. Taking time to enjoy the work allows us to be reminded of what a wonderful gift narrative is.

Overall, we feel privileged to have been a part of such a program. Thinking back over the process while completing this chapter has clarified for us the remarkable effects that have occurred as a result of it. We have used narrative care to facilitate meaning-making, connectedness, and empowerment for those we care for, not to mention for the members of our York Care Centre community and beyond. The effects have arrived subtly and slowly, so much so that it has been difficult at times to grasp them. As we move forward, we do so with an overwhelming respect for this lovely gift bestowed on human nature: narrative and its ripple effect.

NOTE

1 The resource we have chosen is *The LifeBio Memory Journal* (Sanders, 2001), a collection of questions related to four main themes throughout the lifespan: "The People Who Shaped You," "Memories," "The Real World," and "Bringing It All Together." As a tool for gathering information, this resource has proven extremely thought provoking and insightful, and thus far has been enjoyed by all of the participants.

REFERENCES

Bruner, J. (2002). *Making stories: Law, literature, life.* New York: Farrar, Straus and Giroux.

MacKeracher, D. (2004). *Making sense of adult learning* (2nd ed.). Toronto: University of Toronto Press.

Randall, W. (2001). Storied worlds: Acquiring a narrative perspective on aging, identity and everyday life. In Kenyon, G., Clark, P., & deVries, B. (Eds.), *Narrative gerontology: Theory, research, and practice* (pp. 31–62). New York: Springer.

Sanders, L. (2001). *The LifeBio Memory Journal.* Marysville, OH: LifeBio Inc.

Afterword

Toward a Narrative Turn in Health Care

Ernst Bohlmeijer, Gary Kenyon, and William L. Randall

This book is about narrative gerontology. It is also about human development in later life and about care for older adults. Implicitly or explicitly, many of the authors represented in the book write about health care, albeit from very different perspectives. Indeed, one could say that the implications of narrative gerontology for health care constitute one of the book's dominant underlying themes. Our aim in this final chapter is to highlight this theme. In our opinion, all of those who have contributed to the book would support a model of health care that is, at least to some degree, based on narrative knowledge, and on narrative perspectives on both human development and health in later life. Insofar as this is the case, we can ask what would characterize such a model? Further, what kind of knowledge is needed for a "narrative turn" in health care? In what follows, we will formulate some initial answers to these intriguing questions. Our intention is to show how the theoretical considerations (Issues), the research (Investigations), and the approaches to practice (Interventions) described in this book are examples of building blocks of a health care that is based at least partly on narrative principles. We begin, however, with a slightly broader perspective by outlining some general limitations or biases in current perspectives on health care.

CURRENT HEALTH CARE: A THIN STORY

At a conference on reminiscence and life review in Atlanta in 2009, gerontologist Jim Birren (this volume) reflected on the high demand for autobiographical groups by indicating that, while our social structure is becoming increasingly efficient, it is also less personal. This insight is relevant to developments in health care as well. Efficiency and cost-effectiveness have become dominant forces in its organization. With the exception of geriatric specialists, medicine is primarily about symptoms, classifications, and diagnoses. Diagnoses relate symptoms to underlying physical and neurological impairments. Medicine is also about protocolled treatments that have been proven effective in randomized, controlled trials. "Effective" in this case means that, following treatment, the diagnosis cannot be established any longer, or that the symptoms have (largely) disappeared. Moreover, the shorter the treatment, the better; it reduces costs. And "treatment" itself has been segmented into tasks, and these tasks are defined by minutes.

Mental health care has developed analogously with medical health care, in that the focus is on psychopathology. In addition to physical factors, psychological processes offer an explanation for psychopathology. Insurance companies have increasing influence on the duration of treatment. It may not be long before symptoms will be monitored after every session, and funding for treatment will stop as soon as the symptoms drop below a certain cutoff score. Such treatment models rely heavily on positivistic empirical scientific methods in which replicability and testability are central requisites (Davey, 2008). In order to conduct experiments that fulfill these criteria, both reduction and control of context are essential. Overall, there is a fundamental belief that there is an objective reality, independent of the observing subject, in which laws and regularities exist and that can be detected with objective methods.

Let us first stress that this approach has brought humanity considerable good. Numerous physical illnesses that in earlier times would lead inevitably to premature death can now be all but cured. By the same token, medications can be extremely effective in managing severe mental disorders. In a similar vein, we are not arguing that costs should not be taken into account, that we should not classify and implement short, effective treatments, or that we should not do quantitative research or randomized, controlled trials. The demand for health care has expanded so much in the last number of years that efficiency and costs must certainly be taken into account. Moreover, effectiveness studies are without doubt helpful in discovering the impact of treatments on a wide range of outcomes. That said, the most important objection of narrative gerontology to this (medical) model is its exclusiveness (Kenyon & Randall, 2001). In other words, it leads to what may be called a "thin" perception or a thin story of both health and health care alike. To explain this, let us first address certain limitations or biases of the positivistic, empirical approach within health care at present.

FOUR IMPORTANT BIASES WITHIN HEALTH CARE

Health as More Than Absence of Illness

The focus in much of current health care is on the treatment of illnesses and pathology. Yet, in mental health care at least, there is growing recognition that health is more than merely the absence of illness. The World Health Organization (2004) defines mental health in positive terms as "a state of well-being in which the individual realizes his or her own abilities, can cope with the normal stresses of life, can work productively and fruitfully, and is able to make a contribution to his or her community" (p. 12). The two-continua model of mental health states that positive mental health is related to, though different from, mental illness (Keyes, 2005). In empirical studies, different measures of emotional, psychological, and social well-being load on a distinct factor that relates to a second factor that accounts for measures of psychopathology. In other words, an individual may be suffering from mental illness (e.g., a panic disorder) but, at the same time, have a high, positive state of mental health. The two-continua model has been confirmed in adolescent and adult samples in the United States (Keyes, 2005, 2006, 2007). Positive mental health can be linked to the Aristotlean concept of *eudaimonia* (Verduin, 2007), which refers to the ability to develop our talents and our virtues in harmony with our environment. Happiness in terms of eudaimonia can be defined as the subjective experience of living one's life in a meaningful way. Contemplation and logos (e.g., understanding, or ordering facts into stories) enable us to reflect on our experiences and to understand what our lives are all about. Randall and McKim (2008) refer to this as the ability to read our lives. Eudaimonia is "the ability to take decisions in full freedom and responsibility and to develop oneself in harmony with living reality as one sees or reads it" (Verduin, 2007, p. 70; trans. EB). Praxis, or learning by doing and acting, is a necessary condition for the presence of eudaimonia. A model of health care that has eudaimonia as its goal empowers people to answer the question of what is happening to them in the moment. It helps them to see what possibilities and potentialities are present to respond to in the given situation (e.g., coping with an illness or some other restriction), to choose between these possibilities, and to actualize their choices in real life.

The Premise of Control over Life

Overcoming suffering is a central aim in current health care. It is built on the belief that, with the help of rational, scientific methods and technology, we will ultimately be able to understand and control the underlying processes of various illnesses and thus find a cure or a fix for any problem. In an inspiring book on health care, philosopher Pieter Verduin (1998) challenges this premise. Building on the concept of the body-subject proposed by the philosopher Merleau-Ponty, Verduin discusses a fundamentally different conception of life—as ambiguous, as finite or transitory, and as infinite.

Simply put, life is ambiguous in the sense that experiences can be interpreted in several different ways. It is finite on the basis of our mortality and because experiences (thoughts, feelings, sensations) come and go. In other words, life is a chain of moments that is always in motion. Finally, life is infinite in that it is a process that transcends our personal life-span. On the one hand, such infiniteness is historical in nature, insofar as our life is influenced by a long history of events and developments that precede it; by the same token, it influences events that will happen long after we have died. On the other hand, infiniteness is spiritual in nature as well, in the sense both that there is a consciousness that transcends our personal consciousness and that everything is related to everything else.

When we acknowledge these core existential conditions, they have a huge impact on our lives. For instance, ambiguity will make us modest (e.g., in our claims to own the truth). These conditions also make us realize the value of consciousness, in that our mental abilities allow us to notice the chain of moment-to-moment experiences and to observe how our own mental activities, such as evaluation, have an effect on these experiences. In addition, finiteness bestows a sense of urgency on the here and now. Furthermore, the experience of infiniteness promotes solidarity, not only in our sense of connectedness throughout the ages but also in our shared contingency vis à vis the conditions of life. One important implication, in other words, is that an existing human being is always a coexisting human being. "We exist in a dynamic of reciprocal influence of everything and everybody" (Verduin, 1998, p. 50).

Building on these three notions of finiteness, infiniteness, and ambiguity, Verduin contrasts current health care with the philosophy of Friedrich Nietzsche. According to Nietzsche, suffering is an integral part of life. The art of living is the ability to say "yes" to the three conditions of life with full commitment. It is the ability to both enjoy life and suffer life. Sympathy and compassion support this art of living; feeling sorry for one's self diminishes it.

The art of living is also the knowledge (as with the heroes in the Greek tragedies) of what one has to do in life. Spiritually, life can be experienced as a creative vitality in our being. From this perspective, the process of coping with a chronic illness, for instance, always involves questions about how to live one's life and trying to understand what one's life is about. It is knowing when to emphasize change and control, and when to actively accept a life situation as it is (see also Kenyon, this volume).

The Need for Narratives

A third bias of current health care, with its focus on illness and curing, is that it overlooks the importance of meaning and storytelling. Society has, at least in part, moved from modern to postmodern times. The self has become a reflexive project (Giddens, 1991). In the confrontation with illnesses, whether curable or not, whether chronic or not, there is a need for identity work (finding one's voice) and for testimonials. In the words of Arthur Frank (1995), "The illness story faces a dual task. The narrative attempts to restore an order that the interruption fragmented, but it must also tell the truth that interruptions will continue. Part of this truth is that the tidy ends are no longer appropriate to the story. A different kind of end—a different purpose—has to be discovered" (p. 59).

In general hospitals, one could be satisfied perhaps with a focus on curing. As long as no mistakes are made and one is cured effectively, why complain? The healing of one's wounds as a storyteller (Frank, 1995) can be done later with fellow-sufferers, with social workers, or with a psychologist. But what about mental health care, where the loss of stories and rediscovering one's voice may be the central issue? And what about those settings where one will be living for a long time, or where one knows it is one's last home before dying?

There Is No Ultimate Truth

The positivistic scientific method has become so dominant in the social sciences that we may forget that it still is a model based on particular assumptions. A different approach can be envisioned, however, based on social constructionism (e.g., Burr, 1995). Central to this model is the assumption that there is no such thing as a basic truth that we can discover with the aid of scientific methods. Rather, knowledge is always a form of construction based on subjective perspectives and contingent upon specific cultural and historical contexts. From this perspective, the discovery of replicable and generalizable laws in human behavior comes with a high price: a reduction of the experience of the multileveled, radical connectedness of coexistence to more generic, causal relationships between individuals as "isolated" objects. Put in narrative terms, reality as we can know it is, by definition, storied and, therefore, so is truth. Systematic methods for research, based on a reconstructive framework, are studies based on phenomenological and qualitative principles (see, e.g., various chapters in the second part of this volume).

A THICKER STORY OF HEALTH CARE

If the limitations in current health care were removed, a much thicker story would emerge. Inspired by philosophers such as Nietzsche, Heidegger, Merleau-Ponty, and Habermas, Verduin (1998, 2007) would describe this as the transformation of "small health care" toward "large health care." From a narrative perspective, it could be called a "narrative turn in health care." The following description is inspired by Verduin's work, central to which is the idea that cure and care are always embedded in a broader perspective on the art of living. Health care is, by nature, emancipatory—that is, it involves enabling another person to make sense of their own experiences in a given situation and to express themselves, to tell their story. It is rooted in a sense of solidarity. Caregiver and care-receiver are both "co-existent." The caregiver may have specific knowledge that is very helpful in a given situation at a given time, but this does not make him or her an expert on issues of life in general or, more importantly, on the life of another person. Caregiver and care-receiver are co-authors in a biographical encounter (Randall & Kenyon, 2002). Further, the idea of "large health" implies that there is always an ethical or moral dimension: for example, "How do I make the best of this situation?" One of the underlying central issues is the need to find a wise answer to the dilemma of change versus acceptance. "Symptoms" of large health are joy for living, life-courage, a clear mind, the experience of solidarity, the wish and ability to discuss the "slow questions" about life (Ubels, this volume), and having arrangements or commitments that show how one is connected and helpful to others (Verduin, 2007). And, large health is very much possible even in the presence of severe physical or mental illness.

It is important to note that "large health care" may take very different forms depending on the different domains of health care. The context of intensive care—discussing the slow questions of life here could be slightly disastrous—is very different from the context of plastic surgery. The context of primary care is very different from that of care in nursing homes.

The concept of large health care could be elaborated for all the domains in health care. However, the underlying principles remain the same.

Building on this thicker description of health care, we can try, in a nutshell and only preliminarily, to characterize a health care based on a thicker conception of aging and health. Large health care, we would say, has its roots in philosophy: for example, humanism. Central are questions about what makes us human beings human. What is the essence of being human? Ethical questions and questions about values are always implied. A large health care emphasizes the human ability to grow psychologically and spiritually. In treatment, there is a focus on development as well as on illnesses and symptoms. Professionals and clients are both knowledgeable and co-create decisions about optimal care. In general, treatment has a more integrative approach, with more room for meditation, body awareness, and other creative interventions. The attitude of the professional is one of solidarity. There is a basic interest in the client as a person, and a basic principle of treatment consists in informing the client of what might be helpful. The professional has a strong ethical consciousness. Treatment is much more question oriented, with a special interest in the slow questions (again, see Ubels, this volume). A large health care is built on both quantitative and qualitative research. There is a special interest in studies of meaning. There is also interest in a wide range of outcomes such as meaning in life, mastery, psychological well-being, and ego-diversity, as well as inquiries into illnesses and disorders themselves. A large health care is coordinated by management that balances productivity in relation to finances with an interest in optimizing care in relation to the needs of both patients and workers.

Large health care is inclusive of small health care, with its focus on cost-effective treatment, but broadens it. Large health care involves the ability to shift from applying "expert" knowledge to "solidarity" knowledge, from helping with control to helping with acceptance, and vice versa. The psychologist Hulsbergen (2009, p. 180) has written a short case study that illustrates this well.

Working as a psychologist in a general hospital, Hulsbergen received a request to consult a young man, 30 years of age, who had been admitted to internal medicine. The day before, he had been diagnosed with incurable stomach cancer and was told that he would die in the very near future. Since that moment, no aftercare had taken place. The nurses noticed that the young man was overwhelmed with anxiety. On her way to see him, Hulsbergen was very anxious herself. Confronted with anxiety about her own death, she felt an urge to return to her department and transfer the consult to a colleague. She then decided to notice her anxiety and to accept it.

While keeping in touch with her anxiety, she shook the young man's hand. While shaking hands and looking into his eyes, she experienced a strong sense of connectedness with him. A sense of quietness arose in both of them. For a long time, he talked about his fear of leaving his wife and child behind and about his good relationship with his parents. Hulsbergen listened attentively and continued to keep in touch with her inner sensations. She then went on to discuss how this was a turning point for her in helping people with serious illnesses, how thereafter she felt the importance of making real contact with the other, and how this was only possible by making real contact with herself. After their meeting, the young man was able to discuss his concerns with his wife and parents. Not much later, he died.

This testimony demonstrates that the concept of large health care is consistent with a narrative perspective on health care, and a narrative gerontological perspective on health care in later life in particular (Kenyon & Randall, 2001). A narrative turn in health care would imply that health care professionals (e.g., physicians, psychologists, nurses, social workers) develop narrative competencies and use these competencies in daily practice. Rita Charon (2004) has defined narrative competence as the "set of skills required to recognize, absorb, interpret, and be moved by the stories one hears or reads. This competence requires a combination of textual skills (identifying a story's structure, adopting its multiple perspectives, recognizing metaphors and allusions), creative skills (imagining many interpretations, building curiosity, inventing multiple endings), and affective skills (tolerating uncertainty as a story unfolds, entering the story's mood)" (p. 862; see also Rishi & Charon, this volume). One way to train narrative competencies, of course, is by way of reading literary texts.

Within the context of health care for older adults, Gass (2001) defines narrative competence as the ability to co-create health care decisions that take into account both scientific knowledge and metaphoric or narrative knowledge. Gass builds on work by Nussbaum (1990), who identifies four characteristics of narrative knowledge: fine perception of particular detail, the role of surprise and uncontrolled events, emotions and belief, paradox and noncommensurable qualities. For Gass (2001), narrative competence includes the ability to establish "a relationship that moves beyond objective scientific observation to create a space in which the patient's voice can be expressed" (p. 229).

The increase of narrative practices in health care may initially increase costs because of the time needed to address the stories of care-receivers. In the long run, however, it may also decrease costs, as a result of such things as increased compliance with the chosen therapy, enhanced feelings of mastery and self-efficacy that may reduce the use of health care services, and increased engagement and decreased burnout of health care professionals themselves. Future studies should address the benefits, as well as the costs, of narrative practices in health care.

THE KIND OF KNOWLEDGE NEEDED FOR A NARRATIVE TURN IN HEALTH CARE

How then, do narrative gerontologists keep the idea of large health care alive? Or, to put it more ambitiously, what knowledge and practices are needed for a narrative turn in health care? We will end this concluding chapter by sketching some preliminary answers to these important questions and linking the conditions just outlined to a number of the contributions in this book.

Philosophy

Human history has brought about so many great sources of philosophical wisdom, in both classical and modern times. Philosophers keep these sources alive and available to us by linking older ideas and concepts to new developments. In many ways, they show us and remind us of the infiniteness of our being in the world that was mentioned earlier. They let us stand back from our daily routines and contemplate societal developments, organizational structures, and personal interactions. In this way, they help us to sharpen and to story our ideas about what we want—and don't want—in health care, that is, to formulate our personal ethics. A good philosopher prevents narrow-mindedness, which is a central characteristic of large health and an insight exemplified in the chapter by Frits de Lange (this volume). And what goes for philosophy, goes for the study of literature as well (Rishi & Charon, this volume).

Theories

Science in general, and practice based on science in particular, cannot do without good ideas and theories. For one thing, we need theories about human development in later life. They guide us in what to look for when studying the lives of older adults. In his thought-provoking book, *The Force of Character and The Lasting Life*, eminent psychologist James Hillman (1999) pleas for a paradigm shift when we study oldness: "The move from lasting to leaving changes our basic attitude from holding on to letting go" (p. 53).

He depicts oldness as an adventure in its own right. It is the period, he claims, when our true nature emerges the most. Our final years serve an important purpose: the fulfillment and confirmation of one's character. "To be fully old, authentic in our being and available in our presence with its gravitas and eccentricity, indirectly affects the public good and thereby the good. This makes oldness a full-time job from which we may not retire" (p. 47). That is what good ideas and theories do: they place phenomena in a different perspective. They show us what to look for. In really advanced age, urges Hillman, we have to look for character. The study of character invites phenomenological approaches, so don't show up with questionnaires. Show up with good questions, with observations, and with a curious mind. This is a direction well understood by Linda Caissie in writing about the Raging Grannies (this volume). Of course, narrative gerontology is itself a theory that directs us to hermeneutical research in the first place. Within this grand theory, all kinds of (sub)theories that explain various phenonema are possible. A good example is the chapter by Mark Freeman (this volume), in which he discusses the concept of narrative foreclosure.

Research

Theories are closely linked to research, and this linkage can be considered in two ways. First, explorative research can help construct new theories. An often-adopted example is qualitative research based on the methods of grounded theory. Cappeliez and Webster (this volume) have used this approach in exploring the content of involuntary memories, which can help build theories about the functions of spontaneous reminiscence in daily life. Second, research can also serve to test theories and hypotheses based on theories. Such research can have implications for large health as well. The intervention "Dear Memories," described by Steunenberg and Bohlmeijer (this volume), is based on many years of research into the autobiographical memory system. The study of narratives and master narratives of older adults is the core business in narrative gerontology. Based on her study of narratives of aging bodies, Cassandra Phoenix (this volume) demonstrates how new narrative maps of aging can be developed and offered to younger people and thus contribute to healthy aging. The availability of a wide diversity of master narratives about aging in a society is of vital importance for large health. They open up possibilities for eudaimonia in later life that were not thought of before. Narrative research can reveal which master narratives are currently dominant in society and their possible impact on health. It can also give voice to previously unheard master narratives so that they become more available in the public domain, and thereby "thickened" in practice.

As is the case with theory, research in the narrative gerontological domain has a reciprocal relationship with interventions. Narrative inquiries can inform the development of new interventions. In their study of the management and integration of memories of traumatic war experiences, Burnell, Coleman, and Hunt (this volume) were able to show the important role of social support. Their research challenges professionals to develop new interventions that facilitate social support and thereby the integration of difficult and painful memories into the lifestories of war veterans. Conversely, research can show the effects of interventions based on narrative perspectives. A good balance of qualitative and quantitative methods is particularly suited to this context. Moreover, combining qualitative and quantitative methods in one design is a promising route to follow. Qualitative methods are excellent for measuring individual changes in meaning and behavior and they are sensitive to personal narratives, but by systematic coding and analysis of these narratives one is able to use statistics as well. Using this strategy, Tromp (this volume) was able to show that the use of lifestory books had significant effects on narrative coherence for older adults with Alzheimer's disease. But even within a narrative perspective, effectiveness studies alone are useful as well. If researchers can show that meaning in life and depression in older adults are significantly affected by narrative interventions (Westerhof, Bohlmeijer, Beljouw, & Pot, 2010), then why not make use of such approaches? We must remember, however, that within a framework of large health care, the reduction of health to an analysis of illnesses and symptoms of distress is not a primary goal as such, and that outcomes related to eudaimonia and human development are equally relevant. Moreover, we must remember that (randomized) controlled trials are in many ways about averages and not about real people. So the real challenge for a narrative turn in health care arises when decisions about evidence and finances are based only on quantitative studies and on randomized controlled trials in particular.

Interventions and Professional Attitude

In Part 3 of this volume, a wide range of interventions for different populations and in different settings has been presented. Following from this discussion, a common thread running through these interventions is that they are helpful in facilitating the living of a meaningful life. Reminiscence and storytelling interventions aim at finding ego-integrity, at discovering what projects still have to be taken up or finished to complete one's life cycle in a meaningful way. They may be helpful in accepting and expressing one's peculiar character and also, importantly, in social bonding and in resolving conflicts. Noonan (this volume) discusses the potential ripple effect of narrative interventions in nursing homes on families and workers. It will be interesting, and significant, to study this effect more systematically in the near future. Social relations and mutual understanding are central in inter-generational interventions as well (Westerhof, this volume). On the topic of relationships and mutual understanding, Singer and Messier (this volume) present a very helpful case study of the use of memories in couples therapy. The use of self-defining memories in the context of therapy is an exciting new road to take within the domain of narrative therapy. However, explicitly narrative or reminiscence interventions are not the only ones that fit well in large health care. Tai Chi (Kenyon, this volume), mindfulness (Hulsbergen, 2009), and other creative forms of therapies are examples of interventions particularly suited to a large health care. Such interventions directly empower caregivers to see, and both caregivers and care-receivers to experience and express, their unique vitality.

Along with the interventions just mentioned, a biographical encounter that deserves particular attention is that of the daily interaction between care-receivers and caregivers. From what perspective does one approach the other? What aspects of the encounter are given attention? How does one communicate? Asking the right questions is of vital importance. Marie-Elise van den Brandt-van Heek and Daphne Noonan clearly demonstrate the fundamental importance of and the need to realize large health within the interactions that characterize health care on a day-to-day basis—interactions between care-receivers, between care-receivers and caregivers, and between caregivers. This notion leads us directly to the important role of education.

Education

Professional attitude is formed primarily during one's years of formal education. We think that for students in psychology, gerontology, social work, and nursing, to mention just a few fields, there should be more empha-sis on education in philosophy, ethics, and narrative. Such education should be more practical than theoretical in nature, confronting students with real situations as they arise in practice. They should be encouraged to really dis-cover and discuss their own values and motives for working in their chosen domain. During their education, they should also become well acquainted with narrative perspectives on aging and with interventions based on these perspectives. It is our experience that teachers in the field of education are especially interested in narrative perspectives on aging and in large health care. This could turn out to be a very strategic, "silent" transformation that could have a significant impact on transforming health care.

Policy and Implementation

Last, but certainly not least, researchers and practitioners can have as many good ideas and theories and as much evidence as they like, but if politicians and managers are unwilling to invest in them, health care will not be transformed. One important strategy is to analyze current public policies and to uncover implicit discourses. Clark (this volume) demonstrates the importance of this issue in his chapter on facts and values in policies on home care. National associations of care organizations play an important role in the innovation of health care. Quality guidelines could prove to be a useful strategy for implementing narrative perspectives in health care. In this regard, Ubels (this volume) gives a good example of how she and her colleagues are moving slowly but steadily toward a large health care.

CONCLUSION

In this afterword, we have attempted to sketch the contours of the transformation of a thin story of health care toward a thicker story—that is, toward a narrative turn in health care. We have also indicated that what is needed for this transformation is a dynamic interplay between philosophers, theorists, practitioners, care-receivers, researchers, and policy makers. Thus, this narrative turn must, by definition, be multidisciplinary.

In addition, we have considered the issue that no single scientific method can claim exclusivity in determining the content and outcomes of health care. An urgent question remains as to how we can facilitate this transformation in practice, given the dominance of a thin economic perspective on current health care. One important strategy remains to be mentioned: that is, to show that large health care may in many ways be more capable of reducing costs than is current health care. In large health care, much responsibility is given back to the care-receiver. The philosophy of large health care would initiate reflection on aspects of life where medicine and psychology could or should be more limited. In other words, perhaps less emphasis should be placed on aspects of living that are too quickly "medicalized" or "psychologized" possibly because of a tendency to not accept suffering and the trend of claiming that a life without physical and psychological pain is natural. Dehue (2007), for example, conducted a thorough critical study of the origins of our current epidemic of depression. On the basis of her analysis, she concluded that at the heart of this epidemic are the ever-growing demands on people for productivity—i.e., the need to be "successful." "Depression" is a label for not being able to meet the demands of modern politics—that is, to be fully responsible for one's own destiny (see also de Lange, this volume).

In any case, a sudden, radical turn toward narrative in health care is not to be expected. However, if we continue to work on new theories, new interventions, and new policies, and if we continue to point out the counterproductive effects of current (small) health care and the meaningful effects of alternative interventions and policies, then who knows what turns health care will take in the future. We certainly hope that this volume, which demonstrates that substantial progress can indeed be made through use of narrative, proves helpful in the process.

REFERENCES

Burr, V. (1995). An introduction to social constructionism. London: Routledge.

Charon, R. (2004). Narrative and medicine. *New England Journal of Medicine, 350*, 862–864.

Davey, G. (2008). *Psychopathology, research, assessment, and treatment in clinical psychology*. Chichester, UK: John Wiley & Sons.

Dehue, T. (2007). *De depressie epidemie* [The depression epidemic]. Amsterdam: Uitgeverij Augustus.

Frank, A. (1995). *The wounded storyteller, body, illness, and ethics*. Chicago: University of Chicago Press.

Gass, D. (2001). Narrative knowledge and health care of the elderly. In G. Kenyon, P. Clark, & B. de Vries (Eds.), *Narrative gerontology: Theory, research, and practice* (pp. 215–236). New York: Springer.

Giddens, A. (1991). *Modernity and self-identity: Self and society in the late modern age*. Cambridge, UK: Polity Press.

Hillman, J. (1999). *The force of character and the lasting life*. New York: Random House.

Hulsbergen, M. (2009). Mindfulness. *De aandachtsvolle therapeut* [The therapist's full attention]. Amsterdam: Uitgeverij Boom.

Kenyon, G., & Randall, W. (2001). Narrative gerontology: An overview. In G. Kenyon, P. Clark, & B. de Vries (Eds.), *Narrative gerontology: Theory, research, and practice* (pp. 3–18). New York: Springer.

Keyes, C. (2005). Mental illness and/or mental health? Investigating axioms of the complete state model of health. *Journal of Consulting and Clinical Psychology, 73*(3), 539–548.

Keyes, C. (2006). Mental health in adolescence: Is America's youth flourishing? *American Journal of Orthopsychiatry, 76*(3), 395–402.

Keyes, C. (2007). Promoting and protecting mental health as flourishing: A complementary strategy for improving national mental health. *American Psychologist, 62*(2), 95–108.

Nussbaum, M. (1990). *Love's knowledge.* New York: Oxford University Press.

Randall, W., & Kenyon, G. (2002). Reminiscence as reading our lives: Toward a wisdom environment. In J. Webster & B. Haight (Eds.), *Critical advances in reminiscence: Theoretical, empirical, and clinical perspectives* (pp. 233–253). New York: Springer.

Randall, W., & McKim, A. (2008). *Reading our lives: The poetics of growing old.* New York: Oxford University Press.

Verduin, P. (1998). *De vraag naar het lichaam: Filosofie van lichamelijkheid in de gezondheidszorg.* [The demand for the body: On the philosophy of bodily health]. Maarssen, The Netherlands: Elsevier/de Tijdstroom.

Verduin, P. (2007). *Chronisch ziek en toch gezond: Theorie en praktijk van de integratieve gezondheidszorg* [Chronically ill and still healthy: Theory and practice of integrative healthcare]. The Hague, The Netherlands: Uitgeverij Lemma.

Westerhof, G., Bohlmeijer, E., Beljouw, I., & van Pot, A. (2010). Improvement in personal meaning mediates the effects of a life-review intervention on depressive symptoms in a randomized controlled trial. *The Gerontologist.* Advance online publication: doi:10.1093/geront/gnp168.

World Health Organization (2004). *Promoting mental health: Concepts, emerging evidence, practice* (summary report). Geneva, Switzerland: Author.

Index

Acceptance, 243–44, 279

Accountable Care, 322–24

Activism

empowerment and, 139

feminism and, 126–27

humor and, 137

past and, 138

by Raging Grannies, 128

social identity and, 130

Activity theory, 29–30

ActiZ, 320, 326, 328, 331, 335

Acute-care services, 87

Adults, 308

Affect, 199

Affective skills, 373

Affect regulation hypothesis, 295

Age

gender identity crossover and, 152–53

narrative and, 143–44

segregation, 307–9

social policies and, 308

stereotypes, 309–10

Aged by Culture (Gulette), 113

The Ageless Self (Kaufman), 239

Agency, 14, 146

Aging, 242–43

alternative storylines about, 120

arrested, 116

autobiographical memory and,
297–98

community subtext, 91–92

growing while, 29–30

inner v. outer, 238–40

meaning to, 113

metaphor, wisdom and, 31–34

narrative fate of, 116

narrative mapping of, 118–20

physical, 30

portrayal of, 214

reminiscence and, 187, 254

successful, 191

temporal dimension of, 75

wisdom and, 31–34

working memory and, 298

*Aging and Biography: Explorations in Adult
Development* (Birren, Kenyon,
Ruth, Schroots, & Svensson), xiv

À la recherche du temps perdu (Proust),
68, 180

Alzheimer's disease, 240–41, 248

Ambiguity, 369

Amends making, 30

American Psychological Association, 311

Amsterdam Longitudinal Aging
Study, 309

Anamnēsis, 178–79, 186, 191, 192n1

Androgyny, 146, 154

Aristotle, 67, 178, 192n1

Army Corps of Engineers, 172

Art, 5–6, 7–8, 275, 350–52

Artist/God, 6

Assisted living, 14

Athletes, 112

Athletic bodies, 116–18

older, 120–23

young, 113–16

Autobiographical memory, 21, 292–95
    aging and, 297–98
    assessment of, 300–302
    depression and, 296–97, 302–3
    episodic, 297
    importance in restorying of, 302
    overgeneral, 295–96
    personality traits and, 300–301
    positive events in, 300
    protocol, 298–99
    retrieval, 296, 297
    sample questions, 298–99
    self and, 294
    specific, 295
Autobiographies, 28, 164. *See also* Memoirs
    expression through , 30
    groups, 276
    guided, 26, 143, 147–49, 297
    through interview, 255–56
Autonomy, 312, 340
Awareness, 161
    critical, 123
    of finiteness, 239
    memory loss and, 17
    shifts, 333

Bachelard, Gaston, 69
Bakhtin, M. M., 69
Baldwin, Christina, 34
Barclay, Craig, 26
Barnes, Djuna, 78
Baudrillard, Jean, 69
Baumann, Zygmunt, 55
Beck, Ulrich, 55
Beer, Gillian, 71
Benevolence, 260
Bergson, Henri, 68
Berman, Harry, 27
Bern Sex Role Inventory (BSRI), 145
Best practices, 332–33
Biographers, 357
    connectedness with, 361
    empowerment and, 363
    meaning-making and, 359
    training of, 357
Biographical aging, 22

Biographical capital, 29
Biographical construction, 39
    definitional consequences of, 40
    play of, 40–42
    shared understandings and, 49
Biographical diversity, 45–49
Birren, James, xiii–xiv, xvii, 147, 366–67
Birthday charts, 349f
Black, Helen, 242, 244
Blogging, 275
Blue Highways: A Journey into America
    (Moon), 20–21
Bodies, 111. *See also* Athletic bodies
    high-performance, 112
    predictability of, 119
Bodybuilding, 112, 120–21, 124
Bohlmeijer, Ernst, xiv, xvi, 31
Böszörményi-Nagy, Iván, 59
Bourdieu, Pierre, 69
Brain
    attributes of, 30
    exercises, 238
    rearrangements of, 32
BSRI. *See* Bern Sex Role Inventory
Bunyan, John, 58
Burnell, Karen, xv
Burnout, 374
Butler, Robert, 273–74, 291

Caissie, Linda, xv, xvii, 375
Canada, 85–86
Canada Health Act, 88
    counterstories and, 93
    ethical imperative of, 94
    principles of, 89–90
    Romanow Commission Report and, 89
Canadian Association on Gerontology, 91
Canadian Journal on Aging, 91
Cappeliez, Philippe, xvi, 192
Caregivers
    as characters, 321
    dementia and, 338
    organization of, 329–30
    skills of, 327
Care organizations, 321, 329–30, 378
Cather, Willa, 70

"Celebrating Our Stories" program,
    355–57
Center for Psychogerontology of Radboud
    University, 312
Chandler, Sally, 31
Change
    learning and, 332
    suffering and loss and, 240–43
Characters, caregivers as, 321
Charmé, Stuart, 28
Charon, Rita, xiii, xv, 332, 373
Children, 308
    affective relationship with, 278–79
    independence and, 281
    life review and, 280
    rearing, 146
Christian Association of Healthcare
    Organization, 270
Clark, Phillip, xv, xvi
Client Quality Index, 323, 335
Clients
    lifestories and, 324–25
    orientation, 323
Cognitive-behavioral therapy, 277
Cognitive impairments, 299
Cognitive psychology, 178
Cognitive therapy, mindfulness-based, 297
Cohen, Gene, 30, 32
Coherence. See also Narrative coherence
    autobiographical memory and, 293
    externalization and, 268
    integration v., 263
    life review and, 263t, 264t, 279
    in lifestories, 256–57
    social support and, 201–3
    trauma and, 195, 197–98
Cole, Thomas, 31
Coleman, Peter, xv
Collaboration, 356
Collages, 282, 284
Columbia University, 332
Comments, reflective, 123
Communal traits, 146, 155
Communication
    age stereotypes in, 309–10
    comradeship and, 203–4

cross-generational, 316
    patterns, 220–21
Communism, 284
Community care, 88
Compassion, 225, 369
Competition, 121
Compliance, 334
Comradeship, 203–4
Concentration camps, 9, 109
Conflict resolution, 279, 292
Connectedness, 360–62, 373
Contact, cross-generational, 312–13
Contemplation, 368
Content, 163
Context, 143, 173
Continuity
    autobiographical memory and, 293
    identifying, 292
    theory, 277
Control
    locus of, 156
    premise of, 369–70
    societal, 52
Conversations
    with persons with dementia, 346–47
    soulful, 28
Core care, xv, 321
Cost-effectiveness, 334, 372
Counterstories, 86, 91–93, 122
    disability community, 92–93
    narrative of decline and, 139
    public policy analysis and, 94
    of Raging Grannies, 129–30
Couples therapy, 221–22
Creative skills, 373
Crisis intervention, 220
Critical narrativity, 86–87
Crossley, Michelle, 197
Csikszentmihalyi, Mihaly, 19
Cultural storylines, 4
    deconstructing, 14–15
    internalizing, 6, 10
    reification of, 117
Culture
    shifts, 333
    vision and, 332

Daily care, for persons with dementia, 347–48

Day-to-day activities, 354

"Dear Memories" program, 375

Death, 273
  life review before, 292
  preparation, 182

The Death of Ivan Ilych (Tolstoy), 11–12

De Beauvoir, Simone, 239

De Certeau, Michael, 69, 76

Dedication, 364

Deinstitutionalization, of society, 60

De Lange, Fritz, xv

De Medeiros, Kate, xvi, 31

Dementia, 4–5, 240–41
  appropriate questions in, 342–46
  art exhibitions and, 350–52
  basic needs for, 341
  caregivers and, 338
  constraints of, 341
  conversations with persons with, 346–47
  daily care for persons with, 347–48
  depression and, 350
  hidden-and-succumbed stage of, 340
  language and, 340–41
  lifestories and, 341
  lost me stage of, 340
  painting and, 350–51
  privacy and, 349
  spirituality and, 248
  stages of, 339–40
  threatened me stage of, 339–40
  triggers and, 343
  visualized stories and, 348
  well-being and, 339–40

Demystification, 8

Depression
  autobiographical memory and, 296–97, 302–3
  characteristics of, 56
  collective, 108
  contamination memories and, 223
  dementia and, 350
  epidemic of, 379
  identity construction and, 51–52
  interventions for, 290
  life review and, 291–92
  Looking for Meaning in Life and, 281–83
  prevalence of, 291
  prevention, 325–26
  reminiscences and, 275
  rumination and, 296
  "Searching for Meaning" and, 326

Depressive symptoms, 281
  life review for, 291
  reduction in, 301–2

Desocialization, 8

Dialogue, 330–32

Diaries, 180

Dionigi, Rylee, 122

Disengagement theory, 29–30

Drawing, 284

Drouin, Héloïse, 192

The Drowned and the Saved (Levi), 9–11

Dubar, Claude, 57–58

Eakin, Paul John, 26

Economic paradox, 324

Education, 377–78
  adult, 308
  gender stereotypes and, 154–55
  stereotypes and, 316

Ego-integration, 253, 255, 269

Ehrenberg, Alain, 56

Eichberg, Henning, 115

Eldercare
  lack of respect for, 327
  life review and, 252–54
  narrative care in, 335
  narrative focus in, 321
  in Netherlands, 319–20

Elderspeak, 309

Embodiment, 118

Emotional management
  negative memories and, 184–85
  reminiscence and, 183

Emotions
  focus on, 343–44
  gender and, 144
  mutual reminiscences and, 216–17
  narrative coherence and, 198–99
  processing, 293

questions regarding dementia
        and, 345–46
re-creation of, 282
regulation, 276
reminiscence and, 187
self-defining memories and, 222
spontaneous reminiscences and, 181
storytelling and, 342
Empowerment, 139, 362–65
Engagement, 374
Enjoyment, 365
Envy, 4–5
Episodic characteristics, 259
Episodic memory, 214, 293–94, 297
Equanimity, 47–48
Erikson, Erik, 53, 252–53, 338
Ethics, 372
    language, 86
    public, 86
Etymologies (Isidore of Seville), 67
Eudaimonia, 368
Eurobarometer study, 308–9
Evaluative function, 258
Existential despair, 11–12
Existentialism, 53
Existential psychoanalysis, 28
Experience
    of competition, 121
    critical, 184
    feminism and, 138
    individual, 44
    recreation of, 282
Expressive traits, 145*f*
Externalization, 267–68, 267

Facts
    narrative frame and, 85–86
    public policy analysis and, 94
Family
    connectedness and, 361
    empowerment, 363
    genealogy, 275
    intergenerational solidarity, 278
    meaning-making and, 359
    memories of, 183
    narrative coherence and, 204

self-defining memories and, 223
    support, 209
Feminine traits, 151, 152*f*
Feminism, 126–27
    experience and, 138
    gerontology and, 128
Finiteness, 239, 369
First Ministers' Health Accord, 89–90
The Force of Character and the Lasting Life
        (Hillman), 374–75
Forgetting, intentional, 188–89
Formal organization, 257
Forster, E. M., 70
Fortunoff Video Archive for Holocaust
        Testimonies, 108–9
Foucault, Michel, 57
Fragmentation, 201, 257
Frank, Arthur, 111
Frankl, Viktor, 241
Freeman, Mark, xiii, xv, 21–22, 116,
        249, 375
Free recall, 297
Freud, Sigmund, 53
Friedman, Susan Stanford, 69
Friendships, 204, 282, 284
Frye, Northrop, 261
Fundamental projects, 28

Galen, 67
Ganzevoort, R. Ruard, 269
Gardner, Howard, 32
Gender
    identity crossover, 146–47, 152–53
    narrative and, 143–44
    norms, 144–46
    role ideologies, 149–51
    roles, 144–46
    stereotypes, 148–49, 153–56
    trait development, 156
General events, 294
Generations, xiii
Generativity, 30, 184
Genette, Gérard, 68
Genres, 162–63, 164
Geography, 154
Geriatrics, 80

German Wehrmacht, 103–4
Germany, 101–3
Gerontology
    feminist, 128
    hermeneutical, 27
    literary, 21
    multidisciplinary aspect of, xvi
    urgency of spaces and, 79–80
Gerotranscendence, 269
Geschichte und Erinnerung, 105
Getzels, J. W., 19
Giddens, Anthony, 55
Glavey, Brian, 78
Goldberg, Elkhonon, 33
Goldman, Emma, 136
Governmentality, 60
Goyal, Rishi, xv
"Green and Gray" program, 307, 312–16
Greimas, A. J., 69
Group-defining moments, 166–69
Growth
    involuntary reminiscences and,
        190–91
    ripple effect and, 358–60
Guided imagery, 26
Guided imaginative recall, 282–83
Guilt, 9
Guindon, Marilyn, 192
Gulette, Margarette Morganroth, 113
Gulf War Syndrome (GWS), 199–200
Guttman, David, 146
GWS. *See* Gulf War Syndrome

Habits
    role identity and, 61
    spatial attachment and, 80
Haight, Barbara, 279
Hamilton, Margaret, 226
Hampl, Patricia, 25, 31
Health Canada, 88
Health care
    biases within, 368–71
    Canadian, 86
    current, 366–68
    future of, 371–74
    large, 371–72

moral authority within, 88
    narrative turn in, 374–78
Health Council of Canada, 90
Hen Co-op, 139
Herman, David, 69
Hillman, James, 374–75
Historical understanding, 280
History, 71, 108, 275
Hitler, Adolf, 103
Hochschild, Arlie Russell, 42–44
Holocaust, 107, 241
Holocaust (film), 102–3
Holocaust Memorial, 103
Home care
    advantages of, 89
    background, 87–88
    disability community and, 92–93
    expansion of, 90–91
    NACA and, 92
    policy, 85
    values, 88–89
Homes, 282
Hope, 10, 12
Horace, 67
Huizing, Wout, 339, 343
Hulsbergen, Monique, 372–73
Humanism, 372
Humility, 246
Humor, 136–38
Hunt, Nigel, xv
Hussey, Mark, 72

Identity, 17. *See also* Narrative identity
    acceptable , 132–33
    amalgams, 59
    bodies and, 111
    decaying, 340
    final, 53
    forms of*t*, 59
    gender crossover, 146–47, 152–53
    generative, 206
    as holistic desire, 53–54
    life events and, 302
    life review and, 253
    maintaining, 207
    narrative and, 21–22

personal, 52–53
  reflexive, 57
  reminiscences and, 187, 190
  renegotiation, 206
  role, 58, 60–61
  salience, 63
  social, 130
  societal, 57
  societal control and, 52
  status, 58, 144–46
  symbolic, 62
  typology, 57–58
  virtual, 63
Identity construction
  depression and, 51–52
  pressure of, 54–56
  as self-reflexive project, 55
Illegal substances, 124
Imagination, loss of, 117
Independence, 281
Infiniteness, 369
Information gain, 276
Inner life, 144
  Integration, 199, 257
  internalization and, 268
  in life review, 263t, 264t
  narrative coherence v., 263
  narrative length and, 260
Intergenerational legacy, 280
Interiority, 144
Internalization, 267–68, 267f
*International Institute for Reminiscence
  and Life Review*, xiv
Interpersonal relations
  inequities in, 218
  reminiscence and, 187
Interplay, 41–42, 49
Interventions, xiv, 366
  for depression, 290
  moral deliberation and, 328
  narrative-based, xv
  peer support, 208
  professional attitude and,
    376–77
  reminiscence, 273
  research and, 376

Interviews
  active, 129
  autobiographies through, 255–56
  between children and parents, 278
  life review, 276
  narrative form of, 161
  with Raging Grannies, 129
  taboo and, 105–6
Intimacy maintenance, 182
Introspection, 172–73
Investigations, xiv
Iraq War, 196
Irrevocability, 8–12
Isidore of Seville, 67
Isolation, 76

The Jack-Roller (Shaw), 40
James, Henry, 68
Johnson, Myrtle, 46–47
Jones, Jana, 355
Josselson, Ruth Ellen, 21
Journal of Aging Studies, xiii
Journey to life, 238, 243–45
Judgment, 347
Jung, Carl, 146

Kahn, Stephen P., 19
Kaufman, Sharon, 239
Kaufmann, Jean-Claude, 53
Kenyon, Gary, xiv, xvi
King's Centre for Military Health
  Research, 208
Knipscheer, Kees, 61
Knowledge, 370
  basis for, 370–71
  for narrative turn in health care, 374–78
  ongoing accumulation of, 120
  questions regarding dementia and,
    344–45
  solidarity, 372
  storytelling and, 342
Kordelaar, Karen van, 315
Kunneman, Harry, 329

Labouvie-Vief, Giselle, 32
L'Amour, Louis, 20

Language, 299
  age stereotypes and, 309–10
  in conversations with persons with
      dementia, 346
  dementia and, 340–41
  ethics, 86
  in guided autobiographies, 148
Laub, Dori, 108–9
Lawton, Mortimer Powell, 80
Learning
  change and, 332
  lifelong, 120, 308
Leo Hayes High School, 362
Letters, 164
Levi, Primo, 9–12
Lévi-Strauss, Claude, 57
Life-as-story, 23, 237
The LifeBio Memory Journal
      (Sanders), 365n1
Life curve model, 115–17, 115f
Life events
  age-related, 277, 302
  disruptive, 277
  identity and, 302
  meaning from, 185–86
  painful, 31
  processing, 184
  recalling, 188
Life experiences. See Experience
Life review, 183, 274, 276–77, 279
  benefits of, 279–80
  central hypothesis, 255
  before death, 292
  depression and, 291–92
  development of, 253–54
  eldercare and, 252–54
  historical understanding and, 280
  independence and, 280
  integration in, 263t, 264t
  narrative coherence in, 263t, 264t, 279
  opportunities for, 286
  overlap with reminiscence, 278
  participation in, 264–67
  positive effects of, 301–2
  research, 254
  as self-help, 278–83

solidarity and, 280
theory, 252–53
therapy, 277
training, 286
well-being and, 291–92
wisdom environment and, 285
"The Life Review: An Interpretation of
      Reminiscence in the Aged" (Butler),
      273–74
Life satisfaction, 185
Life-Space Assessments, 80
Life stages, 66–67
Lifestories, 25, 197
  age differences in, 215–16
  clients and, 324–25
  coherent, 177, 183
  components of, 185
  cross-generational contact through, 313
  dementia and, 341
  diversity of, 45
  fluid structure of, 195
  narrative coherence in, 256–57
  needs assessments, 307–12
  research, 325
  schemas, 294
  social relations and, 307
  source of, 244
  spoken v. written, 163
  transference of, 280
Lifestory books, 254, 343, 376
  "Mapping My Life" and, 326
  standardized, 255
Lifetime periods, 294
Literary competence, 33–34
Literary gerontology, 21
Literature, 6, 127
"Living and Working with a Story" method,
      340–41, 344–45
Living conditions, 322
LOC, 331
Logos, 368
Long-term care
  biographical diversity in, 45–49
  home care v., 87–88
  narrative care and, 354
Looking for Meaning in Life, 281–83, 286

Loss, 237–38
  acceptance and, 243
  age-related, 302
  suffering, change and, 240–43
Loss-deficit model, 213
Love, lack of, 283–84
Lukács, Georg, 68

Magical mastery, 269
Management, 329–30, 332
Mann, Thomas, 68
"Mapping My Life," 326
Marks, Stephan, xv
Markus, Hazel, 60
Martial arts, 245
Masculine traits*f*, 150, 151*f*
Mastery, 269, 276, 373–74
The Mature Mind (Cohen), 30
McAdams, Dan, 21, 25–26, 55
McKim, Elizabeth, 21–22, 80
Meaning, 18, 22–25
  to aging, 113
  from life events, 185–86
  life review and, 276, 279, 292
  in narratives, 256–62
  over time, 27–29
  in particulars, 48
  plasticity of, 23
  process of, 24
  suffering and, 242
  from trauma, 197–98, 207
Meaningful order, 260
Meaning-making, 196
  bodies and, 111
  research, 207
  ripple effect and, 358–60
  storytelling and, 112
The Measure of My Days (Scott-Maxwell),
    244–45
Medications, 238, 367
Meditation, 245
Memoirs, 163, 164. *See also* Autobiographies
Memorability, 18
Memory, 22–25. *See also* Autobiographical
    memory; Self-defining memories
  categorical, 295

childhood, 226
as compost heap, 106
contamination, 223
contextualizing, 184
conveying metaphors, 25–26
descriptors, 295
episodic, 214, 293–94, 297
extended, 295
fading, 349
of family, 183
generic, 33
involuntary, 178
long-term, 292–93
loss, 17
mechanics of, 22
metaphors evoking, 26–27
multiple systems of, 292–93
negative, 184–85
positive, 276
priming system, 293
procedural, 293
relationship-defining, 217, 227
repisodic, 33
research, 214
searches, 296
semantic, 214, 293
spatial attachment and, 79–80
specificity of, 299
triggers, 180
voluntary, 178
working, 298
"Memory and Imagination" (Hampl), 31
Men, 145–46
Mental health
  care system, 367
  definition of, 368–70
  functions of reminiscence and, 273–75
  two-continua model of, 368
Mental illness, 368
Messier, Beata Labunko, xvi
Metamemory, 189–90
Metamorphosis (Ovid), 67
Metaphor, 22–25
  aging, wisdom and, 31–34
  evoking memories, 26–27
  memories conveying, 25–26

Metaphoric competence, 32

Metaphorizing process, 24

Metaphors of Aging in Science and the Humanities (Kenyon, Birren, & Schroots), xiv

Metaphors of Self (Olney), 23–24

Metropolitan Museum of Art, 80

Middle age

   gender stereotypes and, 154–55

   old age v., 146

Mindfulness, 297, 377

Mini Mental State Exam (MMSE), 164, 165*t*

Mitscherlich, Alexander, 108

Mitscherlich, Margarethe, 108

MMSE. *See* Mini Mental State Exam

Mnëmë, 178–79, 188–89, 191, 192n1

Mnemonic interlock, 296

Moon, William Least Heat, 20–21

Moral authority, in health care system, 88

Moral deliberation, 328

Moral suasion, 92

Morrison, Mary, 242–43

Moser, Tilman, 109

Motivation, 6–7

Multiple memory systems, 292–93

Music, 136–38

My Life in Fragments (van den Brand-van Heek & Huizing), 338, 343

NACA. *See* National Advisory Council on Aging

Names, 59–60

Narrating process, 258

Narrative care

   as core care, xv, 321

   in eldercare, 335

   enhancing, 324–30

   future of, 335–36

   guidelines, 364

   long-term care and, 354

   stories in, 249

   Tai Chi and, 245–50

Narrative ceremonies, 357, 360

Narrative coherence

   analysis protocol, 202*t*

   comradeship and, 203–4

   criteria, 200*t*

   defined, 198–99

   friends and family and, 204

   societal support and, 204–5

Narrative Discourse (Genette), 68

Narrative events, 39–40, 49

Narrative exposure therapy (NET), 208

Narrative Fiction: Contemporary Poetics (Rimmon-Kenan), 69

Narrative foreclosure, 3–4, 269

   athletic bodies and, 116

   history of, 5–7

   hope in, 12

   identity and, 54

   older athletic bodies and, 120–23

   young athletic bodies and, 116–18

Narrative frame, 85

   developing, 85–87

   emergence of dominant, 87–91

   in public policy analysis, 93–94

   redefining, 269

Narrative gerontology, 366

   exclusiveness of, 367–68

   focus of, 320

   premise of, 24

   reminiscences and, 183

   suffering and loss and, 237–38

Narrative Gerontology: Theory, Research, and Practice (Birren), xiii

Narrative identity, 51

   construction, 56–58

   disruption of, 206

   history of, 58

   integrative role of, 58–62

   social support and, 205–6

   version light, 62–64

Narrative inquiry, 198–201, 376

Narrative intelligence, 197

Narrative Knowing and the Human Sciences (Polkinghorne), 22

Narrative mapping, 118–20, 139, 326

Narrative Matters, xiii

Narrative occasions, 41

Narrative order, 262

Narrative organization, 257–58*f*, 257, 258*f*

Narrative psychology, 24

Narratives
    age and, 143–44
    communities, 321
    competence, 373
    connectedness and, 360–61
    damage caused by, 10–11
    of decline, 24, 113, 139
    density, 259
    dialogue and, 331
    dominant cultural, 122
    epiphenomenal level of, 259–60
    exchange of, 361
    fate, 116
    focus in eldercare of, 321
    forces, 8, 68
    form, 161
    freedom, 8
    gender and, 143–44
    identity and, 21–22
    of inexorable decline, 15
    lengths of, 260
    levels in, 258
    meaning in, 256–62
    metaphenomenal level of, 260
    need for, 370
    origins of, 177
    patterns, 263f, 264f
    phenomenal level of, 259
    policy, 84
    poor dear, 42–45
    progress, 134
    quality, 256–57
    of Raging Grannies, 128–29
    of self-sufficiency, 15
    shared structure, 44
    templates, 23
    therapies, 56, 277
    written, 162–63
    written v. spoken, 172–73
Narrativity, critical, 86–87
Narratology, 68–69
National Advisory Council on Aging
    (NACA), 92
National Conference on Home
    Care, 88
National Health Service (UK), 208

National Partnership on Depression
        Prevention (Netherlands), 326
National Socialism, 102
Nazi Party, 101–3, 105
Needs assessments, 307–12
Neisser, Ulrich, 33
Nelson, Hilde, 122
NET. *See* Narrative exposure therapy
Netherlands, xvi, 299, 308
    eldercare in, 319–20
    Looking for Meaning in Life in, 286
    obligatory retirement age in, 308
    reminiscence interventions in, 273
Networking, 329
Network program, 328–29
Neugarten, Bernice, 146
Neurogenesis, 30
Nietzsche, Friedrich, 55, 369
Nightwood (Barnes), 78
Noonan, Daphne, xvi–xvii
Novels, 68
NSDAP. *See* Nazi Party
Nursing homes
    as hotel, 48
    as life event, 292
    patronizing behavior in, 311
    stereotypes, 310

Old age
    duration of, 67
    loss of self in, 74
    middle age v., 146
    reclaiming, 131–33
    trauma in, 196
    Woolf and, 71
Older adults, 308
    autonomy of, 312
    demographics, 213
    frail, 338
    stereotypes, 309–11
    well-being in, 291–92
Olney, James, 23–24
O'Neill, Patricia, xvii
Oneness, 16
On Genesis Against the Manichees
        (Saint Augustine), 67

On Rhetoric (Aristotle), 67
Open Cards, 255
Openness, 314–15
Opinions
    focus on, 343–44
    questions regarding dementia and,
        345–46
    storytelling and, 342
Oral histories, 275
Organization, 329–30
Organized modernity, 52–53
Orientating function, 258
Ovid, 67

Pain, 240, 379. *See also* Suffering
Painting, 350–51
Parent, Marion, 136
Parent-child relationship, 278
Parents, 278–80
Participants, finding, 333
Parva Naturalia (Aristotle), 178
Passive mastery, 269
Past, 3–4, 28, 138
Pathos, 179
Patience, 347, 364
Patronizing behavior, 311
Pattern recognition, 33
Peer support, 208
Persona, 132–33
Personal identity. *See* Identity
Personality
    reminiscence and, 183
    traits, 300–301
Personal subjectivity, 52
Pet therapy, 248
Philosophic homework, 30
Philosophy, 372, 374
Phoenix, Cassandra, xv, 375
Photographs, 284
Piaget, Jean, 32
Pilgrim's Progress (Bunyan), 58
Pinnacle event of life, 197
Play, 41–42, 49
Plot, 261
Poetics, 21, 70, 78
The Poetics of Space (Bachelard), 69

Poetry, 164
    first-person story v., 170t
    self-refining moments in, 167
Polkinghorne, Donald, 22–23, 27
Poor dear hierarchy, 43–45
Positivity effect, 276
Possibility, 8
Postformal thought, 21, 32
Practice of Everyday Life (de Certeau), 76
Praxis, 368
Pride, 364
Privacy, 349
Process
    narrating, 258
    self-expression and, 163
    of self-presentation, 173
Professional attitude, 376–77
Professionals, 310–11, 327–29, 372
Professional settings, 310–11, 316
Program in Narrative Medicine, 332
Protestant Theological University, 269
Protoselves, 26
Proust, Marcel, 68, 180
Psychotherapy, 213, 296
Public exhibitions, 350–52
Public policy, xvi, 84, 378
    analysis, 93–94
    discourse, 88–89
    frame, 87

Quality Assurance Framework for
        Responsible Care, 322–23, 335
Quality guidelines, 378
Quality of care, 322–24
Questions, 377
    appropriate, 342–46
    autobiographical memory, 298–99
    ethical, 372
    leading, 347
    slow, 320–21, 330, 334–35, 371

Raging Grannies, xv, xvii, 126–28, 375
    discussion about, 129–30, 129–38
    humor and, 137
    narratives of, 128–29
Randall, L. William, xiv, xvi, 80, 106

Rau, Johannes, 104
Ray, Ruth, 31–32
Reconciliation, of trauma, 200, 207
Redemption, 222
Referential function, 258
"Reflect-on," 330
Reflexivity, habits v., 61
Religion
    suicide and, 46–47
    symbolic identity and, 62
    totality and, 53–54
Remembering, 179
Reminiscence, 162
    aging and, 254
    avoiding, 196
    bump, 25, 180, 214
    death preparation, 182
    defined, 188, 274
    escapist, 182
    etymology of, 192n1
    framework for implementing, 275–78
    functions of, 260, 273–75
    impact of, 188–89
    instrumental, 181
    integrative, 182
    interventions, 273
    intimacy maintenance and, 182
    involuntary, 179–80, 190–91
    as life review, 183
    metamemory and, 189–90
    mutual, 216–17
    narrative, 181–82
    narrative approach to, 183–86
    obsessive, 182
    opportunities for, 286
    overlap with life review, 278
    reconstructive nature of, 274
    research, 286
    simple, 276
    spontaneous, 180–83, 253
    structured, 253–54
    taxonomy of, 178
    themes, 187, 187t
    theories, 186–88
    transmissive, 181
    triggers, 189

    voluntary, 274
    wisdom environment and, 285
Reminiscence and the Self in Old Age
    (Sherman), 22
Reminiscence Functions Scale, 178
Reminiscence groups, 159, 165
    group-defining moments in, 168–69
    self-presentation in, 166
    writing groups v., 169–72
Research, 366
    empirical, 94
    hermeneutical, 375
    large health care and, 372
    life review, 254
    lifestories, 325
    mixed methods, 286
    for narrative turn in health care,
        375–76
    self-defining memories, 214–16
Restorying, 239, 297
    guided, 292
    importance of autobiographical
        memory in, 302
    journey to life and, 243–44
    through Tai Chi, 238
Retirement
    age, 308
    role identity in, 61
Rewriting the Self (Freeman), 22
Ricoeur, Paul, 23, 68, 178, 192n1
Rimmon-Kenan, Shlomith, 69
Rinehart, Peter, 42, 46–49
Ripple effect, 357–62, 358f, 377
Roles
    distance, 60
    gender, 144–46
    gender, ideologies, 149–51
    identity, 58
    playing, reverse, 217
Romanow Commission Report, 86,
        89–91
A Room of One's Own (Woolf), 71
Rowles, Graham, 79–80
Rubenstein, Robert, 80
Rumination, 296
Ruth, Jan-Erik, xiv

Saint Augustine, 67
Salvation Army, 290
Sanders, Beth, 365n1
Sangha, 247
Sarton, May, 27
Sartre, Jean-Paul, 28
Schroots, Johannes, xiv
Scientific methods, 370
Scott-Maxwell, Florida, 244–45
Scrapbooking, 275
"Searching for Meaning," 326
Secularization, 67
Self
    actual, 63
    autobiographical memory
        and, 294
    complementary, 161
    conceptual, 294
    defining, 160–62
    defining one's, 130–31
    expressions of, 159
    externally presented, 161
    hypothesized, 243
    idealized, 63
    long-term, 294
    loss of, 74
    nominal, 59–60
    plurality of, 58–62
    possible, 118
    reflective, 114–16
    settled, 114–15
    sporting, 114–15
    unified, 160
    universal, 160
    working, 62, 294
Self-acceptance, 276
Self-actualization, 55
Self-aging, 113–16
Self-concept, 144
Self-creation, myth of, 56–58
Self-defining memories, 25, 214–15
    application of, 228
    in couples therapy, 221–22
    criteria, 221
    examples, 229–31
    exchange of, 224–25

interpreting, 222–24
    research, 214–16
Self-defining moments, 166–68
Self-efficacy, 373–74
Self-esteem, 144
Self-expression, 163
Self-forgetfulness, 15
Self-forgiveness, 10
Self-help, life review as, 278–83
Self Memory System (SMS), 294
Self-perception, 6, 339–40
Self-presentation, 160
    in group work, 162–63
    influences on, 173
    spoken v. written, 166
Self-reporting, 147
Self-schemata, 60
Self-sufficiency, 15
Self-understanding
    crisis of, 24
    horizon of, 27
    independence and, 281
    life review and, 279
    wisdom and, 25
Self-worth, 261
Sensei, 247
Shame, 9–10
Shaw, Clifford, 40
Sherman, Edmund, 22, 243
Signal Corps, 172
Signature stories, 25
Silence, 41, 108
Sin, 10
Singer, Jefferson, xvi
The Singing of the Real World
    (Hussey), 72
Sitedness, 69
Skills development, 332
Slow questions, 320–21, 330, 334–35, 371
SMS. See Self Memory System
"Snapshots of Life" exhibition,
    351–52, 352f
Social constructionism, 370
Socialization, 118
Social links, 189
Social networks, 308–9

Social participation, 322
Social policies, 308
Social relations, 307
Social responsibility reports, 322
Social return on investment (SROI), 324
Social role theory, 145
Social support
    narrative coherence and, 201–3
    narrative identity and, 205–6
    trauma and, 196–97
    for trauma integration, 198
    value of, 207
Social workers, 310–11
Societal support, 204–5, 312
Socioemotional selectivity theory, 184, 276
Solidarity, 280–81, 369
    among professionals, 372
Space, 70, 76
    public, reclaiming, 133–34
    time v., 77
    trust and, 332
    urgency of, 79–80
Sparkes, Andrew, 111
Spatial attachment, 79–80
Spatial ordering, 75
Speaking, 161–62
Spiritual confession, 28
Spirituality, 245, 248, 261
SROI. See Social return on investment
St. Thomas University, 355
Stability, 190–91
Steinem, Gloria, 126
Stereotypes
    age, 309–10
    education and, 316
    gender, 148–49, 153–56
    gender role, 150–51
    made by professionals, 310–11
    reinforcing, 133
    of women, 126
Steunenberg, Bas, xvi
Stichting Sluyterman van Loo, 312
Stimulation program, 324
STING, 331
Stories
    about bodies, 111

celebrating, 355
factors, 197
first-person, v. poetry, 170t
first-person v. third-person, 163
individual vs. societal, 106–8
multilayered model of, 259f
in narrative care, 249
order in, 261
redemptive, 185
slow questions and, 320–21
third-person, 164
visualized, 348
Storying moment, 244
Storylines
    alternative, 120
    identifying, 6–7
    long, 269
Storytelling
    emotions and, 342
    knowledge and, 342
    meaning-making and, 112
    opinions and, 342
    rules, 68
    spoken v. written, 161–62
    well-being and, 342
Structure
    of lifestories, 195
    narrative coherence and,
        198–99
    self-expression and, 163
    of self-presentation, 173
    shared, 44
    written, 172
Subinstruments, 258–61
Substance abuse, 216
Subtexts, 91–93, 94
Suffering, 237–38
    accelerated, 11–12
    change, loss and, 240–43
    disconnection from, 244
    overcoming, 369
Suicide, 9, 46–47, 107
Svensson, Torbjorn, xiv
Symbolic ordering, 260
Symbolic organization, 257, 268
Sympathy, 369

Taboo, 105–6

Tai Chi, xiv, 377
  narrative care and, 245–50
  restorying through, 238

TAT. *See* Thematic Apperception Test

Temporal ordering, 75

Temporal organization, 257–58

Ten-Year Plan to Strengthen
      Health Care, 90

Text interpretation, 32

Textual commentaries, 89

Textual skills, 373

Thematic Apperception Test
      (TAT), 146–47

Thematic qualitative analysis, 206

Themes, 160
  books, 343
  in "Green and Gray" program, 314
  life, 26
  lifestories and, 185
  narrative coherence and, 201
  reminiscence, 187, 187t

Theoretical considerations, 366

Theories, 374–75

Thierse, Wolfgang, 104

Third Way, 245–46

Time
  disposable, 29
  experience of, 66–67
  meaning over, 27–29
  narrative, 239–40
  space v., 77

Time and Free Will (Bergson), 68

Time and Narrative (Ricoeur), 68

Tolle, Eckhart, 243

Tolstoy, Leo, 11–12, 68, 70

Totality, 53–54

Trauma
  integration of, 197
  meaning from, 197–98, 207
  narrative coherence and, 195, 197–98
  narrative inquiry and, 198–201
  in old age, 196
  reconciliation, 200, 207
  throughout life course, 196–97

Traveling, 48

Treatment models, 367

Triggers
  dementia and, 343
  memories, 180
  reminiscence, 189
  for structured reminiscence, 254
  visualized stories and, 348

Trimbos Institute, 326

Tromp, Thijs, xvi, 326

Trust, 219, 332

Truth, 370–71

Tulle, Emmanuelle, 122

Ubels, Gerdienke, xv

Understanding, shared, 43, 49

The Unexpected Community
      (Hochschild), 42

University of Education in Freiburg, 105

Values, 18
  ethical questions and, 372
  home care, 88–89
  narrative frame and, 85–86
  public policy analysis and, 94
  social, 130

Van den Brandt-van Heek, Marie-Elise,
      xvi–xvii, 339, 343

Van Gastel, Lena, 330

Vanier, Jean, 240, 242

Verduin, Pieter, 369

Vergemeinschaftung, 57

Veterans, 203t

Vietnam War, 107

Vilans, 328, 330–31

Violence, 132

Vision, culture and, 332

Visualization, 348

Vlak, Astrid, 315

Vulnerability, 219, 273

Wandering Self, 6

War, 196–97

War and Peace (Tolstoy), 70

The Waves (Woolf), 70–75, 77

Webb, Theodore, 243

Web community, 329

Weber, Max, 57

Webster, Jeff, xvi

We-consciousness, 218–19

Wehrmachts-Ausstellung, 103

Welfare state, 334

Well-being, 163
    coherent lifestories and, 183
    dementia and, 339–40
    life review and, 291–92
    mental, 322
    physical, 322
    storytelling and, 342

Westerhoff, Gerben, xvi

Wheelock, John Hall, 33

"Who Am I" exhibition, 350–51, 351f

Wikis, 329

Wilson, Gail, 131

Winner, Ellen, 32

Wisdom
    aging, metaphor and, 31–34
    critical life experiences, 184
    environment, 238, 250, 285
    as generic memory, 33
    pattern recognition and, 33
    reminiscence and, 183
    self-understanding and, 25

The Wizard of Oz, 226

Women
    agentic qualities and, 146
    community, 134–36
    emotion and, 144
    gender roles and, 145
    older, 128
    social issues and, 135
    stereotypes of, 126

Woolf, Virginia, xv, 70–75, 77

Work, 146

World War II, 171–72, 196, 283

Writing, 161–63
    about self-defining memories, 221
    introspection and, 172–73

Writing groups, 159, 164–65
    reminiscence groups v., 169–72
    self-defining moments in, 166–68
    self-presentation in, 166

The Years (Woolf), 70–71

Yielding, 246

Yin energy, 246

York Care Centre, 355–56, 362

Younger generation, 312–13

ZonMw, 270